W9-BRZ-020

ACUTE CORONARY SYNDROMES

ACS ESSENTIALS

Third Edition

Robert M. Califf, MD

Vice Chancellor for Clinical Research
Duke University Medical Center
Director
Duke Translational Medical Institute
Durham, North Carolina

Matthew T. Roe, MD, MHS

Associate Professor of Medicine
Duke Clinical Research Institute
Duke University Medical Center
Durham, North Carolina

2010

PHYSICIANS' PRESS
AN IMPRINT OF JONES AND BARTLETT PUBLISHERS
Sudbury, Massachusetts
BOSTON   TORONTO   LONDON   SINGAPORE

World Headquarters
Jones and Bartlett
  Publishers
40 Tall Pine Drive
Sudbury, MA 01776
978-443-5000
info@jbpub.com
www.jbpub.com

Jones and Bartlett
  Publishers Canada
6339 Ormindale Way
Mississauga, ON L5V 1J2
Canada

Jones and Bartlett
  Publishers International
Barb House, Barb Mews
London W6 7PA
United Kingdom

Jones and Bartlett's books and products are available through most bookstores and online booksellers. To contact Jones and Bartlett Publishers directly, call 800-832-0034, fax 978-443-8000, or visit our website at www.jbpub.com.

Substantial discounts on bulk quantities of Jones and Bartlett's publications are available to corporations, professional associations, and other qualified organizations. For details and specific discount information, contact the special sales department at Jones and Bartlett via the above contact information or send an email to specialsales@jbpub.com.

The authors, editor, and publisher have made every effort to provide accurate information. However, they are not responsible for errors, omissions, or for any outcomes related to the use of the contents of this book and take no responsibility for the use of the products and procedures described. Treatments and side effects described in this book may not be applicable to all people; likewise, some people may require a dose or experience a side effect that is not described herein. Drugs and medical devices are discussed that may have limited availability controlled by the Food and Drug Administration (FDA) for use only in a research study or clinical trial. Research, clinical practice, and government regulations often change the accepted standard in this field. When consideration is being given to use of any drug in the clinical setting, the healthcare provider or reader is responsible for determining FDA status of the drug, reading the package insert, and reviewing prescribing information for the most up-to-date recommendations on dose, precautions, and contraindications, and determining the appropriate usage for the product. This is especially important in the case of drugs that are new or seldom used.

Production Credits
Executive Publisher: Christopher Davis
Sr. Acquisition Editor: Alison Hankey
Editorial Assistant: Sara Cameron
Production Editor: Daniel Stone
V.P., Manufacturing and Inventory Control: Therese Connell
Composition: diacriTech, Chennai, India
Printing and Binding: Cenveo
Cover Printing: Cenveo
Cover Design: Kristin Parker

ISBN-13: 978-0-7637-6862-1

Printed in the United States of America
13 12 11 10 09   10 9 8 7 6 5 4 3 2 1

ABOUT THE AUTHORS

Robert M. Califf, MD

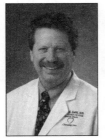

Dr. Califf was born in Anderson, South Carolina, in 1951 and attended high school in Columbia, SC, where he was a member of the 1969 AAAA South Carolina Championship basketball team.

He graduated from Duke University, summa cum laude and Phi Beta Kappa, in 1973 and from Duke University Medical School in 1978, where he was selected for Alpha Omega Alpha. He performed his internship and residency at the University of California at San Francisco and his fellowship in cardiology at Duke University. He is board-certified in internal medicine (1984) and cardiology (1986) and is a Master of the American College of Cardiology (2006).

He is currently Vice Chancellor for Clinical Research, Director of the Duke Translational Medicine Institute (DTMI), and Professor of Medicine in the Division of Cardiology at the Duke University Medical Center in Durham, North Carolina. For 10 years he was the founding Director of the Duke Clinical Research Institute (DCRI), the premier academic research organization in the world. He is the editor-in-chief of Elsevier's *American Heart Journal*, the oldest cardiovascular specialty journal. He has been author or coauthor of more than 900 peer-reviewed journal articles and a contributing editor for theheart.org, an online information resource for academic and practicing cardiologists. He was recently acknowledged as one of the 10 most cited authors in the field of medicine by the Institute for Scientific Information (ISI).

Dr. Califf led the DCRI for many of the best-known clinical trials in cardiovascular disease. With an annual budget of over $100 million, the DCRI has more than 1000 employees and collaborates extensively with government agencies, the medical-products industry, and academic partners around the globe in all therapeutic areas. In cooperation with his colleagues from the Duke Databank for Cardiovascular Disease, Dr. Califf has written extensively about the clinical and economic outcomes of chronic heart disease. He is considered an international leader in the fields of health outcomes, quality of care, and medical economics.

Dr. Califf's role as Director of the Duke Translational Medicine Institute, which is funded in part by an NIH Clinical and Translational Science Award (CTSA), includes service as co-chairman of the Principal Investigators Steering Committee of the CTSA. Dr. Califf has served on the Cardiorenal Advisory Panel of the U.S. Food and Drug Administration (FDA) and the Pharmaceutical Roundtable of the Institute of Medicine (IOM). He served on the IOM committees that recommended Medicare coverage of clinical trials as well as the removal of ephedra from the market and on the IOM's Committee on Identifying and Preventing Medication Errors. He is currently a member of the IOM Forum in Drug Discovery, Development, and Translation and a subcommittee of the Science Board of the FDA. He was the founding director of the coordinating center for the Centers for Education & Research on Therapeutics™ (CERTs), a public/private partnership among the Agency for Healthcare Research and Quality, the FDA, academia, the medical-products industry, and consumer groups. This partnership focuses on research and education that will advance the best use of medical products. He is now the co-chairman of the Clinical Trials Transformation Initiative (CTTI), a public private partnership focused on improving the clinical trials system.

Dr. Califf has been married to Lydia Carpenter since 1974, and they have three children— Sharon Califf Boozer, a graduate of Elon College; Sam, a graduate student at the University of Colorado-Boulder; and Tom, a recent graduate of Duke University—and one grandchild. Dr. Califf enjoys golf, basketball, and listening to music.

Matthew T. Roe, MD, MHS

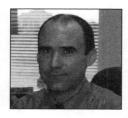

Dr. Matthew Roe is an Associate Professor of medicine in the Division of Cardiovascular Medicine at Duke University Medical Center and the Duke Clinical Research Institute. Dr. Roe has had numerous leadership roles in prospective registries that have evaluated treatment patterns for acute MI patients in the United States including the CRUSADE registry (2001–2006) and the ACTION Registry®–GWTG™ (2007–2009). Additionally, Dr. Roe has been the principal investigator for a number of clinical trials evaluating anti-platelet therapies for acute MI patients and reperfusion injury agents for STEMI patients. Dr. Roe serves as a co-director of the DCRI Clinical Research Fellowship Program and has an ongoing interest in the training and mentorship of clinical investigators.

DEDICATION

We dedicate this volume to the memory of our Duke colleague, Gary Dunham, PharmD, whose knowledge about the pharmacopoeia made us all better doctors and was surpassed only by his caring about the patients we all shared.

TABLE OF CONTENTS

CONTRIBUTORS

Robert M. Califf, MD
Vice Chancellor for Clinical Research
Duke University Medical Center
Director, Duke Translational Medical Institute
Durham, NC

S. Michael Gharacholou, MD
Fellow in Cardiovascular Medicine
Duke Clinical Research Institute
Duke University Medical Center
Durham, North Carolina

Renato D. Lopes, MD, MHS
Adjunct Professor of Medicine
Division of Cardiovascular Medicine
Duke Clinical Research Institute
Duke University Medical Center
Durham, North Carolina

Jonathan P. Piccini, MD, MHS
Fellow in Cardiovascular Medicine
Duke Clinical Research Institute
Duke University Medical Center
Durham, North Carolina

Matthew T. Roe, MD, MHS
Associate Professor of Medicine
Division of Cardiovascular Medicine
Duke Clinical Research Institute
Duke University Medical Center
Durham, North Carolina

ACKNOWLEDGMENTS

To accomplish the task of presenting the data compiled in this reference, a small, dedicated team of professionals was assembled. This team focused their energy and discipline for many months into typing, revising, designing, illustrating, and formatting the many chapters that make up this text.

I would like to thank Penny Hodgson, director of communications, Duke Clinical Research Institute, for researching information, coordinating communication between contributors, and handling the logistics of the revisions.

The editors would like to acknowledge the significant efforts put forth by Dr. Jonathan P. Piccini, Dr. Renato D. Lopes, and Dr. Shahyar Michael Gharacholou for their expert reviews, updates, and edits to chapters contained in this handbook.

Robert M. Califf, MD
Matthew T. Roe, MD, MHS

NOTICE

ACS Essentials has been developed as a concise, practical, and authoritative guide for the treatment of patients with unstable angina and acute myocardial infarction. The clinical recommendations set forth in this book are those of the authors and are offered as general guidelines, not specific instructions for individual patients. Clinical judgment should always guide the physician in the selection, dosing, and duration of drug therapy for individual patients. Not all medications have been accepted by the US Food and Drug Administration for indications cited in this book, and drug recommendations are not necessarily limited to indications in the package insert. The use of any drug should be preceded by careful review of the package insert, which provides indications and dosing approved by the US Food and Drug Administration. The information provided in this book is not exhaustive, and the reader is referred to other medical references and the manufacturer's product literature for further information. Clinical use of the information provided and any consequences that may arise from its use is the responsibility of the prescribing physician. The authors, editors, and publisher do not warrant or guarantee the information herein contained and do not assume and expressly disclaim any liability for errors or omissions or any consequences that may occur from use of this information.

ABBREVIATIONS

ACC	American College of Cardiology	LAFB	left anterior fascicular block
ACE	angiotensin-converting enzyme inhibitor	LBBB	left bundle branch block
ACLS	advanced cardiovascular life support	LDL	low-density lipoprotein
ACS	acute coronary syndrome	LMWH	low molecular-weight heparin
ACT	activated clotting time	LOS	length of stay
ADP	adenosine diphosphate	LPFB	left posterior fascicular block
AF	atrial fibrillation	LV	left ventricular; left ventricle
AHA	American Heart Association	LVEF	left ventricular ejection fraction
AIVR	accelerated idioventricular rhythm	LVH	left ventricular hypertrophy
APC	atrial premature contraction	max	maximum
aPTT	activated partial thromboplastin time	mcg	microgram
ARDS	adult respiratory distress syndrome	mcL	microliter
AV	atrio-ventricular	mg	milligram
BP	blood pressure	MI	myocardial infarction
BUN	blood urea nitrogen	min	minute
CABG	coronary artery bypass grafting	mL	milliliter
CAD	coronary artery disease	MR	mitral regurgitation
CCS	Canadian Cardiovascular Society	NSAID	nonsteroidal anti-inflammatory drug
CCU	coronary care unit	NCEP	National Cholesterol Education Program
CK-MB	creatine kinase-MB isoform	NNT	number needed to treat
CNS	central nervous system	NPO	nothing by mouth
CO	cardiac output	NYHA	New York Heart Association
COPD	chronic obstructive pulmonary disease	O_2	oxygen
CPK	creatine phosphokinase	PA	pulmonary artery
CPR	cardiopulmonary resuscitation	PAI	plasminogen activator inhibitor
ECG	electrocardiogram	PaO_2	pulmonary artery oxygen saturation
Echo	echocardiogram; echocardiography	PAR	plasminogen activator receptor
EF	ejection fraction	PCI	percutaneous coronary intervention
e.g.	for example	PCWP	pulmonary capillary wedge pressure
EP	electrophysiology	PE	pulmonary embolism
ET	endotracheal	PET	positron emission tomography
g	gram	PO	per os—by mouth; oral
GI	gastrointestinal	PTCA	percutaneous transluminal coronary
gm	gram		(balloon) angioplasty
GP	glycoprotein	PVR	pulmonary vascular resistance
HDL	high-density lipoprotein	q__h	every __ hours
HIT	heparin-induced thrombocytopenia	q__d	every __ days
IABP	intra-aortic balloon pump	qmonth	once a month
ICD	internal cardioverter defibrillator	qweek	once a week
ICH	intracranial hemorrhage	QTC	corrected QT interval
INR	international normalized ratio	RA	right atrium; right atrial
ISA	intrinsic sympathomimetic activity	RAP	right atrial pressure
IV	intravenous	RBBB	right bundle branch block
IVCD	intraventricular conduction delay	RBC	red blood cell
kg	kilogram	RCA	right coronary artery
L	liter	rPA	recombinant plasminogen activator
LAD	left axis deviation		(Reteplase)

Abbreviations

RV	right ventricular
RVH	right ventricular hypertrophy
SaO$_2$	systemic arterial oxygen saturation
SK	streptokinase
SL	sublingual
SQ	subcutaneous
SVG	saphenous vein graft
SVR	systemic vascular resistance
SVT	supraventricular tachycardia
TEE	transesophageal echocardiography
TFPI	tissue factor pathway inhibitor
TLR	target lesion revascularization
TNK-tPA	TNK-tissue plasminogen activator (Tenecteplase)
tPA	tissue plasminogen activator (Alteplase)
TTP	thrombotic thrombocytopenic purpura
TVR	target vessel revascularization
UFH	unfractionated heparin
V/Q	ventilation/perfusion
VF	ventricular fibrillation
VPC	ventricular premature contraction
VSD	ventricular septal defect
VT	ventricular tachycardia
WPW	Wolff-Parkinson-White
yrs	years

ACRONYMS

A-to-Z	Aggrastat to Zocor
ACUTE	Antithrombotic Combination Using Tirofiban and Enoxaparin
ADMIRAL	Abciximab Before Direct Stenting in Myocardial Infarction Regarding Acute and Long-Term Follow-Up
APRICOT	Antithrombotic in the Prevention of Reocclusion in Coronary Thrombolysis
ASPECT	Asian Paclitaxel-Eluting Stent Clinical Trial
ASSENT	Assessment of the Safety and Efficacy of a New Thrombolytic
BARI	Bypass Angioplasty Revascularization Investigation
BRAVE	Bavarian Reperfusion Alternative Evaluation
CACHET	Comparison of Abciximab Complications with Hirulog Events Trial
CADILLAC	Controlled Abciximab and Device Investigation to Lower Late Angioplasty Complications
CAMIAT	Canadian Amiodarone Myocardial Infarction Arrhythmia Trial
CAPRICORN	Carvedilol Postinfarct Survival Control in LV Dysfunction
CAPRIE	Clopidogrel Versus Aspirin in Patients at Risk of Ischemic Events
CAPTURE	Chimeric c7E3 Antiplatelet Therapy in Unstable Refractory Angina
CARS	Coumadin Aspirin Reinfarction Study
CHAMP	Combination Hemotherapy and Mortality Prevention
CLASSICS	Clopidogrel Aspirin Stent International Cooperative Study
CONSENSUS	Cooperative New Scandinavian Enalapril Survival Study
COOL-MI	Cooling as an Adjunctive Therapy to Percutaneous Intervention in Patients with AMI
CREATE	Clinical Trial of Metabolic Modulation in Acute Myocardial Infarction Treatment Evaluation
CREDO	Clopidogrel for the Reduction of Events During Observation
CRUISE	Clinical Revascularization Using Integrilin Simultaneously with Enoxaparin
CURE	Clopidogrel in Unstable Angina to Prevent Recurrent Events
DANAMI	Danish Trial in Acute Myocardial Infarction
DAVIT	Danish Verapamil Infarction Trial
DIGAMI	Diabetes Mellitus Insulin Glucose Infusion in Acute Myocardial Infarction
DINAMIT	Defibrillator in AMI
ELUTES	European Evaluation of Paclitaxel-Eluting Stent
EMERALD	Enhanced Myocardial Efficacy and Recovery by Aspiration of Liberalized Debris
EMIAT	European Myocardial Infarct Amiodarone Trial
ENRICHD	Enhancing Recovery in Coronary Heart Disease
EPHESUS	Eplerenone Post-MI Heart Failure Efficacy and Survival Study
EPIC	Evaluation of c7E3 Antiplatelet Therapy in Unstable Refractory Angina
EPILOG	Evaluation in PTCA to Improve Long-Term Outcome with Abciximab GP IIb/IIIa Blockade
EPISTENT	Evaluation of Platelet IIb/IIIa Inhibitor for Stenting
ESPRIT	Enhanced Suppression of Platelet IIb/IIIa Receptor with Integrilin Therapy
ESSENCE	Efficacy and Safety of Subcutaneous Enoxaparin in Non-Q-Wave Coronary Events
EUROPA	European Trial on Reduction of Cardiac Events in Stable Coronary Artery Disease
FRAXIS	Fraxiparine in Ischemic Syndromes
FRESCO	Florence Randomized Elective Stenting in Acute Coronary Occlusions
FRIC	Fragmin in Unstable Coronary Artery Disease
FRISC	Fragmin During Instability in Coronary Artery Disease
GIPS	Glucose Insulin Potassium Study
GISSI	Gruppo Italiano per lo Studio della Sopravvivenza nell'Infarto Miocardico
GRACE	Global Registry of Acute Coronary Events
GRACIA	Grupode Analisis de la Cardiopatia Isquemica Aguda

GUSTO	Global Use of Strategies to Open Occluded Coronary Arteries
HERO	Hirulog and Early Reperfusion or Occlusion
HOPE	Heart Outcomes Prevention Evaluation
IMPACT-AMI	Integrilin to Manage Platelet Aggregation to Combat Thrombosis
IMPACT HF	Integrilin to Manage Platelet Aggregation to Combat Thrombosis—Heart Failure
INTEGRITI	Integrilin and Tenecteplase in Acute Myocardial Infarction
INTERACT	Integrilin and Enoxaparin Randomized Assessment of Acute Coronary Syndromes Treatment
ISAR	Intracoronary Stenting and Antithrombotic Registry
ISAR-COOL	Intracoronary Stenting and Antithrombotic Registry—COOL
ISAR-REACT	Intracoronary Stenting and Antithrombotic Registry—Rapid Early Action for Coronary Treatment
ISIS	International Study of Infarct Survival
LIDO	Levosimendan Versus Dobutamine in Several Low-Output Heart Failure
MADIT	Multicenter Automatic Defibrillation Implantation Trial
MAGIC	Magnesium in Coronary Disease
MDPIT	Multicentre Dilitiazem Postinfarction Trial
MERLIN	Middlesbrough Early Revascularization to Limit Infarction
MIRACL	Myocardial Ischemia Reduction with Aggressive Cholesterol Lowering
MUSTT	Multicenter Unsustained Tachycardia Trial
NICE	National Investigators Collaborating on Enoxaparin
NRMI	National Registry of Myocardial Infarction
OASIS	Organization to Assess Strategies for Ischemic Syndromes
OAT	Open Artery Trial
ON-TIME	Ongoing Tirofiban in Myocardial Infarction Evaluation
PACT	Plasminogen Activator Angioplasty Compatibility Trial
PAMI	Primary Angioplasty in Myocardial Infarction
PARADIGM	Platelet Aggregation Receptor Antagonist Dose Investigation and Reperfusion Gain in Myocardial Infarction
PARAGON	Platelet IIb/IIIa Antagonism for the Reduction of Acute Coronary Syndrome Events in a Global Organization Network
PASTA	Primary Angioplasty and Stent Implantation in Acute MI
PCI-CURE	Percutaneous Coronary Intervention—Clopidogrel in Unstable Angina to Prevent Recurrent Events
PEACE	Prevention of Events with Angiotensin-Converting Enzyme Inhibitor
PRAGUE	Primary Angioplasty in Patients Transferred from General Community Hospitals to Specialized PTCA Units With or Without Emergency Thrombolysis
PRISM-PLUS	Platelet Receptor Inhibition in Ischemic Syndrome Management in Patients Limited by Unstable Signs and Symptoms
PROVE IT	Pravastatin or Atorvastatin Evaluation and Infection Therapy
PURSUIT	Platelet Glycoprotein IIb/IIIa in Unstable Angina: Receptor Suppression Using Integrilin Therapy
RALES	Randomized Aldactone Evaluation Study
RAPPORT	ReoPro and Primary PTCA Organization and Randomized Trial
RAVEL	Randomized Double-Blind Study with the Sirolimus-Eluting Bx Velocity Balloon-Expandable Stent in the Treatment of Patients with de novo Native Coronary Artery Lesions
REACT	Rescue Angioplasty Versus Conservative Treatment or Repeat Thrombolysis
REPLACE	Randomized Evaluation in PCI Linking Angiomax to Reduce Clinical Events
RESTORE	Randomized Efficacy Study of Tirofiban for Outcomes and Restenosis
RITA	Randomized Intervention Treatment of Angina
SADHART	Sertraline Antidepressant Heart Attack Randomized Trial
SCD-HeFT	Sudden Cardiac Death in Heart Failure Trial
SHOCK	Should We Emergently Revascularize Occluded Coronaries for Cardiogenic Shock
SIAM	Southwest German Study in Acute MI

SECTION 1
OVERVIEW OF ACS

Chapter 1

Acute Coronary Syndromes (ACS)

Acute coronary syndromes (ACS) comprise a continuum of biological events progressing from plaque instability to plaque rupture, coronary thrombosis, reduced coronary blood flow, myocardial ischemia, and ultimately, myocardial necrosis. It is a term used to encompass the spectrum of clinical disorders caused by acute ischemic heart disease, including unstable angina, non-ST-elevation myocardial infarction, and ST-elevation myocardial infarction, which account for over 1.5 million hospitalizations and around 30% of all deaths in the United States each year and many millions more worldwide. Despite major advances in diagnosis and treatment, tens of thousands of lives are lost each year due to delays in diagnosis, failure to implement potent pharmacological and interventional strategies, and inconsistent applica-tion of secondary preventive measures. *ACS Essentials* integrates the latest clinical guidelines recommendations and results from recently published clinical trials into a concise, practical, and authoritative guide to the management of acute coronary syndromes.

INITIAL CLASSIFICATION

Therapeutic decisions are required before patients with ACS can be categorized into unstable angina or acute myocardial infarction (MI) based on serum cardiac markers and serial electrocardiograms (ECGs). To facilitate early management, patients are classified into ST-elevation MI (STEMI) or non-ST-elevation ACS (NSTE-ACS) based on the presence or absence of persistent ST-elevation ≥1 mm in two or more contiguous leads on initial ECG. Clinical features and management of ACS are summarized in Table 1.1 and Figure 1.1.

Table 1.1. Clinical Features of Acute Coronary Syndromes

Feature	STEMI	NSTE-ACS
Clinical syndromes	STEMI.	Unstable angina or non-ST-elevation MI (NSTEMI).
Prevalence (U.S.)	330,000 cases per year.	1.5 million cases per year.
Presentation	Typical chest, neck, or jaw discomfort (pressure, burning, squeezing) lasting >30 minutes. Atypical symptoms (weakness, dizziness, dyspnea) are more common in women, diabetics, and the elderly. Acute MI is silent in 20%, most often in diabetics with autonomic dysfunction.	Same as STEMI. Early risk stratification is important for prognosis and therapy (Chapters 6, 7).

Table 1.1. Clinical Features of Acute Coronary Syndromes (cont'd)

Feature	STEMI	NSTE-ACS
ECG	Persistent ST elevation ≥1 mm in at least two consecutive leads. LBBB and posterior MI are treated the same as ST-elevation ACS. Q-waves develop in 80% without reperfusion.	ST depression >0.5 mm and/or T wave inversion >2.0 mm indicate high risk. Nonspecific ST-T changes or a normal ECG can be present. Complete coronary occlusion with persistent ST-elevation develop in some during hospitalization. Q-waves develop in 20%.
Pathophysiology	Plaque rupture with occlusive thrombus. Most ruptures develop in moderate stenoses with soft, lipid-rich cores and thin fibrous caps. Complete coronary occlusion develops in 90% of patients.	Plaque rupture with microvascular embolization of platelet aggregates from nonocclusive thrombus in most. Complete coronary occlusion develops in 10% to 40% of patients. Intermittent thrombosis and dynamic vasoconstriction cause symptoms in unstable angina.
Initial therapy	Primary PCI with stents. Fibrinolytic therapy if a cath lab with a skilled interventionalist and team is not available in a timely fashion. Prehospital fibrinolysis reduces treatment delay by ~1 hour compared to in-hospital fibrinolysis and is associated with improved survival and less progression to acute MI.	PCI with stents plus antithrombin therapy, clopidogrel, and a GP IIb/IIIa inhibitor for high-risk and some intermediate-risk patients. Antithrombin therapy for all other hospitalized patients followed by cath/PCI for recurrent ischemia or high-risk findings on noninvasive testing.
Prognosis	Acute mortality in 25% to 30% of patients, including those who die from sudden cardiac death before hospitalization. In-hospital survival depends on the speed and adequacy of reperfusion.	In-hospital MI or death in unstable angina varies from 1% to 5%, depending on risk class. NSTEMI has lower hospital mortality than STEMI but higher 1-year mortality due to more late events.

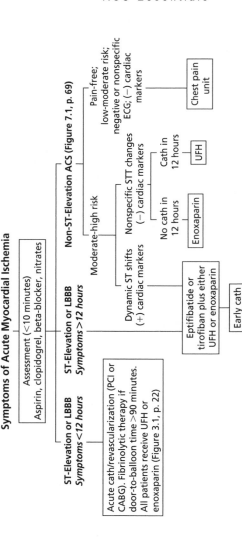

Figure 1.1. Overview of Management of ACS

(−) = negative, (+) = positive, ACS = acute coronary syndromes, CABG = coronary artery bypass grafting, ECG = electrocardiogram, LBBB = left bundle branch block, PCI = percutaneous coronary intervention, UFH = unfractionated heparin.

ST-ELEVATION MI (STEMI)

A. Clinical Syndrome. STEMI has also been labeled "reperfusion-eligible" ACS because prognosis is improved by early reperfusion with percutaneous coronary intervention (PCI) or fibrinolytic therapy. Patients with new left bundle branch block (LBBB) or posterior MI on initial ECG (manifest by anteroseptal ST-segment depression) are considered to be STEMI equivalents also benefit from reperfusion therapy. Approximately 30% to 40% of the ACS patients are classified as STEMI.

B. Prevalence. There are approximately 330,000 cases in the United States annually.

C. Clinical Presentation. The most common presentation for STEMI is abrupt-onset chest, neck, or jaw discomfort, which is usually described as pressure, burning, or squeezing in character. Symptoms typically last for more than 30 minutes and can occur de novo or in patients with antecedent angina. A precipitating factor is present in 50% of patients. Atypical presentations—weakness, dyspnea, heart failure, and dizziness—are more common in women, diabetics, and the elderly.

D. Classification. Patients with STEMI are identified by eligibility for reperfusion therapy (see Table 5.2, p. 47), infarct location, and associated mechanical, ischemic, or electrical complications (e.g., lytic-eligible patient with anterior MI complicated by ischemic papillary muscle dysfunction with acute mitral regurgitation and heart failure).

E. Electrocardiogram. ST-segment elevation ≥ 1 mm in two or more contiguous leads is required for the diagnosis. Unless reperfusion occurs rapidly, Q-waves develop in 80%. Patients with LBBB (new or presumably new) or posterior MI (with anteroseptal ST-segment depression) caused by left circumflex coronary artery occlusion also benefit from reperfusion therapy. If hyperacute (giant upright) T-waves are present, the ECG should be repeated in 15 minutes to identify ST-segment elevation because hyperacute T-waves often precede ST elevation early after symptom onset. For patients with fully paced rhythms, it is often difficult to identify ST-elevation and determine eligibility for reperfusion.

F. Pathophysiology (see Figures 3.2 and 3.3, pp. 25, 26). The most common cause of STEMI is an occlusive thrombus that develops at the site of a ruptured or fissured atherosclerotic plaque. Most ruptures develop in moderate ($<70\%$) stenoses with soft, lipid-rich cores and thin fibrous caps. Without coronary reperfusion, myocardial necrosis begins in the subendocardium and spreads to the epicardium, resulting in transmural infarction, and Q-waves develop on ECG. Even with coronary reperfusion, embolization of atherothrombotic debris can prevent myocardial tissue reperfusion and recovery of left ventricular (LV) function. On coronary angiography, 40% of STEMI patients without prior MI or angina have single-vessel disease, 30% have two-vessel disease, 15% have three-vessel disease, and 10% to 15% have no significant obstruction. In contrast, 50%

of patients with prior MI or angina have three-vessel disease and 15% have significant left main obstruction. Ruptured plaques in nonculprit vessels are often evident during angiography for STEMI, consistent with a growing body of evidence suggesting that plaque rupture and ACS are local manifestations of a systemic inflammatory disease affecting the entire vascular tree.

G. **Management** (Figure 3.1, p. 22). Acute, rapid reperfusion therapy with PCI or fibrinolysis is recommended for all STEMI patients, depending on the availability of a skilled interventionalist and lytic eligibility. Primary stenting is preferred over balloon angioplasty (percutaneous transluminal coronary angioplasty, or PTCA). Adjunctive pharmacotherapy includes aspirin, adenosine diphosphate (ADP) inhibitors, heparin, beta-blockers, ACE inhibitors, a statin, and nitrates; the routine use of glycoprotein (GP) IIb/IIIa inhibitors is reasonable. Prehospital fibrinolysis reduces treatment delay by approximately 1 hour compared to in-hospital fibrinolysis and is associated with improved survival and less progression to acute MI. Transfer to a PCI center may be preferred to onsite fibrinolytic therapy if the total door-to-balloon time can be achieved in less than 90 minutes. Facilitated PCI with upstream use of partial or full-dose fibrinolytics with or without adjunctive GP IIb/IIIa inhibitors may be harmful and therefore should be avoided.

H. **Prognosis.** Many patients with STEMI die before seeking medical attention, and another 10% die during hospitalization, for an overall acute mortality rate of 25% to 30%. The majority of hospital deaths occur within the first 2 days, emphasizing the importance of early intervention. Most deaths that occur in the first year do so within the first 12 weeks, usually in patients with LV dysfunction (EF <0.40), symptomatic heart failure, complex ventricular arrhythmias, significant residual coronary artery disease, or LV aneurysm. Restoration of coronary blood flow within the first 12 hours of symptom onset results in improved myocardial salvage, enhanced preservation of LV function, fewer in-hospital complications (heart failure, pulmonary emboli, arrhythmias), and better survival. The benefits of reperfusion, however, are time dependent: If coronary blood flow is reestablished within 1–2 hours of symptom onset, the relative risk of hospital death is reduced by 50%. Optimal prognosis depends on prompt restoration of epicardial and microcirculatory (tissue-level) blood flow.

UNSTABLE ANGINA AND NON-ST-ELEVATION ACS (NSTE-ACS)

A. **Clinical Syndromes.** Unstable angina and NSTEMI.

B. **Prevalence.** Responsible for 1.5 million hospital admissions in United States each year, being 570,000 cases of NSTEMI and 670,000 of unstable angina.

C. **Clinical Presentation.** Unstable angina can present as rest angina, new-onset severe angina, or increasing severity and frequency of angina. Symptoms are similar to

STEMI (p. 7) and usually last less than 30 minutes and often wax and wane. Atypical presentations—weakness, dyspnea, heart failure, dizziness—are more common in women, diabetics, and the elderly. Symptoms >30 minutes in duration are often associated with elevated serum cardiac markers consistent with a NSTEMI. NSTE-ACS can occur de novo or in patients with antecedent angina, and a precipitating factor is present in 50%. Up to 20% of NSTEMIs go unrecognized by the physician or patient.

D. Classification. Patients are initially divided into risk categories (high-, intermediate-, or low-risk of short-term death or MI) based on clinical characteristics, presentation features such as heart rate and blood pressure, ECG findings, and serum cardiac markers (see Table 6.2, p. 65). Risk stratification can identify patients most likely to benefit from aggressive treatments such as antiplatelet therapies (GP IIb/IIIa inhibitors and clopidogrel) and the early invasive approach to management.

E. Electrocardiogram. The ECG for NSTE-ACS patients can show transient ST-segment elevation with rapid resolution, ischemic ST-segment depression, T-wave inversion, non-specific ST-T changes, or no changes at all. Evolution to Q-wave MI is uncommon (~25%).

F. Pathophysiology. The most common cause of NSTE-ACS is microvascular emboliza-tion of platelet aggregates from nonocclusive thrombus at the site of atherosclerotic plaque rupture. In contrast to STEMI, total occlusion of an epicardial coronary artery by intracoronary thrombus is less common in NSTE-ACS, myocardial necrosis is less extensive, and Q-waves develop in a minority of cases. Symptoms in unstable angina are due to transient reductions in coronary blood flow caused by periodic thrombosis and dynamic vasoconstriction from platelet activation and endothelial dysfunction. Occlusive thrombus is present in 10% to 20% of patients with unstable angina, 20% to 40% of patients with NSTEMI, and more than 80% of patients with STEMI. Compared to STEMI, NSTEMI is associated more commonly with normal epicardial flow in the infarct artery, better collaterals, older age, and greater comorbidity (prior MI, multivessel disease, hypertension, heart failure, diabetes mellitus, peripheral vascular disease).

G. Management (see Figure 7.1, p. 69). Initial therapy for NSTE-ACS depends on the risk category of the patient. High-risk patients are best treated with an early invasive strategy (typically coronary angiography within 48 hours of hospital presentation) plus a GP IIb/IIIa inhibitor. Intermediate-risk patients are treated with antithrombin therapy with or without a GP IIb/IIIa inhibitor and either an early conservative or early invasive strategy. Both high-risk and intermediate-risk patients should also receive clopidogrel. Low-risk patients are treated medically, often as outpatients in an observational area typically known as a chest pain unit, in a manner similar to patients with chronic stable angina. Hospitalized patients without contraindications should also receive aspirin, beta-blockers, nitrates, antithrombin therapy, a statin, and cardiac monitoring. Patients initially treated medically should be triaged to an early invasive management strategy for second-positive troponin or ECG at 4–6 hours, recurrent ischemia, LV dysfunction (EF <0.40), prior PCI or coronary artery bypass graft (CABG) surgery, or a high-risk finding on stress testing. Fibrinolytics should be avoided in NSTE-ACS due to the lack of clinical benefit and possible detrimental effect.

H. Prognosis

1. **Unstable angina.** Prior to the availability of potent antiplatelet and antithrombin regimens and contemporary interventional techniques, medical therapy for unstable angina was associated with hospital mortality in 1% to 4% and nonfatal MI in 7% to 9% at 4–6 weeks. At 1 year, cardiac death occurred in 8% to 18%, nonfatal MI in 14% to 22%, and repeat hospitalization in 28% to 40%. Early use of clopidogrel, GP IIb/IIIa inhibitors, antithrombins, and the early invasive management strategy has improved clinical outcomes, although patients still remain at increased risk for adverse cardiac events.

2. **NSTEMI.** Compared to STEMI, NSTEMI is associated with smaller infarcts, better preservation of LV function, and lower in-hospital mortality rates. However, because NSTEMI is often associated with high-grade nonocclusive stenosis of the infarct-related artery, residual viable myocardium, and multivessel disease, reinfarction rates are higher and, by 1 year, mortality rates are higher than with STEMI because patients with NSTEMI are older and typically have more comorbidities compared with STEMI patients.

SECTION 2

ST-ELEVATION MI (STEMI)

Chapter 2

Diagnosis and Evaluation of ST-Elevation MI (STEMI)

DIAGNOSIS

The diagnosis of acute MI is made based on the rise and fall of cardiac markers (troponin or CK-MB) *plus* one of the following: symptoms of ischemia, Q-waves or ischemic changes on ECG, or coronary intervention. There are important limitations to these criteria: Acute MI patients can present with atypical symptoms, noncardiac disorders can manifest ischemic-type chest pain and ST-segment changes, and the rise and fall in cardiac markers are time dependent and not readily assessed within the first few hours after patient arrival at the hospital. In addition, there is a need for new definitions for: MI postcoronary artery bypass graft surgery (based on postoperative CK-MB and troponin values), threatened infarction, aborted MI, silent MI, and sudden ischemic cardiac death.

SYMPTOMS

A. **Typical Presentation.** The most common presentation for a patient with STEMI is chest, neck, or jaw discomfort, which is usually described as a pressure, burning, or squeezing sensation lasting 30 minutes or longer. It is important to consider nonischemic causes of chest pain at presentation—aortic dissection, pneumothorax, pericarditis, pulmonary embolus, esophageal rupture, ischemia/rupture of an intra-abdominal organ—because these conditions can progress to life-threatening situations without expedient diagnosis and treatment. When the distinction between acute MI and aortic dissection is unclear, imaging studies (e.g., TEE, contrast chest CT/MRI) should be obtained.

B. **Atypical Presentations.** Weakness, dyspnea, heart failure, dizziness, and syncope are more common in diabetics and the elderly, and it is not uncommon for women to present with shortness of breath, fatigue, or jaw pain, stretched out over hours, rather than minutes. Women often experience prodromal symptoms—unusual fatigue, sleep disturbance, dyspnea—in the weeks preceding acute MI. Pleuritic-type symptoms and pain reproduced by palpation are very unusual symptoms but do not exclude the possibility of acute MI.

C. **Silent MI.** Up to 20% of infarcts are silent or go unrecognized, most often in diabetics with autonomic dysfunction.

ELECTROCARDIOGRAM

A. **ST-Segment Shifts** (Figure 2.1). A 12-lead ECG should be obtained within 10 minutes of presentation. ST-elevation ≥1 mm in two or more contiguous leads (anterior, inferior, lateral) is required for the diagnosis of STEMI. ST-elevation is usually convex ("out-pouching") in configuration and can persist from 48 hours to several weeks. For symptomatic patients with nondiagnostic ECGs in whom the suspicion of ST-segment elevation MI is high, serial ECGs every 5–10 minutes or continuous ECG monitoring should be obtained to detect the potential development of ST elevation, if this is not recognized on the presenting ECG. For patients with inferior MI, a right-sided ECG should be obtained to detect RV infarction. Nonischemic causes of ST-elevation can mimic acute MI on ECG, and these "pseudoinfarct" patterns can be seen in acute pericarditis, myocarditis, severe hyperkalemia, ventricular aneurysm, acute CNS disorder, left ventricular hypertrophy, Wolff-Parkinson–White syndrome, early repolarization, and apical hypertrophic cardiomyopathy.

B. Evolution of ECG (see Figure 2.1). Ischemic ECG abnormalities evolve in a relatively predictable fashion after the onset of symptoms for a patient with STEMI who has a complete occlusion of an epicardial coronary artery. Marked, symmetrical peaking of the T-wave ("hyperacute T-waves") in the infarct region is the earliest finding in STEMI but is often missed because it occurs very early (<15 minutes) before patients present to the hospital and converts to ST-elevation within 15–30 minutes. ECGs with hyperacute T-waves should be repeated in 15 minutes to confirm progression to persistent ST-elevation. If transmural ischemia persists for more than 15 minutes, peaked T-waves evolve into convex ST segment elevation, which usually subsides in a few days but can last from hours to weeks. Infarct size and prognosis correlate with the number of ECG leads demonstrating ST-elevation. As the STEMI event continues to evolve, ST-elevation decreases and T-waves begin to invert. The T-waves usually deepen as the ST segments return to baseline, and T-wave inversion can persist indefinitely or regress/disappear in months to years. Abnormal Q-waves develop within hours to days of acute MI, usually while ST segments are still elevated, and persist indefinitely in 60% to 80% of patients.

C. Left Bundle Branch Block (LBBB). The incidence of new LBBB in the setting of acute STEMI is around 2%. Patients with acute MI and presumably new LBBB have high (20% to 25%) in-hospital mortality rates and derive substantial benefit from reperfusion therapy—a 21% reduction in death at 35 days (18.7% versus 23.6%), which translates into 49 lives saved for every 1000 patients treated. Nevertheless, patients with new LBBB are much less likely to receive reperfusion therapy than those with persistent ST-elevation.

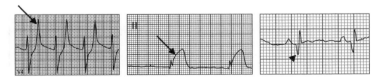

Figure 2.1. Evolution of ECG in STEMI

Left panel: Hyperacute T-waves (transient; may be missed).
Middle panel: Concave upward ST-segment elevation.
Right panel: Abnormal Q-waves (develop in 80% without reperfusion).

Although the diagnosis of acute MI in the presence of LBBB is primarily based on history, three criteria that make acute MI more likely in the setting of LBBB include: (1) ST-segment elevation ≥ 1 mm concordant with (in the same direction as) the major deflection of the QRS complex; (2) ST-segment depression ≥ 1 mm in lead V_1, V_2, or V_3; and (3) ST-segment elevation ≥ 5 mm discordant with (in the opposite direction to) the major deflection of the QRS complex.

D. Posterior MI. Posterior MI from left circumflex coronary artery occlusion presents with dominant R-waves and horizontal ST-segment depression ≤ 2 mm in the anteroseptal precordial leads (V_1–V_2). Posterior infarction is often associated with acute inferior or inferolateral MI but can occur in isolation. ST-elevation in posterior chest leads V_{7-9} may improve the detection of posterior MI in patients with normal or nonspecific ECG changes. Leads V_{7-9} are placed in the same horizontal plane as lead V_6 at the posterior axillary line, scapular angle, and paravertebral line, respectively.

E. Paced Rhythm. If acute MI is suspected in a patient with a pacemaker, the pacemaker can be temporarily reprogrammed to a lower rate to allow the intrinsic rhythm to be observed. ST-elevation is an indication for reperfusion therapy, although pacemaker-induced repolarization abnormalities can persist and mimic myocardial ischemia.

F. Normal ECG. Patients with symptoms of acute MI and a normal or nonspecific ECG should be managed as NSTE-ACS (see Chapter 7), unless posterior chest leads detect true posterior MI, in which case reperfusion therapy is indicated.

SERUM CARDIAC MARKERS

Several biochemical markers of myocardial necrosis can be used to establish the diagnosis of acute MI and estimate prognosis, but it typically takes 1–2 hours to receive the results from initial cardiac marker assessment after hospital arrival. No single cardiac marker is ideal, and each has its own advantages and disadvantages (Tables 2.1 and 2.2). Because cardiac markers may not turn positive for hours, early treatment should be based on clinical presentation and initial ECG.

A. Creatine Kinase-MB. Enzyme levels usually exceed normal range by 4–6 hours and return to normal by 48–72 hours after acute MI. Levels should be obtained every 6–8 hours, and at least three negative values are required to rule out acute MI. In general, CK-MB levels should be between 4% and 25% of total creatine kinase levels in acute MI. Small infarcts can present with elevated cardiac troponin but normal CK-MB levels.

B. Cardiac Troponins (T/I). These cardiac-specific regulatory proteins usually exceed normal range by 3–4 hours and remain elevated for 10–14 days after acute MI. Cardiac troponins are particularly useful to detect small MI, remote MI (>24–48 hours) or acute MI in patients with skeletal muscle injury. At least two measurements should be obtained

Table 2.1. Serum Cardiac Markers

	CK-MB	Myoglobin	Cardiac Troponis
Description	High-energy transfer cytoplasmic protein.	O_2-binding heme protein; rapidly released after myocyte injury.	Regulatory proteins for calcium-dependent interactions between actin and myosin.
Origin	Cardiac and skeletal muscle.	Cardiac and skeletal muscle.	Cardiac muscle.
Release kinetics *Peak rise* *Return to normal*	2–3 hours; sensitivity 94% at 8 hours and ≤50% at 2 hours.	1.5–2 hours.	3–4 hours.
	24–48 hours.	8–12 hours.	10–14 days.
Advantages	Able to detect early reinfarction.	Best marker to detect very early MI.	More sensitive and specific than CK-MB. Best marker for MI with skeletal muscle injury, small MI, or late MI (>2–3 days).
Disadvantages	Low sensitivity for detection of very early (<6 hr) MI, late (>36 hr) MI, small MI; false-positive with skeletal muscle trauma, CPR, cardioversion, cardiac surgery.	Low sensitivity for detection of late MI; false-positive with skeletal muscle trauma, CPR, renal failure.	Low sensitivity for detection of early (<6 hr) MI or late reinfarction.
Comments	Should be between 4% and 25% of total CK in acute MI. With skeletal muscle injury, ratio of CK-MB mass to CK activity ≤3 suggests myocardial source of elevated CK-MB.	Normal value useful for excluding early (4–8 hr) MI. Elevated levels insufficient to diagnose acute MI without elevated CK-MB or troponin levels.	Identifies high-risk NSTE-ACS and helps guide therapy. 30% of ACS patients with negative CK-MB have elevated troponins.

Adapted from: Ryan TJ, Anderson JL, Antman EM, Braniff BA, Brooks NH, Califf RM, Hillis LD, Hiratzka LF, Rapaport E, Riegel BJ, Russell RO, Smith EE III, Weaver WD. ACC/AHA guidelines for the management of pateints with acute myocardial infarction: a report of the American College of Cardiology/American Heart Association Task Force on Practice Guidelines (Committe on Management of Acute Myocardial Infarction). *J Am Coll Cardiol* 1996;28:1328–1428.

Table 2.2. Use of Serum Cardiac Markers

Subset	Total CK	CK-MB	Myoglobin	Cardiac Troponins
MI <4 hours	−	−	+	−
MI 4–12 hours	+	+	+	+
MI >2–10 days	−	−	−	≥
Early reinfarction	+	+	≥	−
Small MI	−	−	−	+
MI after operation or trauma	−	≥	−	+

+ useful; ≥ some value; − not useful.

at 4–8 hour intervals. In NSTE-ACS, elevated levels indicate increased risk of death or MI and identify patients most likely to benefit from GP IIb/IIIa inhibitors and the early invasive approach to management (Chapter 3).

C. **Myoglobin.** This oxygen-binding heme protein is rapidly released after myocyte injury. Levels rise before CK-MB or troponins, but elevated levels can also be seen in skeletal muscle trauma, CPR, and renal failure. Elevated myoglobin levels are insufficient for the diagnosis of acute MI, which requires confirmation by CK-MB or cardiac troponins. A negative value early after symptom onset is useful for ruling out acute MI. Heart fatty acid–binding protein is also of cytosolic origin and has a similar small size and kinetic profile in the blood to that of myoglobin, but is more cardiospecific. However, neither heart fatty acid–binding protein nor myoglobin has achieved widespread use as cardiac biomarkers in clinical practice.

Chapter 3

Overview of Management of ST-Elevation MI (STEMI)

REPERFUSION THERAPY

It is well-established that use of rapid reperfusion therapy with primary PCI or fibrinolysis reduces infarct size, preserves LV function, and improves survival in patients with STEMI or new LBBB when administered within 12 hours of symptom onset. Primary PCI has supplanted thrombolysis as the most frequently used form of reperfusion therapy. However, only 67% of eligible STEMI patients in the GRACE registry, 71% in the NRMI registry and 57% in the Euro Heart Survey received reperfusion therapy. Common reasons for withholding reperfusion therapy included advanced age, absence of chest pain, left bundle branch block, history of heart failure, or prior MI/CABG surgery. Fortunately, with the increased utilization of primary PCI, it is expected that the percentage of eligible STEMI patients who receive reperfusion therapy will increase.

A. **Fibrinolytic Therapy** (see p. 43). Following plaque rupture, circulating blood is exposed to highly thrombogenic constituents of the vessel wall (e.g., tissue factor, cholesterol esters), which rapidly induce intravascular thrombosis via activation of primary and secondary hemostasis (Figures 3.2 and 3.3). Primary hemostasis results in the formation of loosely adherent platelet aggregates at the site of plaque rupture; secondary hemostasis results in the formation of cross-linked fibrin (via activation of the coagulation cascade), which reinforces the primary hemostatic plug to produce fresh clot. By converting plasminogen into plasmin, fibrinolytic agents degrade the fibrin polymer to restore coronary perfusion. For every 1000 patients treated with fibrinolytic therapy, approximately 20 lives are saved at 6 weeks. Furthermore, these benefits are long lasting: in the 10-year follow-up of GISSI-I, 18 lives were saved for every 1000 patients treated with streptokinase. Survival benefit is apparent across all subgroups, regardless of age, gender, or comorbid medical conditions, but the greatest benefit is derived by patients who receive therapy in the first few hours and those at high risk (e.g., heart failure, LBBB). Prehospital fibrinolysis reduces treatment delay by ~1 hour compared to in-hospital fibrinolysis and is associated with improved survival and fewer complications. Despite the benefits of fibrinolytic therapy, important limitations exist: acute patency rates after fibrinolytics are typically only 50% to 60%, life-threatening intracranial bleeding occurs in 0.5% to 1.5% of patients who receive fibrinolytics, recurrent ischemia and vessel reocclusion occur in 15% to 30% of patients after initial successful reperfusion, and limited patient eligibility due to a large number of contraindications to fibrinolytic use including a prior cerebral event or recent bleeding. Current practice guidelines recommend that the "door-to-lytic" time for patients who receive fibrinolytics should be <30 minutes because the benefits of fibrinolysis are clearly time dependent.

B. **Percutaneous Coronary Intervention (PCI)** (Figure 3.4 and p. 27). Primary PCI, either for patients who directly present to a PCI-capable center or interhospital transfer for patients who initially present to a non-PCI center, has replaced fibrinolysis as the treatment of choice for reperfusion therapy in STEMI. Advantages of primary PCI in the hands of experienced interventionalists (>75 interventional procedures per year) at high-volume centers (>200–300 interventional cases per year with >36 primary PCI procedures for STEMI per year) include high (85% to 95%) infarct vessel patency rates; low rates of vessel reocclusion, reinfarction, death, and stroke; avoidance of intracranial bleeding; shortened length of hospital stay; and the ability to treat lytic-ineligible patients. The guidelines-recommended time to reperfusion ("door-to-balloon" time) for patients undergoing primary PCI is under 90 minutes.

C. **PCI Versus Fibrinolysis.** In 1997, 10 clinical trials comparing thrombolysis versus primary PCI were compared in a meta-analysis, which was updated in 2003 to include 23 randomized trials. In those trials, 7739 patients were randomized, comparing primary PCI to either streptokinase (8 studies), 3–4 hour tPA regimens (3 studies), or accelerated tPA (12 studies). A meta-analysis of these trials demonstrated marked benefits for PCI, including 30% to 50% reductions in death, reinfarction, and stroke at 30 days and 6 months and virtual elimination of intracranial bleeding (0.1% versus 1.0% with fibrinolysis) (Table 3.1). This benefit was observed regardless of fibrinolytic agent, balloon angioplasty or intracoronary stenting, or adjunctive antiplatelet therapies. In a meta-analysis of 22 trials, involving 6763 patients, primary PCI was found to reduce 30-day mortality in all increments of presentation delay (0–1 hours: 4.7% versus 6.0%; 1–2 hours: 4.2% versus 6.2%; 2–3 hours: 5.1 versus 7.3%; 3–6 hours: 5.6% versus 9.5% and 6–12 hours: 8.5% versus 12.7%). Primary PCI was shown to be superior even if patients present late after symptom onset. Furthermore, while fibrinolysis has only shown to improve outcomes when started within 6 hours of symptom onset, primary PCI reduces cardiac morbidity and mortality for up to 12 hours after symptom onset.

In the National Registry of Myocardial Infarction (NRMI), which compared primary PCI to fibrinolytic therapy in over 62,000 patients, PCI was associated with 37% lower mortality at high-volume interventional centers but had no impact on survival at low-volume hospitals. Nevertheless, PCI reduced the risk of stroke by 64% (0.4% versus 1.1%) at high- and low-volume hospitals. Combined with the vastly improved experience with primary angioplasty, these results support the superiority of primary PCI over fibrinolytic therapy for reducing death, reinfarction, stroke, and intracranial hemorrhage.

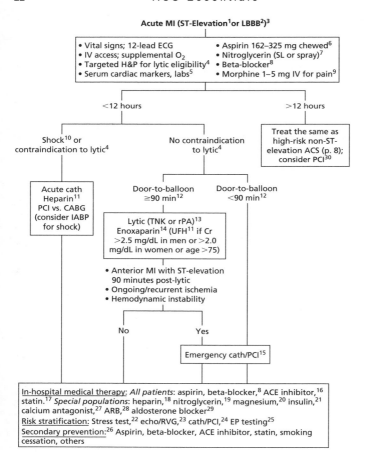

Figure 3.1. Management of STEMI

1. ST-segment elevation ≥1 mm in two or more contiguous leads.
2. LBBB limits the ability to detect ST-elevation. Substantial mortality benefit for MI with new LBBB treated with fibrinolytics or PCI within 12 hours. Mortality rate without reperfusion therapy is high (~25%).
3. Posterior MI from isolated circumflex coronary artery occlusion presents without ST-elevation but benefits from acute reperfusion therapy. A 12-lead ECG may show ST-depression with upright T-waves

Figure 3.1. Management of STEMI (cont'd)

in leads V_{1-2} but can be normal or nonspecific. Posterior chest leads V_{7-9}, placed at the same horizontal plane as V_6 at the posterior axillary, scapular angle, and paravertebral lines, often show ST-segment elevation. Paced ventricular rhythms limit the ability to detect ST-elevation. Consider temporarily reprogramming the pacemaker below the intrinsic heart rate to observe ST-segment shifts, and treat with PCI or fibrinolytics if ST-segment elevation is present.

4. See Table 5.2 (p. 47) for contraindications to fibrinolytic therapy.

5. CK-MB every 6–8 hours × 3, cardiac troponins repeated at least once at 4–8 hours, complete blood count, platelet count, fibrinogen, lipid profile, electrolytes, BUN/creatinine, portable chest X-ray.

6. Buccal absorption of crushed or chewed nonenteric-coated aspirin produces the most rapid antiplatelet effects. Avoid enteric-coated preparations acutely due to delays in GI absorption and platelet inhibition. An aspirin suppository (325 mg) can be given to patients unable to take oral medications. Clopidogrel 300 mg PO loading dose followed by 75 mg PO q24h should be used for aspirin-allergic patients.

7. Administer up to three nitroglycerin tablets (0.4 mg) or three metered doses of nitroglycerin spray (0.4 mg) onto/under tongue at 5-minute intervals. Avoid if systolic BP <90 mmHg, heart rate <50 bpm, or suspected RV infarction. Avoid if sildenafil (Viagra) or vardenafil (Levitra) is used within 24 hours or tadalafil (Cialis) within 48 hours. If sublingual/spray is followed by IV nitroglycerin, discontinue if hypotension during use limits administration of beta-blockers.

8. Avoid beta-blockers acutely if systolic BP <120 mmHg, heart rate <50 bpm, severe heart failure, prolonged PR-interval (>0.24 ms), MI precipitated by cocaine, or history of significant bronchospasm. Patients with an early contraindication to beta-blocker therapy should be reevaluated later in their hospital course for candidacy. See pp. 169–192 for dosing and administration guidelines.

9. Morphine can be repeated in small increments of 2–8 mg IV q5–15 minutes and is the analgesic of choice for pain associated with acute MI. Avoid in severe chronic lung disease (increased risk of respiratory depression). Hypoventilation can be reversed with naloxone (0.4–2.0 mg IV). Hypotension usually responds to leg elevation ≥IV saline (200–300 cc if no pulmonary congestion). Bradycardia, nausea, and vomiting often improve with atropine (0.5–1.0 mg IV).

10. Cardiogenic shock complicates 5% to 7% of acute infarctions, usually within the first few hours. Treatment requires *immediate* angiography, IABP counterpulsation, and revascularization, especially for patients <75 years. Supportive measures include IV fluids to optimize filling pressures, dobutamine to enhance cardiac output, dopamine to maintain vital organ perfusion, and treatment of associated mechanical defects, arrhythmias, and conduction disturbances. A left ventricular assist device (LVAD) may be required as a stabilizing bridge to revascularization. It is important to exclude hypovolemia, RV infarction, papillary muscle rupture, ventricular septal defect, cardiac tamponade.

11. Weight-adjusted IV heparin bolus of 60 U/kg (max. 4000 units) followed by initial heparin infusion of 12 U/kg/hr (max. 1000 U/hr) adjusted to aPTT 1.5–2.0 × control (50–70 seconds). Monitor platelet counts daily. For cath/PCI without GP IIb/IIIa inhibitor, give 60–100 U/kg IV bolus to achieve intraprocedural ACT of 300–350 seconds. For cath/PCI with GP IIb/IIIa inhibitor, give 60 U/kg IV bolus dose to achieve intraprocedural ACT of 200–250 seconds. May not be required in low-risk patients receiving streptokinase or other nonfibrin-specific agents (anistreplase, urokinase), but should be given if the risk for embolism is high (large or anterior MI, atrial fibrillation, prior embolus, known LV thrombus).

12. An interventionalist performs over 75 cases per year at hospitals that perform over 200 PCI procedures per year, of which at least 36 are primary PCI procedures for STEMI. If a skilled interventionalist is not available, consider a transfer to an interventional center for an emergency PCI as long as first door-to-balloon time can be less than 90 minutes. For symptom duration <3 hours, if the expected door-to-balloon time exceeds 90 minutes, consider fibrinolytic treatment with a fibrin-specific agent over PCI. For symptom duration >3 hours, PCI is preferred, with door-to-balloon time as soon as possible.

13. TNK-tPA is administered as a single, weight-adjusted IV bolus over 5 seconds: <60 kg (30 mg); 60–69 kg (35 mg); 70–79 kg (40 mg); 80–89 kg (45 mg); ≤90 kg (50 mg). rPA is administered as a 10 U IV bolus over 2 minutes, repeated in 30 minutes × 1. See Table 5.3 (p. 49) for other fibrinolytic regimens.

Figure 3.1. Management of STEMI (cont'd)

14. Enoxaparin dose: 30-mg IV bolus followed by 1 mg/kg SC q12h × 2–8 days up to hospital discharge (optimal duration unknown).

15. *Primary stenting is preferred over primary PTCA.* Clopidogrel 300 mg or 600 mg PO loading dose is recommended prior to stenting, followed by 75 mg PO q24h × 1 year. For patients at high risk of bleeding (e.g., need for chronic warfarin therapy), clopidogrel should be continued for at least 1 month after bare metal stent implantation and for several months after drug-eluting stent implantation (3 months for sirolimus, 6 months for paclitaxel). Recent reports indicate a special risk of thrombosis in patients who discontinue clopidogrel within the time window just given, and perhaps beyond. Practitioners should investigate the patient's ability and willingness to procure clopidogrel before choosing a drug-eluting stent. Routine use of a GP IIb/IIIa inhibitor is reasonable, starting as soon as possible prior to PCI (see Table 9.4, p. 94 for dose). When a GP IIb/IIIa inhibitor is used, an initial UFH IV bolus of 60 U/kg is recommended to achieve an intraprocedural ACT of 200–250 seconds. When no GP IIb/IIIa inhibitor is used, an initial UFH IV bolus of 60–100 U/kg is recommended to achieve an intraprocedural ACT of 300–350 seconds. Patients with one- or two-vessel disease and successful PCI can be considered for discharge on day 3 if age <70 yrs and EF >45%.

16. Start oral ACE inhibitor at low dose as soon as patient is stabilized from MI (after reperfusion and once blood pressure has stabilized [systolic BP ≥100 mmHg]; usually no sooner than 6 hours but within first 24 hours). Titrate upward over 24–48 hours as tolerated. Continue indefinitely for secondary prevention. See p. 174 for dosing and administration guidelines. An ARB should be administered to patients intolerant to ACE inhibitors with heart failure (radiographic or clinical) or LVEF <40%; valsartan and candesartan have proven efficacy in this setting. (ARBs can be used as an alternative to ACE inhibitors in post-MI patients with heart failure or LVEF <40%, but there is more experience using ACE inhibitors in this setting.)

17. In-hospital initiation (within 10 days and after patient is stable) of intensive LDL-lowering drug therapy (LDL target <70 mg/dL) using a statin is recommended. See discussion on pp. 104–106.

18. In addition to use with acute reperfusion therapy, IV heparin (aPTT 50–75 seconds) is indicated for recurrent ischemia or reinfarction and for patients at high risk of thromboembolism (e.g., large anterior MI, previous embolus, atrial fibrillation, possibly LV thrombus). Subcutaneous heparin 5000–7000 U q12h or enoxaparin 1 mg/kg q12h should be considered in others during periods of prolonged immobilization.

19. IV nitroglycerin is continued × 24–48 hours for large anterior MI, heart failure, hypertension, or recurrent/ongoing ischemia. Tachyphylaxis can develop as early as 24 hours after continuous therapy and may require an increase in dose or a 12-hour nitrate-free interval.

20. Magnesium (1–2 gm IV) is indicated for hypomagnesemia or torsade de pointes.

21. For patients with hyperglycemia, an insulin infusion is recommended during the acute phase of MI to normalize blood glucose, particularly in those with a complicated course.

22. Either of two stress testing approaches is acceptable: (1) submaximal stress test at 4–7 days followed by a symptom-limited stress test at 6 weeks; or (2) symptom-limited stress test at 10–14 days.

23. Echo/RVG is recommended for large MI, prior MI, heart failure, sustained hypotension, murmur, pericarditis, suspected LV dysfunction, or mechanical complication.

24. Cardiac catheterization is recommended for spontaneous or inducible ischemia, heart failure, EF <40%, prior revascularization, VT or VF >48 hours post-MI.

25. EP testing is recommended for VT or VF >2 days from MI for patients with LVEF 31–40% ≤1 month after MI who demonstrate electrical instability (e.g., NSVT) (Figure 12.1, p. 122).

26. Secondary prevention measures include aspirin (75–162 mg), beta-blocker, ACE inhibitor, statin, exercise, smoking cessation, weight control, Mediterranean diet. Consider gemfibrozil, niacin, and/or fish oil (omega-3 fatty acids) for low HDL cholesterol. Control hypertension (blood pressure 130/85 mmHg), diabetes mellitus (HgbAlc <7%), and dyslipidemia (LDL cholesterol 70 mg/dL; HDL-cholesterol >40 mg/dL; triglyceride 150 mg/dL). Provide instructions to patient and family on the use of nitrates for recurrent pain, when to return to the emergency room, the purpose and dose of each discharge medication, and the importance of compliance.

Figure 3.1. Management of STEMI (cont'd)

27. It is reasonable to administer verapamil or diltiazem when beta-blockers are ineffective or contraindicated (bronchospastic disease) to relieve ongoing ischemia or control atrial fibrillation with a rapid ventricular response in the absence of CHF, LV dysfunction, or AV block. Immediate-release nifedipine is contraindicated in acute MI.

28. An ARB should be given to patients who are intolerant of ACE inhibitors and have heart failure (clinical or radiographic) or LVEF <40%; valsartan and candesartan have proven efficacy in this setting. ARBs can also be used as an alternative to ACE inhibitors in this setting, but there is more experience with ACE inhibitors.

29. Long-term aldosterone blockade (eplerenone 25 mg/d titrated to maximum 50 mg/d or spironolactone 25–50 mg/d) should be given to patients already receiving therapeutic doses of an ACE inhibitor who have LVEF ≤40% and either symptomatic heart failure or diabetes. Avoid if creatinine >2.5 mg/dL in men or >2.0 mg/dL in women or K^+ >5.0 mEq/L.

30. It is reasonable to perform primary PCI in patients with symptom onset between 12–24 hours plus either severe heart failure, severe electrical instability, or persistent ischemic symptoms.

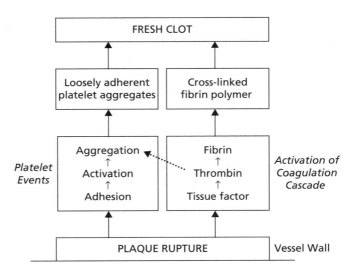

Figure 3.2. Pathophysiology of Acute Coronary Syndromes

Intravascular thrombosis is central to the pathogenesis of ACS. Plaque rupture exposes circulating blood to vessel wall contents, which rapidly include clot formation via activation of two complementary systems: platelets and the coagulation cascade. Abrupt, occlusive, intracoronary thrombosis manifests clinically as acute STEMI. The amount of angiographic thrombus has been correlated with the severity of clinical presentation. Numerous phospholipids, glycoproteins, enzymes, and other factors are involved in the process.

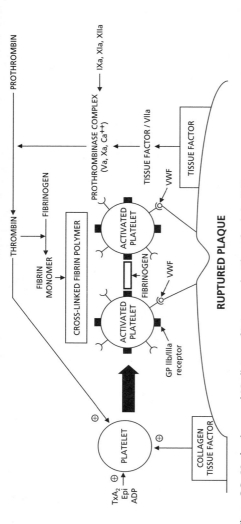

Figure 3.3. Mechanisms and Mediators of Intravascular Thrombosis in ACS

Plaque rupture exposes the highly thrombogenic lipid-rich core to circulating blood, resulting in activation of primary and secondary hemostasis.

Primary hemostasis (platelet plug formation): Plaque rupture induces platelets to proceed through adhesion, activation, and aggregation. Platelet adhesion: Initiated by the binding of von Willebrand factor (vWF), an adhesive glycoprotein released from the injured vessel wall, to the platelet glycoprotein (GP) Ib receptor. Platelet activation: Platelets are exposed to multiple agonists at the same time (e.g., ADP, thromboxane A_2, epinephrine, thrombin), which triggers a series of events within the platelet, including increased cytosolic calcium, cell shape changes, phosphorylation of proteins, release of granules and lysosomes, arachidonic acid metabolism, and conformational change in the GP IIb/IIIa receptor complex so that it becomes expressed and active on the platelet surface. Platelet aggregation: 50,000–80,000 GP IIb/IIIa receptors reside on the surface of activated platelets. Fibrinogen is the most important ligand of the GP IIb/IIIa receptor and can bind two GP IIb/IIIa receptors simultaneously, creating a molecular platelet-to-platelet bridge.

Secondary hemostasis (fibrin formation): The principal mechanism for thrombin generation and fibrin deposition following plaque rupture is exposure of tissue factor, a low molecular-weight glycoprotein concentrated in vessel wall macrophages and vulnerable plaques. Tissue factor initiates the extrinsic pathway of coagulation by forming a high-affinity complex with clotting factors VII/VIIa. Thrombin plays a critical role in clot formation: It converts fibrinogen to fibrin, activates clotting factors V and VIII and protein C, and is a potent stimulus for platelet activation and aggregation. The formation and polymerization of fibrin is crucial to clot stabilization and propagation, converting the unstable primary platelet plug into an adherent "red" thrombus.

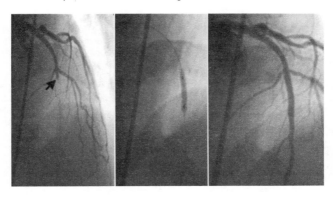

Figure 3.4. Primary Stenting for Acute MI

Left panel: Total occlusion of left anterior descending (LAD) coronary artery (arrow) resulting in acute STEMI.

Middle panel: Balloon-expandable stent.

Right panel: Final result demonstrating no residual stenosis.

D. **PTCA Versus Stents.** In a meta-analysis of 2844 patients in eight randomized trials of PTCA versus stents for acute MI, the composite endpoint of death, reinfarction, and target vessel revascularization (TLR) was reduced by 46% at 6 months with stents (14% versus 26%, p <0.0001), largely driven by a reduction in subsequent TLR. In CADILLAC, the largest of the randomized trials, stents reduced the rate of clinical and angiographic restenosis by ~50% (see Table 4.2, p. 37). Even when a "stent-like" result (e.g., diameter stenosis <30% without dissection) was achieved with balloon angioplasty, primary stenting still resulted in less ischemic TLR and restenosis. These data support the superiority of stents over PTCA (although the entire benefit is in reduction of restenosis; no effect on death or MI has yet been shown) and indicate that primary stenting should be considered the routine reperfusion strategy for acute MI. A large part of repeat revascularization is driven by target vessel revascularization due to in-stent restenosis. In stable CAD, this has been greatly reduced by the use of drug-eluting stents (DES). Indeed, a meta-analysis showed significantly reduced TVR for both paclitaxel- and sirolimus-eluting DES. The MULTISTRATEGY RCT confirmed this for sirolimus-eluting stents. Additionally, the HORIZONS-AMI confirmed this hypothesis for paclitaxel-eluting stents. Using DES in STEMI therefore is reasonable (Stone GW, *TCT* 2008).

E. **Use of Adjunctive Fibrinolytics or Antithrombotics Prior to Primary PCI.** The routine use of GPIIb/IIIa inhibitors peri-procedurally in primary PCI is reasonable and has been extensively researched. The idea of starting lytics, GPIIb/IIIa inhibitors, or both before

PCI to facilitate earlier opening of the IRA is attractive, but has so far been proven either to be harmful, in the case of full- or partial-dose lytics, or not beneficial, in the case of GPIIb/IIIa inhibitors. As of now, this is not recommended. Future research, such as long-term follow-up of the On-TIMI 2 study will have to provide answers to scenarios where upstream antithrombotics may be helpful.

F. Recommendations (Figure 3.1, p. 22). Primary stenting with skilled operators and door-to-balloon times <90 minutes is preferred over fibrinolytic therapy for STEMI. Rapid hospital transfer to an interventional center for primary PCI is preferred to onsite lytic therapy for patients who present to hospitals without PCI capabilities and with systems in place to assure rapid transfer. If expedited transfer for PCI within 90 minutes and within 3 hours after onset of symptoms is not available, lytics should be started with a door-to-needle time of less than 30 minutes if the patient is eligible for lytics. Lytic-eligible patients should be given a fibrinolytic agent, then transferred for emergency PCI for ongoing or recurrent ischemia, labile hemodynamics, or anterior MI with persistent ST-elevation 90 minutes after lytic therapy. Lytic-ineligible patients should be rapidly transferred to an interventional center for PCI or CABG. Adjunctive medical therapy for PCI and non-medical therapies are described on pp. 39–40 and Chapter 11, respectively.

Table 3.1. Meta-analysis of 23 Randomized Trials of Primary PTCA vs. Fibrinolytic Therapy for STEMI*

30-Day Outcomes (%)	Primary PTCA (n = 3872)	Lytic Therapy (n = 3867)	p-Value
Mortality	7.0	9.0	0.002
Reinfarction	3.0	7.0	<0.0001
Stroke	1.0	2.0	0.0004
Hemorrhagic stroke	0.05	1.0	<0.0001
Death, reinfarction or stroke	8.0	14.0	<0.0001

*   From the Primary Coronary Angioplasty Trialists (PCAT) Collaboration.

From: Keeley EC, Boura JA, Grines CL. Primary angioplasty versus intravenous thrombolytic therapy for acute myocardial infarction: a quantitative review of 23 randomised trials. *Lancet* 2003;361(9351):13–20.

Table 3.2. Primary PTCA vs. Fibrinolytic Therapy for STEMI: Subgroup Analysis of 10 Randomized Trials*

| Subgroup | 30-day Death or Reinfarction (%) | | Odds Ratio | Events Prevented per 1000 Patients |
	Primary PTCA (n = 1348)	Lytic Therapy (n = 1377)		
Age <60 years	4.3	8.2	0.48	41
60–70 years	6.3	12.8	0.51	64
>70 years	13.3	23.6	0.43	118
Male	5.7	12.2	0.53	61
Female	11.7	16.4	0.29	82
No diabetes	6.5	11.8	0.45	59
Diabetes	9.2	19.3	0.52	97
No prior MI	6.6	11.5	0.43	58
Prior MI	9.7	22.7	0.57	114
Non-anterior MI	6.2	12.0	0.48	60
Anterior MI	8.2	14.5	0.43	73

*   From the Primary Coronary Angioplasty Trialists (PCAT) Collaboration.

From: Weaver WD, Simes RJ, Ellis SG, et al. Comparison of primary coronary angioplasty and intravenous thrombolytic therapy for acute myocardial infarction. A quantitative review. *JAMA* 1997;278:2093–2098.

GENERAL MEASURES

A. **Emergency Department.** Initial management of STEMI includes the administration of aspirin, nitrates, heparin, and a loading dose of thienopyridine and rapid triage to PCI or fibrinolytic therapy. Bivalirudin is reasonable to use in patients with STEMI according to the HORIZONS-AMI trial. The evaluation process should be streamlined to obtain a "door-to-balloon" time of less 90 minutes or a "door-to-needle" time of less than 30 minutes. Initial assessment should also exclude the presence of a life-threatening condition that can mimic acute MI: aortic dissection, pulmonary embolism, acute pericarditis, pneumothorax, esophageal rupture, or ischemia/rupture of an intra-abdominal organ. Additional measures include IV-line access, supplemental oxygen for respiratory distress or hypoxemia, morphine sulfate for analgesia, vasopressors and possibly intra-aortic balloon pump counterpulsation for hypotension or shock, and control of precipitating factors (e.g., anemia, hypoxemia, hypovolemia, hypotension, hyperthyroidism, infection).

B. Early Hospitalization. Over the first 24 hours of hospitalization, aspirin and heparin are continued. Oral beta-blockers should be started within 24 hours in all stable patients. It is reasonable to start IV beta-blockers immediately to STEMI patients without contraindication, especially if a tachyarrhythmia or hypertension is present. If patients present signs and/or symptoms of acute heart failure, introduction of beta-blockers should be carefully evaluated. Analgesics and antianxiety medications are prescribed as needed. Once reperfusion has occurred and blood pressure has stabilized, an oral ACE inhibitor is started at low dose and titrated upward. Early use of an ACE inhibitor is indicated in the absence of hypotension (systolic BP <100 mmHg or <30 mmHg below baseline) or known contraindications (significant renal failure, bilateral renal artery stenosis, known allergy); early use is discretionary (but generally recommended) for LV ejection fraction >40%. Patients who are intolerant to ACE inhibitors and have heart failure (radiographic or clinical) or LVEF <40% should receive an ARB. Valsartan and candesartan have proven efficacy in this context. IV nitroglycerin and magnesium are recommended for special patient populations (Table 3.4). Monitoring and other general measures include vital signs every 30 minutes until stable, then every 4 hours; pulse oximetry for at least 1 day; bed rest with bedside commode for 12 hours followed by a progressive increase in activity; NPO until pain-free. Patients admitted to the coronary care unit (CCU) who are clinically stable for over 6 hours who were transferred for primary PCI can be transported to their referring hospital. If the patient is stable for 12–24 hours (no recurrent ischemia, heart failure, or hemodynamically significant dysrhythmia) can be transferred to a step-down unit.

C. Late Hospitalization (>24 hours). Aspirin, beta-blockers, and ACE inhibitors are continued throughout hospitalization, and unfractionated or low molecular-weight heparin is usually given for a total of 3–5 days or until revascularization. An insulin infusion is recommended in patients with hyperglycemia to maintain normal blood glucose levels. Statin therapy should be started in-hospital (within 10 days and after patient is stable) and continued long term to reduce mortality and major cardiovascular events, and intensive LDL lowering (target <70 mg/dL) is recommended over standard LDL lowering (target <100 mg/dL) (See the discussion on p. 191.) Early recognition and treatment of mechanical, ischemic, and electrical complications is critical (Chapters 13 and 14). Predischarge risk stratification is used to identify residual ischemia, assess LV function, and identify patients at increased risk for malignant ventricular arrhythmias (Chapter 12).

D. Post-Discharge Measures. Emphasis is placed on implementation of secondary prevention measures, including cardiac rehabilitation; lifestyle modification (Mediterranean diet, smoking cessation, weight control, exercise, stress management); treatment of hypertension (BP 130/85 mmHg), dyslipidemia (LDL cholesterol <70 mg/dL based on PROVE-IT, HDL cholesterol >40 mg/dL, triglyceride <150 mg/dL), and diabetes (Hgb Al$_c$ <7%); and use of aspirin, beta-blockers, statins, and ACE inhibitors (Table 3.5).

Table 3.3. Early Management of STEMI in _All_ Patients Without Contraindications

Treatment	Indications	Dosing and Administration
Aspirin	First dose of 162–325 mg of nonenteric-coated preparation chewed acutely or 500 mg intravenously, followed indefinitely by 75–325 mg (PO) q24h of an enteric or nonenteric preparation. A rectal suppository (325 mg) can be used for patients unable to take medications orally.	p. 177
Clopidogrel / Prasugrel	In primary PCI or low risk for bleeding in lytic: Loading dose 300 or 600 mg PO. Prasugrel is reasonable in primary PCI, loading dose 60 mg PO.	p. 181
Nitrates	Sublingual nitroglycerin tablets (0.4 mg) or aerosol spray (0.5–1.0 seconds) every 5 minutes × 3 to control ischemic pain. Avoid in RV infarction, sildenafil (Viagra) use within 24 hours, severe hypotension, bradycardia, or tachycardia.	pp. 188–189
Beta-blockers	Should be started orally within 24 hours in STEMI patients with no contraindications and without signs/symptoms of acute heart failure. In patients with tachyarrhythmia or hypertension, it is reasonable to administer IV beta-blockers.	pp. 178–179
ACE inhibitors	Started PO at low dose as soon as patient is stable (after reperfusion and once blood pressure has stabilized, usually no sooner than 6 hours post-MI), then titrated upward over 1–4 days, as tolerated. Definite for LV dysfunction; optional for preserved LV function. Ensure adequate hydration prior to initiating therapy.	p. 174
Antithrombin therapy	Used as an adjunct to reperfusion therapy. Unfractionated heparin or low molecular-weight heparin can be used. Bivalirudin is reasonable in patients treated with primary PCI but especially in patients at high bleeding risk. May not be necessary with streptokinase unless at high risk for thromboembolism.	p. 179
Reperfusion therapy	PCI with stenting is preferred over fibrinolytic therapy when available with less than 90 minutes PCI-related delay. Routine use of a GP IIb/IIIa inhibitor is reasonable.	PCI (p. 183); fibrinolytic (p. 184)
Morphine	2–4 mg IV bolus over 1–5 minutes to control ischemic pain; 2–8 mg IV every 5–15 minutes as needed. Also useful in heart failure.	p. 188

Table. 3.3. Early Management of STEMI in _All_ Patients Without Contraindications (cont'd)

Treatment	Indications	Dosing and Administration
Statins	LDL-lowering started in-hospital and continued long-term to reduce mortality and major cardiovascular events.	p. 191
Oxygen	1–4 L/min by nasal cannula for 2–3 hours is given by convention, but data to support its routine use are lacking. Higher doses by different delivery systems for longer durations may be required in hypoxemic patients to keep arterial oxygen saturation >90%.	p. 190

Table 3.4. Early Management of STEMI in _Special_ Patient Populations

Treatment	Indications	Dosing and Administration
Aldosterone antagonist	LVEF ≤40% in patients on therapeutic doses of ACE inhibitors with symptomatic heart failure or diabetes.	p. 175
Angiotensin receptor blockers	Intolerant to ACE inhibitors (or as an alternative to ACE inhibitors) in patients with heart failure (clinical or radiographic) or LVEF <40%.	p. 176
Antiarrhythmics	Adenosine, amiodarone, atropine, lidocaine, magnesium sulfate, procainamide.	Adenosine (p. 174), amiodarone (p. 175), atropine (p. 178), lidocaine (p. 187), magnesium sulfate (p. 187), procainamide (p. 192).
Calcium antagonists	Rate-limiting calcium antagonist for patients with a contraindication to beta-blockers.	p. 180
Dobutamine	Low cardiac output without frank shock when significant RV infarction not responsive to fluids.	p. 182
Dopamine	Severe hypotension.	p. 182
Epinephrine	Cardiac arrest; profound bradycardia or hypotension.	p. 183
Furosemide	Acute treatment of pulmonary congestion associated with LV dysfunction.	p. 184
GP IIb/IIIa inhibitors	Adjunct to PCI.	p. 184
IABP counterpulsation	Cardiogenic shock; as a stabilizing bridge to PCI or surgery in critically ill patients.	p. 116

Table 3.4. Early Management of STEMI in _Special_ Patient Populations (cont'd)

Treatment	Indications	Dosing and Administration
Nitrates (IV)	Heart failure; ongoing or recurrent ischemia; possibly for large anterior MI. Data to support routine use beyond 24 hours are lacking.	p. 188
Nitroprusside	Hypertensive emergencies; acute heart failure; afterload reduction for acute mitral/aortic regurgitation or acute ventricular septal defect.	p. 190
Pacemaker	Prophylaxis against hemodynamic collapse in patients at high risk of progression to complete heart block; treatment of high-grade AV block or bradyarrhythmias not responding to atropine.	pp. 116–118

AV = atrioventricular, LV = left ventricular, PCI = percutaneous coronary intervention, RV = right ventricular.

Table 3.5. Secondary Prevention Measures for Patients with MI

Goals	Recommendations
Smoking cessation	Assess tobacco use. Strongly encourage patient and family to stop smoking and to avoid secondhand smoke. Provide counseling, pharmacological therapy (including nicotine replacement and bupropion), and formal smoking cessation programs as appropriate.
Blood pressure control (<140/90 mmHg or <130/80 mmHg if chronic kidney disease or diabetes)	If BP ≥120/80 mmHg, initiate lifestyle modification (weight control, physical activity, alcohol moderation, moderate sodium restriction, and emphasis on fruits, vegetables, low-fat dairy products). If BP ≥140/90 mmHg or ≥130/80 mmHg for patients with chronic kidney disease or diabetes, add blood pressure medications, emphasizing the use of beta-blockers and inhibition of the renin-angiotensin-aldosterone system.
Lipid management LDL <70 mg/dL. For TG >200 mg/dL, non-HDL cholesterol [total-HDL cholesterol] substantially <130 mg/dL)	Start dietary therapy in all patients (<7% of total calories as saturated fat and <200 mg/d cholesterol). Promote physical activity and weight management. Encourage increased consumption of omega-3 fatty acids. Assess fasting lipid profile in all patients, preferably within 24 hours of MI. Add drug therapy according to the following guide: • LDL-C >70 mg/dL (baseline or on-treatment): Use statins to lower LDL. • LDL ≥100 mg/dL (baseline or on-treatment): Intensify LDL-lowering, giving preference to statins. • TG ≥150 mg/dL or HDL <40 mg/dL: Emphasize weight management and physical activity; advise smoking cessation. • TG 200–499 mg/dL: After LDL-lowering therapy,[†] consider adding fibrate or niacin.[‡] • TG ≥500 mg/dL: Consider fibrate or niacin[‡] before LDL-lowering therapy.[†] Consider omega-3 fatty acids as adjunct for high TG.

Table 3.5. Secondary Prevention Measures for Patients with MI (cont'd)

Goals	Recommendations
Promote physical activity	Assess risk, preferably with exercise test, to guide prescription. Encourage minimum of 30–60 minutes of activity, preferably daily, or at least 3–4 times weekly (walking, jogging, cycling, other aerobic activity) supplemented by an increase in daily lifestyle activities (e.g., walking breaks at work, gardening, household work). Cardiac rehabilitation/ secondary prevention programs, when available, are recommended for patients with MI, particularly those with multiple modifiable risk factors and those moderate- to high-risk patients in whom supervised exercise training is warranted.
Weight management	Calculate BMI and measure waist circumference as part of evaluation; monitor response to therapy. Start weight management and physical activity as appropriate. Desirable BMI range is 18.5–24.9 kg/m². If waist circumference ≥35 inches in women or ≥40 inches in men, initiate lifestyle changes and treatment strategies for metabolic syndrome.
Diabetes management (HbA1c <7%)	Appropriate hypoglycemic therapy to achieve near-normal fasting plasma glucose, as indicated by HbA1c. Treatment of other risks (e.g., physical activity, weight management, blood pressure, cholesterol management).
Antiplatelets/ anticoagulants	Start/continue aspirin 75–162 mg/d indefinitely if not contraindicated. Clopidogrel 75 mg/d in all patients with BMS for minimum of month, 1 year for DES. One year is reasonable for all patients without contra-indications or an indication for anticoagulation with warfarin. Prasugrel is reasonable in patients with clopidogrel resistance. Manage warfarin to INR of 2.5–3.5 post-MI when clinically indicated or for those not able to take aspirin or clopidogrel.
Renin-angiotensin-aldosterone system blockers	ACE inhibitors in all patients indefinitely; start early in stable high-risk patients (anterior MI, previous MI, Killip class ≥II [S_3 gallop, rales, radiographic CHF], LVEF <40%). ARBs in patients who are intolerant of ACE inhibitors and who have either clinical or radiological signs of heart failure or LVEF <40%. Aldosterone blockade in patients without significant renal dysfunction§ or hyperkalemia (K⁺ ≤5.0 mEq/L) who are already receiving therapeutic doses of an ACE inhibitor, have LVEF ≤40%, and have either diabetes or heart failure.
Beta-blockers	Start in all patients; continue indefinitely. Observe usual contraindications.

ACE = angiotensin converting enzyme, ARB = angiotensin receptor blocker, BMI body mass index, CHF = congestive heart failure, HDL = high-density lipoprotein cholesterol, INR = international normalization ratio, LDL = low-density lipoprotein cholesterol, LVEF = left ventricular ejection fraction, TG = triglycerides.

†   Treat to a goal of non-HDL cholesterol substantially <130 mg/dL.

‡   Dietary-supplement niacin must not be used as a substitute for prescription niacin, and over-the-counter niacin should be used only if approved and monitored by a physician.

§   Creatinine ≤2.5 mg/dL in men and ≤2.0 mg/dL in women.

Source: American Heart Association, Inc.

Chapter 4

Interventional Management of ST-Elevation MI (STEMI)

PRIMARY STENTING VERSUS BALLOON ANGIOPLASTY (PTCA)

A. Randomized Trials (Table 4.1). The efficacy and safety of primary stenting has been evaluated in several prospective randomized trials. The largest of these studies, CADILLAC, randomized 2082 patients with acute MI to MultiLink stenting or PTCA (with or without abciximab) in CADILLAC. In contrast to STENT-PAMI, stenting resulted in better event-free survival at 6 months due to less clinical and angiographic restenosis, and was highly cost-effective. In a meta-analysis of 4120 patients in nine randomized trials of PTCA versus stenting for acute MI, the composite endpoint of death, reinfarction, and target vessel revascularization at 6 months was reduced by 41% with stents (13.3% versus 22.5%, $p < 0.001$). Abciximab reduced the rates of recurrent ischemia leading to early-repeat target vessel revascularization after PTCA or stenting and, in a systematic overview of RAPPORT, ISAR-2, ADMIRAL, and CADILLAC, reduced the composite endpoint of death, MI, and revascularization at 6 months (Table 4.2). The ACE trial confirmed this with both lower 30-day and 6-month mortality and reinfarction. Sirolimus- and paclitaxel-eluting stents have led to dramatic reductions in restenosis compared to standard stents (<5% versus 20–30%) (Table 4.3). Small studies suggest that drug-eluting stents are safe and effective in ACS. In a meta-analysis of both small and large clinical trials, drug-eluting stents proved superior to bare metal stents in the treatment of STEMI patients (see Table 4.3). The role of stents versus PTCA for culprit lesions in small (<2.5 mm) diameter vessels and saphenous vein grafts awaits definition.

B. Recommendations. Primary stenting in conjunction with a GP IIb/IIIa inhibitor should be considered the routine reperfusion strategy for patients with acute STEMI, when available.

Table 4.1. Randomized Trials of Stenting vs. PTCA for Acute MI

Trial	N	Stent	Results (Stent vs. PTCA)
CADILLAC	2082	MultiLink, MultiLink-duet	Stents resulted in less clinical and angiographic restenosis, even with an "optimal" PTCA result, but had no effect on death or MI. Abciximab prevented early thrombotic events but had no impact on restenosis.
STOPAMI	162	Stent + abciximab vs. tPA+ abciximab	Compared to tPA, stents resulted in smaller infarct size ($p < 0.05$), better myocardial salvage ($p = 0.001$), and a trend toward less death or MI at 6 months (7.4% vs. 17.3%, $p = 0.053$).
STENTIM-2	211	Wiktor	Stents resulted in less ARS (23.3% vs. 39.6%, $p < 0.05$) but no difference in procedural success, EFS, or TLR at 6 and 12 months.

Table 4.1. Randomized Trials of Stenting vs. PTCA for Acute MI (cont'd)

Trial	N	Stent	Results (Stent vs. PTCA)
FRESCO	150	GR	Stents resulted in less MACE (9% vs. 28%, p <0.01) and ARS (17% vs. 43%, p <0.001) at 6 months.
STENT-PAMI	900	HCPSS	Stents resulted in less TIMI-3 flow (89% vs. 93%, p <0.05), less ischemic TVR at 6 months (7.7% vs. 17%, p <0.001) and at 1 year (10.6% vs. 21%, p <0.0001), less ARS at 6 months (23% vs. 35%, p <0.001), and less MACE (17% vs. 24.8%, p <0.01), but higher mortality at 1 year (5.8% vs. 3.0%, p = 0.054).
GRAMI	104	GR	Stents resulted in less MACE (17.3% vs. 35.6%, p <0.05).
Zwolle	227	PSS	Stents resulted in less TVR (3.6% vs. 16.5%, p <0.01) and MACE (5.4% vs. 20.0%, p <0.01).
PSAAMI	44	Wiktor-GX	Reduction in MACE (18.2% vs. 38.2%, p <0.05).
PRISAM	110	Wiktor	Trends toward less TVR and reinfarction (P = NS).
PASTA	136	PSS	Stents resulted in similar success (99% vs. 97%), less in-hospital MACE (6% vs. 19%, p <0.05) and 1-year MACE (22% vs. 49%, p <0.001), and less ARS at 6 months (17% vs. 37.5%, p <0.05).

ARS = angiographic restenosis, EFS = event-free survival, GR = Gianturco Roubin, HCPSS = heparin-coated Palmaz-Schatz stent, TLR = target lesion revascularization, MACE = major adverse cardiac events.

Table 4.2. Abciximab as Adjunct to PCI for Acute MI

Trial	Number of Patients	Death, Recurrent Infarction, or Any Target Vessel Revascularization at 6 Months	
		Abciximab (%)	Placebo (%)
ADMIRAL	300	22.8	33.8
CADILLAC	2082	13.9	16.2
ISAR-2	401	11.9	17.5
RAPPORT	483	28.2	28.1
Combined	3266	16.6*	19.8

*   OR 0.80, 95% CI: 0.67–0.97.

Table 4.3. Drug-Eluting Stent Trials for STEMI

Study	Number of Patients	Design	Primary Endpoint	Results (DES vs. BMS)
Stone GW et al.	3006 (3:1)	PES vs. BMS	Ischemia-driven target lesion revascularization.	4.5% vs. 7.5% (P = 0.002); TVR: 5.8% vs. 8.7% (P = 0.006).
MULTISTRATEGY	745	SES vs. BMS	Composite of death, reinfarction, or target vessel revascularization.	7.0% vs. 14.5% (p = 0.004) at 8 months follow-up.
BASKET-AMI (cardiosource)		PES/SES vs. BMS	Death, myocardial infarction or target vessel revascularization.	7.2% vs. 12.1% (P = 0.02); driven by TVR 4.6% vs. 7.8% (P = 0.08).
HAAMU-STENT (cardiosource)	164	PES vs. BMS	Angiographic late lumen loss.	0.26 mm vs. 0.73 mm; Stenosis 24% vs. 34%; All (P <0.001).
MISSION (cardiosource)	310	SES vs. BMS	Angiographic late lumen loss.	0.12 mm vs. 0.68 mm (P <0.001); TVR 5.1% vs. 13.3% (P = 0.01).
PASSION	619	PES vs. BMS	Composite of death, reinfarction, or target vessel revascularization.	8.8% vs. 12.8% (P = NS).
SESAMI	320	SES vs. BMS	Angiographic binary restenosis.	9.3% vs. 21.3%; TVR 5% vs. 13.1%; MACE 6.8% vs. 16.8%; All P <0.05.
TYPHOON	712	SES vs. BMS	Cardiac death, myocardial infarction or reintervention.	7.3% vs. 14.3% (P = 0.004) because of TVR:5.6% vs. 13.4%.

BMS = bare metal stent; Late loss = difference in minimum lumen diameter immediately after stenting and at follow-up (reflects degree of intimal thickening); MACE = major adverse cardiac events; MI = myocardial infarction; PES = paclitaxel eluting stent; SES = sicolimus eluting stent; TLR = target lesion revascularization.

ADJUNCTIVE PHARMACOTHERAPY FOR PCI

A. **Preprocedural Pharmacotherapy ("Facilitated PCI").** Several trials have evaluated the ability of fibrinolytic therapy, GP IIb/IIIa inhibitors, and combination therapy to improve early patency and clinical outcomes prior to and after primary PCI. In a meta-analysis of 17 trials of 4000 patients, preprocedural treatment with GP IIb/IIIa inhibitors showed no improvement in mortality, reinfarction or TVR, and when given in combination with a lytic, its use was associated with a strong trend toward worse outcomes. More importantly, protocols incorporating just fibrinolytics showed significantly worse outcome in both death, reinfarction, and TVR. The large randomize ASSENT-4 trial compared PCI ± fibrinolysis and had planned to enroll 4000 patients but was terminated early due to concerns over significantly worse outcome in the group receiving lytics. Also confirming the results of the meta-analyis was the FINESSE study, having three study arms comparing PCI with preprocedural abciximab, abciximab plus reduced-dose reteplase, or normal primary PCI, in which the study showed no difference between the three treatment arms. The On-TIME-2 trial, randomized 936 patients to in-ambulance administration of high-dose Tirofiban versus placebo, showing significantly more rapid ST-segment resolution, but long-term follow-up for clinical endpoints has yet to be published.

B. **Intraprocedural Pharmacotherapy**

1. **Aspirin and clopidogrel (pp. 177, 181).** Prior to PCI, all patients should receive 325 mg of nonenteric chewable aspirin followed by 75–162 mg (PO) q24h long-term. (Although 75–162 mg/d is currently recommended, definitive dosing studies have not been performed, nor has the issue of aspirin resistance been revised. Some practitioners may therefore choose to use the 325 mg/d dose.) Patients should also receive clopidogrel 300 mg or 600 mg PO followed by 75 mg PO q24h for 1 year. Analysis of the STEMI cohort of TRITON-TIMI 38 randomized study saw improved outcome using prasugrel (60 mg loading dose, 10 mg q24h for 1 year) compared to clopidogrel. Currently, prasugrel has been approved in the United States for patients with ACS who are treated with PCI. Clopidogrel should be withheld for 5–7 days prior to CABG unless the urgency of revascularization outweighs the risk of bleeding.

2. **GP IIb/IIIa inhibitors (p. 184).** Trials of abciximab as an adjunct to primary PTCA (RAPPORT, CADILLAC, Antonucci) or stenting (ADMIRAL, CADILLAC) have demonstrated a reduction in events. In a randomized trial of 400 patients undergoing primary stenting for acute MI with or without abciximab, abciximab reduced the primary endpoint at 1 month by 57% (4.5% versus 10.5%, p = 0.023) and at 6 months by 59% (5.5% versus 13.5%, p = 0.006). Abciximab also resulted in a

more rapid resolution of ST-segment elevation and in smaller infarcts. Restenosis rates were similar between groups. In a meta-analysis of 1738 patients in three randomized trials of abciximab versus placebo as adjuncts to stenting for acute MI (CADILLAC, ADMIRAL, ISAR-2), the composite endpoint of death, reinfarction, and target vessel revascularization at 6 months was reduced by 28% with abciximab (12% versus 16.6%, p <0.001). If abciximab is used, an IV bolus of 0.25 mg/kg is given at the start of the procedure followed by an IV infusion of 0.125 mcg/kg/min (max. 10 mcg/min) × 12 hours. Small molecule GP IIb/IIIa inhibitors such as eptifibatide and tirofiban can also be used and have been compared with abciximab (MULTISTRATEGY, EVA-MI) in noninferiority trials using surrogate endpoints and have not shown additional benefit. Also, registry studies have shown similar findings (see Table 9.4, p. 94).

3. **Anticoagulation.** Unfractionated heparin is usually given as a weight-adjusted IV bolus of 60–100 U/kg to achieve an intraprocedural ACT of 300–350 seconds. When abciximab is used, an IV heparin bolus of 60 U/kg is recommended to achieve a target ACT of 200–250 seconds. Prolonged heparin infusions following successful PCI are of no proven value. Bivalirudin as the primary anticoagulant during primary PCI was tested versus UFH and abciximab in the HORIZONS-AMI trial and proved to lead to equivalent ischemic events but significantly lower bleeding events on follow-up, leading to significantly lower mortality. Low molecular-weight heparin (enoxaparin) is easier to administer and can be used as an alternative to unfractionated heparin, but there is no method for monitoring the intraprocedual level of anticoagulation with low molecular-weight heparin as there is with unfractionated heparin (via monitoring ACT values).

4. **Investigational therapies.** There have been several trials investigating the use of adjunctive substances to reduce reperfusion injury after coronary revascularization, such as pexilizumab, caldaret, and FX-06. The results of these trials, despite strong results in animal models, have been disappointing. Recently, two compounds were seen to have promising benificial effects on biosignatures in STEMI such as infarct size and ST-segment resolution in STEMI. These compounds are a delta-protein kinase C inhibitor and cyclosporine. Furthermore, exenatide showed a robust reduction of infarct size in a large animal. Further testing in larger randomized trials will have to elucidate whether these compounds will be effective.

5. **Adjunctive devices.** Thrombectomy has now been established as safe and clinically beneficial by the TAPAS trial. This trial enrolled 1071 patients in routine thrombectomy using the export catheter versus conventional treatment and showed improvement in both myocardial blush grade and clinical outcome (1-year mortality 3.6% versus 6.7%, p = 0.02).

Following the successful use of both distal and proximal embolic protection devices in superior vena cava (SVC) interventions, extensive investigations followed to verify whether this would have a beneficial effect in primary PCI. Distal embolization has been linked to poor prognosis, and as such seems to present a worthwhile avenue for adjunct treatment. The EMERALD, PREMIER, DEDICATION, and ASPARAGUS trials failed to show benefit with embolic protection devices when used during primary PCI.

PROCEDURAL TECHNIQUE

A. **Technical Details.** PCI is performed on the infarct vessel to achieve a residual stenosis over 30% and TIMI-3 flow. Routine thrombectomy should be performed before initial balloon inflations in light of the results of the TAPAS trial. Primary PCI is usually limited to the culprit vessel, but multivessel intervention may be indicated for patients with multivessel disease in cardiogenic shock to improve blood flow to the noninfarct zone and stimulate improvements in compensatory hyperkinesis to maintain adequate pump function. Intra-aortic balloon pump counterpulsation is often employed in patients with ischemia, hypotension, pulmonary edema, or LV dysfunction with cardiogenic shock. Following successful PCI, stable, low-risk patients can be managed in a step-down unit and can often be discharged on the third hospital day. Stress testing is not routinely performed after successful PCI.

B. **Deficiencies of PCI**
   1. **Reperfusion arrhythmias.** Ventricular fibrillation and bradyarrhythmias are more common with right coronary artery (RCA) intervention. To minimize this risk, IV beta-blockers (in stable patients), low-osmolar ionic contrast, continuous monitoring of O_2 saturation, and adequate hydration are recommended prior to reperfusion of the RCA.

   2. **Bleeding complications.** Compared to fibrinolytic therapy, PCI is associated with less intracranial hemorrhage but more blood transfusions. Meticulous vascular access techniques, tight control of ACT levels during the PCI procedure, avoidance of postprocedural heparin, and early sheath removal are established methods to minimize procedural-related bleeding complications. In the future, bleeding can be further reduced using other anticoagulants such as bivalirudin and performing primary PCI through a radial approach.

PRIMARY PCI FOR CARDIOGENIC SHOCK

Patients in cardiogenic shock are usually taken to the catheterization laboratory for hemodynamic stabilization with an intra-aortic balloon pump (IABP), angiography, and emergency revascularization. Nonrandomized studies reported survival rates of 40% to 86% after PTCA compared to 30% after lytic therapy and 10% after medical therapy. In GUSTO-I, an aggressive revascularization strategy of PTCA or CABG was independently associated with improved survival at 30 days. In the SHOCK trial, 302 patients were randomized to an early invasive approach of emergency catheterization followed by immediate revascularization (PTCA or CABG) or an early conservative approach of initial medical stabilization followed by revascularization for recurrent ischemia. Revascularization was performed in 87% of patients in the invasive group and 34% of patients in the conservative group. One-year survival was 46.7% in the early revascularization group and 33.6% in the initial medical stabilization group (p <0.03). At 1 year, 83% of survivors were in New York Heart Association (NYHA) heart failure Class I or II. Benefit was apparent only for patients <75 years (survival 51.6% with early revascularization versus 33.3% with initial medical therapy); however, the number of patients >75 years of age evaluated in SHOCK was small (n = 56), and several registries have shown a possible marked survival benefit for select elderly patients undergoing revascularization. These data support the use of IABP counterpulsation, immediate angiography, and emergency revascularization for cardiogenic shock, particularly in patients who develop shock within 36 hours of MI and can undergo revascularization within 18 hours of shock. Most patients should undergo PCI and the primary reperfusion strategy. CABG can be considered for patients with severe three-vessel or left main disease without RV infarction or major comorbidities. For patients who present to a noninvasive center within 3 hours of STEMI, fibrinolytic therapy can be considered if the expected delay to PCI exceeds 90 minutes, followed by prompt transfer to an invasive center.

CORONARY ARTERY BYPASS GRAFT (CABG) SURGERY

CABG is not widely utilized for STEMI as a primary means of reperfusion due to unavoidable delays in establishing perfusion of the infarct vessel with bypass grafting and the general success of PCI as a therapy. However, CABG should be considered as part of an integrated revascularization strategy, especially for patients in cardiogenic shock. Clinically stable patients with LV dysfunction and multivessel disease should have surgery delayed to allow clinical stabilization; if critical anatomy is present, revascularization is recommended before hospital discharge. Patients with preserved LV function who require revascularization can safely undergo CABG within a few days of STEMI. If possible, clopidogrel should be withheld for 5–7 days prior to CABG to minimize the risk of perioperative bleeding. Indications for emergency CABG in the setting of STEMI are shown in Table 4.4.

Table 4.4. Indications for CABG in STEMI

- Left main stenosis >50% with left anterior descending or left circumflex coronary infarct vessel.
- Left main stenosis >75% with right coronary infarct vessel.
- Severe proximal multivessel disease not suitable for PCI, especially if the infarct vessel is patent.
- Severe multivessel or left main disease with cardiogenic shock, especially in patients. <75 years who develop shock within 36 hours of MI and can undergo CABG within 18 hours of shock.
- Failed mechanical reperfusion with infarct duration <6–12 hours, a large area of jeopardized myocardium, and ongoing ischemic pain, especially in the presence of well-developed collaterals.
- At the time of surgical repair of ventricular septal rupture or mitral valve insufficiency.
- Life-threatening ventricular dysrhythmias with left main stenosis >50% or triple-vessel disease.

Chapter 5

Fibrinolytic Therapy for ST-Elevation MI (STEMI)

If a skilled interventionalist is not available, patients with acute MI and ST-elevation or LBBB without contraindications should receive fibrinolytic therapy. Hospital transfer for emergency PCI after lytic therapy is recommended for ongoing or recurrent ischemic symptoms, labile hemodynamics, or anterior MI with persistent ST-elevation with 90 minutes after lytic therapy. As an alternative to onsite lytic therapy, DANAMI-2 demonstrated the safety and efficacy of hospital transfer for primary PCI. Among 1129 patients with severe ($\geq$4 mm ST-elevation) MI <12 hours, hospital transfer resulted in a 40% reduction in the composite endpoint of death, reinfarction, and disabling stroke at 30 days compared to onsite lytic therapy (8.5% versus 14.2%). There were no deaths during hospital transfer, and time from the door of the first hospital to balloon inflation was only 100 minutes. Similar results were reported in the PRAGUE and CAPITAL-AMI trials (Table 5.1). In a meta-analysis of six randomized trials, interhospital transfer for primary PCI reduced the combined endpoint of death, reinfarction, or stroke by 42% compared to onsite fibrinolysis. More recently, the TRANSFER-AMI and CARESS-in-AMI trials showed that for high-risk STEMI patients receiving thrombolysis at non-PCI centers, urgent transfer and PCI within 6 hours is associated with significantly fewer ischemic complications and no excess in bleeding.

OVERVIEW OF FIBRINOLYTIC THERAPY

A. **Primary Goal of Therapy.** The primary goal of fibrinolytic therapy is to achieve early coronary and myocardial reperfusion, which reduces infarct size, preserves LV function, reduces the risk of arrhythmias and heart failure, and improves survival. Fibrinolytic agents differ with respect to side effects, cost, and degree of systemic fibrinolysis (p. 183), which determines the need for conjunctive heparin therapy. Acute (90-minute) patency rates differ among agents, but by 3 hours patency rates are similar. Until GUSTO-I was published in 1993, randomized trials suggested that all agents were equally effective at preserving LV function and reducing mortality. GUSTO-I showed that an accelerated tPA regimen (100 mg infused over 90 minutes) with concomitant IV heparin reduced 30-day mortality by 14% relative to streptokinase (6.3% versus 7.3%, p <0.001). Genetic recombinant technology has developed new fibrinolytic agents in the last few years, including rPA and TNK-tPA, which offer the convenience of IV bolus dosing and achieve similar patency rates as accelerated tPA.

Table 5.1. Management of STEMI at Noninterventional Centers: Randomized Trials of On-site Lytic Therapy vs. Hospital Transfer for PCI

Trial	Design	Results (PCI vs. Lytic)	Comments
DANAMI-2 (2003)	1129 patients with MI <12 hours and ST-elevation ≥4 mm randomized to on-site accelerated tPA or transfer for PCI if transfer time <3 hours.	Death, reinfarction, or disabling stroke at 30 days* (8.5% vs. 14.2%, p = 0.0003); death at 30 days (6.6% vs. 7.6%, p = 0.35); stroke at 30 days (1.1% vs. 2.0%, p = 0.15).	Transport time ~60 minutes. Few complications during transport (VF 1.4%, high-degree AV block 2.3%). Door to-balloon time 100 minutes in transport group. Stents placed in 93%. Low rate (2.5%) of rescue PCI in tPA group.
CAPITAL-AMI (2003)	173 high-risk patients with MI <6 hours randomized to TNK plus transfer for immediate PCI vs. TNK alone.	Death, reinfarction, stroke, recurrent ischemia at 30 days (9.3% vs. 21.4%, p = 0.034).	TNK-only group transferred for rescue PCI, if needed.
PRAGUE-2 (2002)	850 patients with MI <12 hours randomized to streptokinase or immediate transport for PCI.	Death at 30 days* (6.8% vs. 10%, p = 0.12); patients treated at 3–12 hours (6% vs. 15.3%, p <0.02).	Death or VF during transport 1.2%. Transport increased time to treatment by 32 minutes.
PRAGUE (2000)	300 patients with STEMI <6 hours randomized to lytic therapy in community hospital, lytic therapy during transport for PCI, or immediate transport for PCI.	Death, reinfarction, or stroke at 30 days* (23% vs. 15% vs. 8%, p <0.02); reinfarction at 30 days (10% vs. 7% vs. 1%, p <0.03).	VF during transport: 2% with lytics during transport vs. 0% without lytics during transport.
CAPTIM	840 patients with STEMI <6 hours randomized to either prehospital fibrinolysis and liberal rescue PCI vs. transfer for primary PCI.	Death, non-fatal reinfarction, and non-fatal disabling stroke at 30 days: 6.2% vs. 8.2% p <0.05* in favor of primary PCI. Death was 4.8% vs. 3.8%, p = 0.61.	Cut short due to funding problems.

Table 5.1. Management of STEMI at Noninterventional Centers: Randomized Trials of On-site Lytic Therapy vs. Hospital Transfer for PCI (cont'd)

Trial	Design	Results (PCI vs. Lytic)	Comments
CARESS-in-AMI	600 patients <12 hours and one high risk factor randomized to either half-dose retaplase and abciximab with rescue PCI or transfer for primary PCI.	Death, reinfarction, or refractory ischemia at 30 days: 4.4% vs. 10.7%, p = 0.005*; 1 year combined endpoint was 11.4% vs. 16.4%, p = 0.07; recurrent PCI was 14.4% vs. 42.4%, p <0.0001.	
TRANSFER-AMI (cardiosource)	1030 patients <6 hours without access to primary PCI within 60 minutes and one high risk factor; treatment with either full-dose tenecteplase and liberal rescue PCI or transfer for PCI <6 hours.	Death, MI, heart failure, severe recurrent ischemia, or shock: 10.5% vs. 16.5%, p = 0.0013; Reinfarction (3.3% vs. 6.0%, p = 0.044) and recurrent ischemia (0.2% vs. 2.2%, p = 0.02) were significantly lower.	

* Primary endpoint.

B. Time-Dependent Benefits. Mortality rates are cut in half when fibrinolytic therapy is initiated within 1 hour of acute MI and decline thereafter. For every 1000 patients treated, 65 lives are saved when lytics are given within 1 hour of symptom onset, 26 lives are saved between 3–6 hours, and 18 lives are saved between 6–12 hours. Patients with stuttering infarcts may benefit from fibrinolytic therapy for up to 24 hours. In a pooled analysis of 10 randomized trials of fibrinolytic therapy versus primary angioplasty, the combined rate of death, reinfarction, and stroke at 30 days for patients presenting <2 hours, 2–4 hours, and >4 hours from symptom onset was 12.5%, 14.2%, and 19.6%, respectively. Fibrinolytic therapy improves outcomes in all patient subsets, regardless of age, gender, blood pressure (if systolic BP <180 mmHg), site of infarction, history of MI, or presence of diabetes or heart failure. Benefits are greatest for patients with new left bundle branch block or anterior ST-elevation; benefits are reduced in the very elderly due to an increased risk of major bleeding and in low-risk patients with small infarcts (e.g., inferior MI without RV infarction or anterior ST-depression), who have a good prognosis even without fibrinolytic therapy.

C. Limitations of Fibrinolytic Therapy. Important limitations of fibrinolytic therapy include acute patency rates of the infarct vessel of only 50% to 60%, failure to achieve optimal tissue reperfusion in at least 50% of patients, intracranial hemorrhage in 0.5% to 1.5%, recurrent ischemia in 15% to 30%, and limited patient eligibility. Fibrinolytic therapy also activates platelets by exposing clot-bound thrombin.

Table 5.2. Fibrinolytic Therapy: Indications and Contraindications

Indications

- Patients with ST-segment elevation or LBBB who present within 12 hours of symptom onset, regardless of age, gender, site of infarction, presence of heart failure or diabetes, or history of MI.
- Patients with isolated ST-segment depression with upright T waves and dominant R waves in leads V_1–V_2, consistent with posterior MI from left circumflex coronary occlusion.

Absolute Contraindications

- Any prior intracranial hemorrhage.
- Known structural cerebral vascular lesion (e.g., ateriovenous malformation).
- Known malignant intracranial neoplasm (primary or metastatic).
- Ischemic stroke <3 months EXCEPT acute ischemic stroke <3 hours.
- Suspected aortic dissection.
- Active bleeding or bleeding diatheses (excluding menses).
- Significant closed head or facial trauma <3 months.

Relative Contraindications

- History of chronic, severe, poorly-controlled hypertension.
- Severe uncontrolled hypertension on presentation (systolic BP >180 mmHg or diastolic BP >110 mmHg)*.
- History of prior ischemic stroke >3 months, dementia, or known intracranial pathology not covered in contraindications.
- Traumatic or prolonged (>10 minutes) CPR or major surgery <3 weeks.
- Recent (within 2–4 weeks) internal bleeding.
- Recent noncompressible vascular punctures.
- For streptokinase/anistreplase: prior exposure (>5 days ago) or prior allergic reactions to these agents.
- Pregnancy.
- Active peptic ulcer.
- Current use of anticoagulants (the higher the INR, the higher the risk of bleeding).

* Could be an absolute contraindication in low-risk patients.

Adapted from: ACC/AHA Guidelines for the Management of Patients with ST-Elevation Myocardial Infarction. *J AC Coll Cardiol* 2004;44:617–719.

CHOICE OF FIBRINOLYTIC AGENTS

No fibrinolytic agent is ideal for all patients, and each has its own advantages and disadvantages (Table 5.3). tPA, rPA, and TNK-tPA activate plasminogen directly, while streptokinase binds to plasminogen to form an "activator complex" (Figure 5.1). Ultimately, plasminogen is converted to plasmin, which degrades fibrin clots. Fibrin-specific agents (tPA, TNK-tPA) preferentially activate clot-bound plasminogen, promoting clot lysis without inducing a systemic lytic state. In addition to activating clot-bound plasminogen, streptokinase, and to a lesser degree, rPA, activate *circulating* plasminogen, which degrades circulating fibrinogen and other plasma proteins to induce a systemic lytic state, manifest as elevated of fibrin degradation products, low fibrinogen levels, and depletion of clotting factors V and VIII. Compared to streptokinase, tPA resulted in higher acute patency rates (80% versus 50%) and a 1% absolute reduction in early mortality (6.3% versus 7.3%) in GUSTO-I, but tPA requires IV heparin, results in more intracranial hemorrhage, and is more expensive. tPA, rPA, and TNK-tPA appear to be equivalent clinically, but there are differences in the ease of administration (TNK-tPA = single IV bolus; rPA = double IV bolus; tPA = IV bolus plus 90-minute infusion) and the risk of bleeding complications. Compared to tPA, TNK-tPA resulted in fewer major bleeding complications, fewer blood transfusions, less intracranial hemorrhage (ICH) in low-weight elderly women, and a trend toward less ICH in patients >75 years in ASSENT-2. Compared to tPA, rPA resulted in more bleeding complications in low-weight patients in GUSTO-III. TNK-tPA has the most convincing data for clinical benefit and ease of administration; rPA also has acceptable data, and streptokinase is preferred by some for patients at high risk of intracranial bleeding. The choice of the fibrinolytic agent is typically based on ease of administration, cost, and preferences of each institution.

Table 5.3. Fibrinolytic Agents for Acute MI

Agent	Dose	Comments
Streptokinase (SK)	1.5 million units (MU) IV over 30–60 minutes.	Acute patency rate: 50%. Activates circulating plasminogen to induce a systemic lytic state. Allergic reactions are common (most often hypotension). Least likely to cause intracranial bleeding. Acute IV heparin is not necessary for reduction in mortality or reinfarction, and subcutaneous heparin is of questionable benefit. Consider heparin in high-risk settings.‡ Avoid reuse for ≤2 years due to the persistence of neutralizing anti-streptococcal antibodies. Least expensive lytic ($520*).

Table 5.3. Fibrinolytic Agents for Acute MI (cont'd)

Agent	Dose	Comments
Tissue plasminogen activator (tPA) (Alteplase)	100 mg IV maximum in 90 minutes: 15 mg bolus, then 0.75 mg/kg (max. 50 mg) over 30 minutes, then 0.5 mg/kg (max. 35 mg) over next 60 minutes.	Acute patency rate: 50% to 60%. Preferentially activates clot-bound plasminogen; does not induce a systemic lytic state. No allergic potential. Mortality advantage over SK if accelerated dosing regimen and IV heparin are given within 4 hours of symptom onset despite a slight increase in ICH. Greatest benefit is for patients presenting early with large MI and low risk of ICH. Acute IV heparin[‡‡] is essential to maintain coronary patency. Expensive ($2600*).
Recombinant plasminogen activator (rPA) (Reteplase)	10 U IV bolus over 2 minutes, repeated in 30 minutes × 1. Normal saline flush before and after each bolus.	Acute patency rate: 50% to 60%. Preferentially activates clot-bound plasminogen, but not as fibrin-specific as tPA, and fibrinogen is depleted in many patients. No allergic potential. Deletion mutant of wild-type tPA with a longer half-life and reduced fibrin specificity compared to tPA. Convenient bolus dosing. Mortality and ICH similar to accelerated tPA in GUSTO-III. Acute IV heparin[‡‡] is essential to maintain coronary patency. Expensive ($2650*).
TNK-tPA (Tenecteplase)	Single, weight-adjusted IV bolus over 5 seconds: <60 kg (30 mg); 60–69 kg (35 mg); 70–79 kg (40 mg); 80–89 kg (45 mg); ≤90 kg (50 mg).	Acute patency rate: 50% to 60%. Preferentially activates clot-bound plasminogen; does not induce a systemic lytic state. No allergic potential. Developed by altering amino acids of wild-type tPA; longer half-life and increased fibrin specificity compared to tPA. Convenient bolus dosing. Mortality and ICH similar to accelerated tPA in ASSENT-2. Acute IV heparin[‡‡] is essential to maintain coronary patency. Expensive ($2650*).

ICH = intracranial hemorrhage.

*   Pharmacy cost at Duke Hospital.

‡   Consider IV induction of unfractionated heparin at 12–15 U/kg/hr for patients at high risk of thromboembolism (e.g., large anterior MI, previous embolus, atrial fibrillation, LV thrombus). Begin after 4–6 hours or when aPTT <2–3 times control and continue for 2–5 days. Titrate to aPTT of 1.5–2.5 times control (50–75 seconds). Alternatively, subcutaneous heparin can be given at 12,500 U q12h, starting at 4–12 hours and continued for 3–7 days. Patients at low risk of thromboembolism can be treated either without heparin or with low-dose (7500 U) subcutaneous heparin q12h until ambulatory.

‡‡   Unfractionated heparin IV bolus of 60–70 U/kg (max. 5000 units) followed by an IV infusion of 12–15 U/kg/hr (max. 1000 U/hr), adjusted to aPTT of 1.5–2.5 times control (50–75 seconds) × 48 hours. Alternatively, enoxaparin can be administered at 1 mg/kg (SQ) q12h (consider initial bolus dose of 30 mg IV as in ASSENT-3 trial).

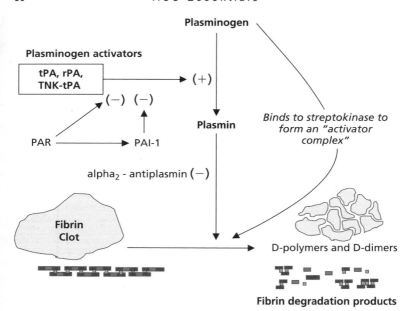

Figure 5.1. Fibrinolytic Therapy and Dissolution of Clot

Fibrinolytic agents activate plasminogen, which degrades thrombus via breakdown of fibrin. tPA, rPA, and TNK-tPA activate plasminogen directly; streptokinase combines with plasminogen to form an "activator complex." Fibrin breakdown results in the release of fibrin degradation products (D-dimers and other D-polymers). PAI = plasminogen activator inhibitor.

ADJUNCTIVE ANTITHROMBIN THERAPY

Fibrinolytic therapy exposes clot-bound thrombin, which is a potent stimulus for further platelet aggregation and fibrin generation. To offset this prothrombotic potential, antithrombin therapy is routinely employed, particularly with tPA, rPA, and TNK-tPA. There is less need for systemic anticoagulation with streptokinase because streptokinase results in the generation of fibrin degradation products and the depletion of clotting factors V and VIII, which confer systemic anticoagulant effects; nevertheless, IV unfractionated heparin (UFH) should be especially considered for patients at high risk of systemic emboli (large or anterior MI, atrial fibrillation, prior embolism, known LV thrombus). Heparin dosing is a balance between the risk of reocclusion and the risk of major bleeding, and current guidelines (for patients >70 kg) recommend an IV bolus of 60 U/kg (max. 4000 units) of UFH followed by a continuous IV infusion of 12 U/kg/hr (max. 1000 U/hr) adjusted to aPTT of 1.5–2.0 times control (50–70 seconds) × 48 hours (Table 5.4). As alternatives to UFH, bivalirudin (direct thrombin inhibitor) and reviparin and enoxaparin (low molecular-weight heparins) have been evaluated during fibrinolytic therapy. As an adjunct to streptokinase in HERO-2, bivalirudin reduced the rate of reinfarction at 96 hours by 30% compared to UFH but did not reduce mortality at 30 days. As an adjunct to streptokinase in CREATE, reviparin reduced the primary endpoint of death, recurrent MI, or stroke by 13% at 7 and 30 days. As an adjunct to TNK-tPA in ASSENT-3, enoxaparin reduced the primary endpoint of 30-day mortality or hospital reinfarction or refractory ischemia by 19% compared to UFH (11.4% versus 15.4%, p = 0.0001). More recently, the Enoxaparin and Thrombolysis Reperfusion for Acute Myocardial Infarction Treatment, Thrombolysis in Myocardial Infarction—Study 25 (ExTRACT-TIMI 25) compared enoxaparin to UFH in patients with STEMI who were eligible to receive fibrinolytic therapy (Antman EM). A total of 20,479 patients from 674 sites in 48 countries were randomized and included in the intention-to-treat final analysis. The median time from symptom onset to initiation of lytic therapy was 3.2 hours, and 97.2% of patients received their assigned therapy within 30 minutes following lytic therapy. The primary endpoint of the study, death, or nonfatal MI at 30 days was significantly lower in patients randomized to enoxaparin (12.0% versus 9.9%), accounting for a 17% relative risk reduction (p <.0001). The benefit was observed as early as 48 hours following therapy (5.2% versus 4.7%; p <.08). In addition, when the endpoint of urgent revascularization was included in the analysis, the difference between the two groups was even more pronounced in favor of enoxaparin at both 30 days and at 48 hours. Overall, use of enoxaparin was associated with an 8% reduction in 30-day mortality, a 33% reduction in nonfatal MI, and a 26% reduction in urgent revascularization rates. The benefit was seen in all groups, except in patients ≥75 years and in patients treated with streptokinase (20% of the fibrinolytics agents used). The benefits of enoxaparin, however, were somewhat offset by a significant increase in major bleeding complications (fatal and nonfatal) and in nonfatal major bleeding complications without an increase in intracranial bleeding.

MANAGEMENT OF LYTIC COMPLICATIONS

A. **Minor Bleeding (puncture site, oral, nasal).** Minor bleeding episodes are treated by local compression. To minimize the risk of bleeding, compressible vascular access sites should be used, vascular access lines should be left in place for several hours after fibrinolytic therapy (especially after streptokinase), and invasive procedures should be kept to a minimum.

Table 5.4. Heparin Dosage Adjustment with Fibrinolytic Therapy for Acute MI*

aPPT (see)	Bolus Dose (units)	Stop Infusion (min)	Rate Changes (mL/hr)	Repeat aPTT
<40	3000	0	+2	6 hours
40–49	0	0	+1	6 hours
50–75	0	0	0 (no changes)	Next AM

Table 5.4. Heparin Dosage Adjustment with Fibrinolytic Therapy for Acute MI* (cont'd)

aPPT (see)	Bolus Dose (units)	Stop Infusion (min)	Rate Changes (mL/hr)	Repeat aPTT
76–85	0	0	−1	Next AM
86–100	0	30	−2	6 hours
101–150	0	60	−3	6 hours
>150	0	60	−6	6 hours

aPTT = activated partial thromboplastin time. Heparin infusion concentration = 50 U/mL.
Target aPTT = 50–70 seconds.

* For standard laboratory reagents with a mean control aPTT of 26–36 seconds. For aPTT obtained <6 hours after fibrinolytic therapy, adjust infusion upward if aPTT <50 seconds, but only down-titrate for aPTT >100 seconds as the aPTT will be affected by the lytic state. For aPTT obtained ≤12 hours after fibrinolytic therapy, use nomogram as above.

Adapted from: Chest 1995;108:258S–275S.

B. **Major Bleeding (GI, intracranial).** The incidence of GI bleeding is 5% and ICH is 0.5% to 1.0% after fibrinolytic therapy. Risk factors for intracranial hemorrhage, which is fatal in 50% to 60%, include older age (especially >70 years), lower body weight, history of cerebrovascular events, hypertension on presentation, and use of a fibrin-specific fibrinolytic agent. Any focal neurological deficit or significant deterioration in mental status during or after reperfusion therapy, especially within the first 24 hours, should be treated as an ICH until excluded by CT scan. STAT blood counts (hemoglobin, hematocrit, platelets, PT/PTT, fibrinogen) should be obtained and treatment should be started before CT results are available. Immediate discontinuation of lytics, heparin, GP IIb/IIIa inhibitors, aspirin, and clopidogrel is mandatory until ICH is excluded by brain imaging. For established ICH, protamine sulfate (20–50 mg IV over 1–3 minutes) can be given to reverse the effects of heparin. Packed RBCs are indicated for bleeding-induced hypotension or hematocrit <25%; platelet transfusions (6–10 units) are indicated to reverse abciximab effects; and cryoprecipitate (10 units IV) is indicated to keep fibrinogen levels >150 mg/dL. (Fibrinogen can be low or dysfunctional 6–8 hours after tPA, rPA, and TNK-tPA, and for up to 30 hours after streptokinase.) For persistent bleeding, fresh frozen plasma (two to three units IV) and repeat cryoprecipitate transfusions are indicated. For continued bleeding despite these measures, additional platelet transfusions (even if the platelet count is normal) are recommended to reverse the effect of aspirin and fibrin split products. Aminocaproic acid may counteract the effect of plasmin but at a risk of severe thrombosis.

C. **Fever.** Fever occurs in 5% of patients receiving streptokinase and is treated with aspirin or acetaminophen.

D. Hypotension. Hypotension occurs in 10% to 15% of patients during streptokinase infusions and is treated with IV fluids and by slowing or temporarily discontinuing the streptokinase infusion until BP >90 mmHg, then resuming the normal infusion rate. Hypotension is not an allergic reaction unless it is associated with anaphylaxis.

E. Rash. A rash occurs in 2% to 3% of patients receiving streptokinase and is treated by discontinuing the streptokinase infusion and giving benadryl 50 mg (IV or PO) and hydrocortisone 100 mg (IV) q6h (if severe). If a full lytic dose was not received, 50 mg tPA or acute PCI should be considered.

F. Anaphylaxis. Anaphylaxis occurs in 0.1% of patients receiving streptokinase and is treated by discontinuing the streptokinase infusion, securing an airway, and giving epinephrine 1–5 cc of 1:10,000 solution IV, hydrocortisone 100–200 mg IV q4–6h × 24h, and IV fluids. IV dopamine 5–20 mcg/kg/min or norepinephrine 0.5–30 mcg/min is indicated for persistent hypotension, and albuterol 0.5 cc of 0.5% solution in 2–5 cc normal saline as an aerosolized mist is useful for bronchospasm.

G. Rigors. Rigors can occur during plasminogen breakdown and are treated with demerol 25 mg IV.

H. Reperfusion Arrhythmias

   1. Bradycardia, 3° AV block. Occurs most often with acute reperfusion of the RCA and usually resolves within minutes. Symptomatic episodes are treated with atropine 0.5–1.0 mg IV every 3–5 minutes and IV fluids. Transcutaneous pacing is rarely needed.

   2. Bezold-Jarish reflex. Presents as profound hypotension with bradycardia in response to activation of vagal afferent fibers following acute reperfusion of the RCA. Treated with atropine 0.5–1.0 mg IV every 3–5 minutes, IV fluids, and possibly temporary pacing. Persistent episodes may require norepinephrine 0.5–30 mcg/min IV.

   3. Idioventricular rhythm. No treatment is required for rates <120 bpm in the absence of hypotension.

   4. Ventricular tachycardia (VT). No specific treatment is required for runs of non-sustained VT, which are common and usually abate over time. Beta-blockers are the first-line therapy for non-sustained ventricular tachycardia (NSV) (which in most of the cases they will already be prescribed because of the acute MI). However, if NSVT is present 4 days after the STEMI with an EF <40%, an electrophysiologic testing is indicated with or without ICD implantation. For pulseless VT or ventricular fibrillation, immediate defibrillation is required. For refractory VT/VF, amiodarone or lidocaine are reasonable options.

PCI AFTER FIBRINOLYTIC THERAPY

Several interventional approaches are available for the management of acute MI after lytic therapy, including rescue, immediate, and delayed PCI (Table 5.5). Most randomized trials evaluating these approaches were conducted prior to the widespread availability of stents and GP IIb/IIIa inhibitors, which have greatly improved the safety and efficacy of PCI.

A. **Rescue (Salvage) PCI for Failed Fibrinolysis.** In small randomized trials of PTCA versus medical therapy for failed lytic therapy, successful PTCA improved regional and global LV function, and there was a trend toward less recurrent ischemia, heart failure, shock, and death in high-risk patients. However, early mortality was high (30% to 40%) when rescue PTCA was unsuccessful. Stenting appears to improve the results of rescue PCI. In 83 patients who underwent rescue stenting, TIMI-3 flow was achieved in 93%, and there were low rates of major adverse cardiac events (death, reinfarction, CABG, or target lesion revascularization) during hospitalization (3.6%) and at 1 year (18.8%), similar to results obtained with primary stenting for acute MI. In the GUSTO-III substudy (nonrandomized), there was a trend toward lower 30-day mortality when abciximab was used during rescue angioplasty (3.6% versus 9.7%, p = 0.076). More recently, in REACT, rescue PCI significantly reduced the primary composite endpoint of death, reinfarction, stroke, or significant heart failure at 6 months by almost 50% (15.3% versus 29.8% for conservative therapy with IV heparin versus 31% for repeat fibrinolysis). In contrast, MERLIN failed to demonstrate a benefit for rescue PCI; however, there were longer delays to PCI and less use of GP IIb/IIIa inhibitors and stents in MERLIN. However, it should be noted that expedited PCI after fibrinolysis has shown superior results over rescue strategies and should be employed in situations where there is no nearby interventional facility rather than rescue PCI in failed thrombolysis.

Table 5.5. PCI Approaches After Fibrinolytic Therapy for Acute MI

Approach	Description
Rescue (salvage) PCI	PCI after failed fibrinolysis (TIMI 0–1 blood flow in the infarct vessel).
Immediate PCI	PCI for significant residual stenosis immediately after successful fibrinolysis.
Delayed (deferred) PCI	PCI for significant residual stenosis 1–7 days after fibrinolysis (prior to discharge).

PCI = percutaneous coronary intervention.

B. Immediate PCI After Successful Fibrinolysis in Asymptomatic Patients. Older studies suggested that immediate PTCA for significant residual stenosis in asymptomatic patients resulted in higher rates of blood transfusion, emergency CABG, and death compared to no intervention, but these studies were limited by inconsistent use of preprocedural aspirin and ACT monitoring. In contrast, contemporary small studies (PACT, CAPITAL-AMI, SIAM) suggest that angioplasty can be performed safely immediately following fibrinolytic therapy, and results from GRACIA and AALK indicate a trend toward improved survival at 1 year for routine PCI after fibrinolysis compared to an ischemia-driven PCI strategy (PCI at mean of 17 hours in GRACIA and 24 days in AALK). The large randomized ASSENT-4 compared PCI $\pm$ fibrinolysis and was terminated early due to concerns over significantly worse outcome in the group receiving lytics. Also, the FINESSE study compared three study arms of PCI with preprocedural abciximab, abciximab plus reduced dose reteplase, or normal primary PCI. It showed no difference between the three treatment arms. Recently, the CARESS-in-AMI showed in 600 patients that performing primary PCI after thrombolyis is superior to a strategy with rescue PCI by reducing the composite endpoint of all-cause mortality, reinfarction, and refractory myocardial ischaemia within 30 days (4.4% versus 10.7%, p = 0.004). The strategy of transferring STEMI patients for PCI within 6 hours of receiving thrombolysis at a non-PCI center was shown to be superior to the more standard wait-and-see strategy in the Angioplasty and Stenting After Fibrinolysis to Enhance Reperfusion in Acute Myocardial Infarction (TRANSFER-AMI) study. In this study, 1030 patients with high-risk STEMI were randomized to either standard treatment after fibrinolysis (rescue PCI for failed reperfusion, with elective PCI encouraged for successfully reperfused patients after 24 hours) or a pharmacoinvasive strategy (transfer for PCI within 6 hours of fibrinolysis). In summary, TRANSFER-AMI trial showed that for high-risk STEMI patients receiving thrombolysis at non-PCI centers, urgent transfer and PCI within 6 hours is associated with significantly fewer ischemic complications and no excess in bleeding when compared with standard treatment after fibrinolysis.

C. Delayed (1–7 days) PCI After Successful Fibrinolysis in Asymptomatic Patients. Randomized trials (TIMI-2B, SWIFT) comparing invasive (routine PTCA before discharge) and conservative (PTCA for spontaneous or inducible ischemia) approaches following successful fibrinolysis showed no difference in death, reinfarction, or LV ejection fraction. However, in TIMI-2B, intraprocedural ACT was not monitored, total occlusions were not dilated, and intention-to-treat analysis may have attenuated the beneficial effect of PTCA, since only 54% of patients in the invasive arm received PTCA and the majority of deaths in the invasive arm occurred prior to revascularization. It is reasonable to consider predischarge angiography in patients with LV dysfunction, severe ventricular arrhythmias, heart failure during acute episode even if LV function is preserved on subsequent evaluation, known multivessel disease, or prior PCI/CABG. This should be followed by stenting with a GP IIb/IIIa inhibitor for high-grade stenoses supplying moderate or large areas of viable myocardium or by CABG for severe multivessel disease. Especially in the light of the Occluded Artery Trial (OAT), discussed more in depth later, the angiography and treatment of asymptomatic patients is not advised.

D. Delayed PCI of an Occluded Vessel After Failed Fibrinolysis in Asymptomatic Patients. TAMI-6 reported improved ejection fraction at 6 weeks in patients treated with PTCA at 48 hours compared to those treated medically, but 40% of vessels were reoccluded at 6 months. Nonrandomized studies reported better survival after successful PTCA, possibly due to improved ventricular remodeling, better recovery of viable but hibernating myocardium, and fewer arrhythmias. Late PCI of occluded infarct vessels was tested in the OAT, which showed no improvement in death, reinfarction, or stroke compared to optimal medical treatment, and only slightly lower revascularization rates (18.4% versus 22.0%, p = 0.03). As such, late revascularization of patients with an occluded infarct-related artery is not recommended.

E. PCI for Recurrent Ischemia After Fibrinolysis. Compared to a strategy of PTCA for refractory symptoms only, PTCA for spontaneous or inducible ischemia after fibrinolytic therapy reduced the incidence of MI, unstable angina, and use of anti-ischemic drugs in DANAMI, and there was a trend toward a reduction in death long term. Patients with postinfarct angina or an abnormal stress test should undergo cardiac catheterization and revascularization based on anatomy.

ALTERNATIVE REPERFUSION STRATEGIES FOR ACUTE MI

Fibrinolytic therapy exposes clot-bound thrombin, which is a potent platelet activator, and TIMI-3 flow rates are achieved in only 50% to 60% of infarct vessels after fibrinolytic therapy. Furthermore, microvascular embolization of platelet aggregates may impair myocardial reperfusion despite good epicardial blood flow. To offset the prothrombotic potential of fibrinolytic therapy, recent trials have evaluated the role for GP IIb/IIIa inhibitors and/or enoxaparin as adjuncts to fibrinolytic therapy.

A. Full-Dose Fibrinolysis plus GP IIb/IIIa Inhibitor. TAMI8 evaluated the safety of tPA (100 mg), aspirin, and graded doses of abciximab in patients with acute MI and demonstrated a dose-dependent reduction in platelet aggregation with increasing doses of abciximab. In IMPACT-AMI, the addition of eptifibatide to tPA increased the speed and frequency of reperfusion, without an increase in bleeding. In PARADIGM, there was no improvement in clinical outcome and more bleeding complications with the addition of lamifiban to tPA or streptokinase, but ST-segment monitoring indicated that lamifiban resulted in more rapid reperfusion.

B. Low-Dose Fibrinolysis plus GP IIb/IIIa Inhibitor. The TIMI 14a pilot study found that half-dose tPA combined with standard-dose abciximab resulted in TIMI-3 flow in 79% at 90 minutes. In SPEED, half-dose rPA plus standard-dose abciximab resulted in TIMI-3 flow in 73% at 90 minutes. In INTEGRITI, compared to full-dose TNK, reduced-dose TNK plus double-bolus eptifibatide tended to improve angiographic flow and ST-segment resolution but was associated with more bleeding. Results of the large, randomized, multicenter ASSENT and GUSTO-V trials have now been published.

1. **ASSENT-3.** In this trial, 6095 patients with acute MI <6 hours and ST-elevation or LBBB were randomized to one of three drug regimens: (1) full-dose TNK-tPA plus unfractionated heparin (UFH); (2) half-dose TNK-tPA plus abciximab plus UFH; (3) full-dose TNK-tPA plus enoxaparin. Compared to TNK-tPA plus UFH, the primary efficacy endpoint (30-day mortality or in-hospital reinfarction or refractory ischemia) was reduced in the enoxaparin and abciximab groups (15.4% versus 11.4% versus 11.1%, respectively; p = 0.0001). The composite endpoint of primary efficacy, in-hospital intracranial hemorrhage, and major bleeding complications was reduced with enoxaparin but not with abciximab. Abciximab was associated with worse outcome in elderly patients (age >75 years), no benefit in diabetics, and increased bleeding complications in diabetics and the elderly. Although fewer patients needed urgent PCI with abciximab and enoxaparin, clinical outcomes after urgent PCI (n = 716) were less favorable in these groups, especially with abciximab. Clinical outcomes after elective PCI (n = 1064) were similar between groups.

2. **GUSTO-V.** In this trial, 16,588 patients with acute MI <6 hours and ST-elevation or LBBB were treated with UFH and randomized to full-dose rPA or half-dose rPA plus abciximab. There was no difference in 30-day mortality (primary endpoint), but half-dose rPA plus abciximab resulted in less death or reinfarction at 30 days (7.4% versus 8.8%, p = 0.0011), less need for urgent PCI (5.6% versus 8.6%, p <0.0001), less reinfarction (2.3% versus 3.5%, p <0.0001) or recurrent ischemia (11.3% versus 12.8%, p = 0.004) at 7 days but more major bleeding complications (1.1% versus 0.5%, p <0.0001). Patients over age 75 had a higher rate of intracranial hemorrhage with half-dose rPA plus abciximab (2.1% versus 1.1%), but those under age 75 had a lower rate of intracranial hemorrhage (0.4% versus 0.5%). At 1 year, mortality rates were identical between groups (8.4%), although there was a trend toward lower mortality in patients <75 years with anterior MI who received half-dose rPA plus abciximab (7.1% versus 8.0%, p = 0.21).

   Combining these data with the outcome of recent meta-analyses shows there is no benefit of combining full-dose fibrinolytics with GP IIb/IIIa inhibitors, mostly due to the excess in bleeding seen with this treatment.

C. **Full-Dose Fibrinolysis plus Low Molecular-Weight Heparin (LMWH).** LMWH has several advantages over unfractionated heparin (UFH) (p. 186), and enoxaparin was associated with less death or MI compared to UFH in randomized trials of non-ST-elevation ACS (p. 174). Compared to UFH in ASSENT-3, the addition of enoxaparin to TNK-tPA for STEMI reduced the primary composite endpoint (30-day death or in-hospital reinfarction or refractory ischemia) by 26% (11.4% versus 15.4%, p = 0.0001), with only a modest increase in major bleeding but with need for additional data, especially in the elderly. The ENTIRE-TIMI trial showed reduced ischemic events using enoxoparine compared to UFH, with no excess in bleeding. The ExTRACT-TIMI 25 trial, however, showed that overall benefits of enoxaparin over UFH (8% reduction in 30-day mortality, 33% reduction in nonfatal MI, and 26% reduction in urgent revascularization rates) were offset by a significant increase in major bleeding complications.

D. Fibrinolysis plus Clopidogrel. The CLARITY-TIMI trial showed that the addition of a loading dose of clopidogrel (300 mg) and maintenance dose (75 mg/24 hr) for patients treated with full-dose fibrinolytic therapy significantly reduced the likelihood of infart vessel reocclusion after fibrinolysis (11.7% versus 18.4%, p <0.001) and cardiovascular death, MI, or recurrent ischemia was reduced at 30 days (11.6% versus 14.1%, p = 0.03). Similar findings were seen in the COMMIT-CCS 2 trial, in which 45,852 patients in China were randomized to either clopidogrel or placebo following ST-elevation myocardial infarction: 50% of these patients received thrombolysis. The primary endpoint of in-hospital death was significantly reduced (7.5% versus 8.1%, p = 0.03). Additionally, clopidogrel treatment reduced the coprimary endpoint of in-hospital death, reinfarction, or stroke (9.2% versus 10.1%, p = 0.002) by reducing reinfarction.

E. Recommendations. Reperfusion strategies combining standard- or low-dose fibrinolytic therapy with enoxaparin, or a direct thrombin inhibitor may enhance reperfusion and reduce ischemic complications in STEMI, and thienopyridine treatment should be administered in all patients at low-bleeding risk.

SECTION 3

UNSTABLE ANGINA AND NON-ST-ELEVATION ACS (NSTE-ACS)

Chapter 6

Diagnosis and Evaluation of Unstable Angina and Non-ST-Elevation ACS (NSTE-ACS)

UNSTABLE ANGINA AND NON-ST-ELEVATION ACS (NSTE-ACS)

Patients with unstable angina (UA) and the NSTE-ACS represent a continuum of ACS with similar underpinnings of pathophysiology, presentation, and considerations for management strategies. Distinguishing the presence of NSTE-ACS requires an assessment of serum cardiac biomarkers to evaluate for evidence of myocardial necrosis. If elevated serum cardiac biomarkers are present, NSTE-ACS becomes the appropriate categorization for this condition. In both instances (UA and NSTE-ACS), the diagnostic and management strategy is selected to reduce the risk for future adverse cardiovascular events.

DIAGNOSIS

A. **Unstable Angina.** Unstable angina is a clinical diagnosis. Based on the onset, duration, and frequency of chest pain, unstable angina can be categorized into rest angina, new-onset severe angina, or increasing angina. ECG changes may or may not be present, and serum cardiac markers are normal.

1. **Rest angina.** Angina that occurs at rest, usually within 1 week of presentation. Episodes are often prolonged (>20 minutes).

2. **New-onset severe angina.** New onset of class III–IV angina. Angina occurs after walking ≤1–2 blocks on a flat surface or climbing ≤1 flight of stairs at normal pace.

3. **Increasing angina.** Previously diagnosed angina that is distinctly more frequent, longer, or lower in threshold. There is at least one functional class increase to class III or IV severity.

B. **NSTE-ACS.** The diagnosis of acute MI requires one of two criteria. The first criterion requires the rise and fall of cardiac markers (troponin or CK-MB) *plus* one of the following: symptoms of ischemia, Q-waves or ischemic changes on ECG, or coronary intervention. The second criterion is pathological findings indicative of acute MI. There are important limitations to these criteria: acute MI can present with atypical symptoms, noncardiac disorders can manifest ischemic-type chest pain and ST-segment changes, and the rise and fall in cardiac markers is time-dependent and can be missed.

SYMPTOMS

The most common presentation for NSTE-ACS is chest, neck, or jaw discomfort, which is usually described as pressure, burning, or squeezing in character. Symptoms typically last <30 minutes in unstable angina and >30 minutes in NSTE-ACS. Atypical presentations—weakness, dyspnea, heart failure—are more common in diabetics, the elderly, and women may present with dyspnea or jaw pain stretched out over hours, rather than minutes. Women often experience prodromal symptoms—unusual fatigue, sleep disturbance, dyspnea—in the weeks preceding acute MI. Pleuritic-type symptoms and pain reproduced by palpation are very unusual presentations but do not exclude the possibility of ACS. Up to 20% of infarcts are "silent" or go unrecognized by the physician or patient. Silent MI occurs most often in diabetics with autonomic dysfunction.

ELECTROCARDIOGRAM

Patients with NSTE-ACS can present with ischemic ST-segment and T-wave changes, nonspecific ST-T changes, or a relatively normal ECG. An interesting group will have transient ST-segment elevation followed by one of the aforementioned patterns. ECG changes can be persistent, evident only during chest pain, or they may not occur at all. Classic ischemic changes include horizontal or downsloping ST-depression ≥0.5 mm and/or symmetrically inverted T-waves >2.0 mm (Figure 6.1). Deep T-wave inversions across the precordial leads strongly suggest severe stenosis of the proximal left anterior descending (LAD) coronary artery. Ischemic T-waves can also be biphasic or upright and peaked (hyperacute). Patients with dynamic ST-T changes are at increased risk of death or MI and are managed more aggressively than patients without ECG changes or other high-risk markers. It is important to obtain serial ECGs in patients with ongoing chest pain and normal or nonspecific changes on initial ECG, since some patients develop complete coronary occlusion and ST-elevation during hospitalization and benefit from reperfusion therapy. Continuous ECG monitoring with attention to ST-segment shifts can be used for this purpose. "Ischemic" ECG changes lack specificity for coronary artery disease and can be seen in a variety of nonischemic conditions (Table 6.1).

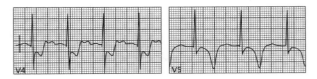

Figure 6.1. ST and T-Wave Changes in NSTE-ACS

Table 6.1. Differential Diagnosis for "Ischemic" ECG Changes

ST-Segment Depression	Deeply Inverted T-Waves	Tall Peaked T-Waves
• Myocardial ischemia • Repolarization changes secondary to ventricular hypertrophy or IVCD • Digitalis effect • "Pseudodepression" from superimposition of atrial flutter waves or prominent atrial repolarization wave on the ST segment, as seen in atrial enlargement, pericarditis, or atrial infarction • CNS disorder • Hypokalemia • Quinidine effect • Mitral valve prolapse	• Myocardial ischemia • LVH • RVH • CNS disorder • WPW syndrome • Hypertrophic cardiomyopathy (apical variant) • Stress-induced (takotsubo) cardiomyopathy	• Acute MI (hyperacute T-waves) • Angina pectoris • Normal variant (usually mid-precordial leads) • Hyperkalemia (more common when acute) • Intracranial bleeding • LVH • RVH • LBBB • Pseudopeaked T-waves from superimposition of P-waves on the T-wave, as seen with APCs, sinus rhythm with marked 1° AV block, or complete heart block • Anemia

APC = atrial premature contraction, AV = atrio-ventricular, CNS = central nervous system, IVCD = intraventricular conduction delay, LBBB = left bundle branch block, LVH = left ventricular hypertrophy, MI = myocardial infarction, RVH = right ventricular hypertrophy, WPW = Wolff-Parkinson-White.
Source: The ECG Criteria Book. Eds: O'Keefe J, Hammill S, Freed M, Pogwizd S. Physician's Press, Royal Oak, MI 2002

SERUM CARDIAC MARKERS

CK-MB and cardiac troponin levels are used to differentiate unstable angina from acute MI, assess prognosis, and guide therapy. Cardiac markers should be obtained on admission and repeated at least once (troponin) or twice (CK-MB) at 6–8 hour intervals. Elevated cardiac troponin levels are associated with a three- to eightfold increased risk of death or MI and identify patients most likely to benefit from GP IIb/IIIa inhibitors and the early invasive approach to management. No single cardiac marker is ideal, and each has its own advantages and disadvantages. The upper limit of normal (ULN) for each cardiac biomarker represents the 99th percentile from a reference population without myocardial necrosis; however, most hospital laboratories may not report the 99th percentile but rather the reference ranges based on their local values. The coefficient of variation (CV) of the assay should be 10% or less. Because cardiac markers may not turn positive for hours after the initial ischemic insult (e.g., plaque rupture), patients who arrive at the hospital soon after symptom onset may initially have negative cardiac biomarker results.

OTHER STUDIES

Hemoglobin, platelet count, serum lipids, and other routine serum chemistries should be obtained in the emergency department. A chest X-ray is recommended on admission in hemodynamically unstable patients and within 48 hours in stable patients.

RISK STRATIFICATION

All patients with NSTE-ACS should be classified according to their risk of short-term death or nonfatal MI (Table 6.2). In addition to providing prognostic information, risk categories serve as the basis for initial management decisions, which range from immediate angiography, GP IIb/IIIa inhibitors, and PCI (if indicated) for high-risk patients to outpatient management similar to chronic stable angina for low-risk patients. Validated and simple-to-use risk prediction scores for NSTE-ACS, such as the TIMI risk score or the GRACE risk score, may also be useful in guiding the selection of management strategies in unstable angina and/ or NSTE-ACS.

Table 6.2. Short-Term Risk of Death or MI in Unstable Angina

High Risk	Intermediate Risk	Low Risk
At least one feature must be present: • Prolonged (>20 min) ongoing rest pain • Angina at rest with dynamic ST-depression ≥0.5 mm or new bundle branch block • Angina with new or worsening MR murmur • Angina with S$_3$, new or worsening rales, or pulmonary edema • Angina with hypotension, bradycardia, or tachycardia • Age ≥75 years • Elevated cardiac troponins (>0.1 ng/mL) • Sustained ventricular tachycardia	No high-risk features but must have one of the following: • Prolonged (>20 min) rest angina, now resolved, with moderate or high likelihood of coronary heart disease • Rest angina (<20 min) relieved with rest or sublingual nitroglycerin • Angina with dynamic T-wave changes >2.0 mm or abnormal Q-waves • Aspirin use prior to hospitalization • Prior MI or CABG • Peripheral vascular disease or cerebrovascular disease • Slightly elevated cardiac troponins (>0.01 ng/mL but <0.1 ng/mL) • Age >70 years	No high- or intermediate-risk features but may have any of the following: • New-onset angina or progressive CCS class III–IV angina without prolonged (>20 min) chest pain but with moderate or high likelihood of coronary heart disease • Normal or unchanged ECG during chest discomfort • Cardiac markers not elevated

CCS = Canadian Cardiovascular Society, MR = mitral regurgitation.
Source: Adapted from ACC/AHA Guideline Update for the Management of Patients with Unstable Angina or Non-ST-Elevation Myocardial Infarction, March 2002.

Chapter 7

Overview of Management of Non-ST-Elevation ACS (NSTE-ACS)

EMERGENCY DEPARTMENT MEASURES

All patients with NSTE-ACS should be triaged to an invasive or conservative management strategy based on their risk category. The use of an early invasive strategy (diagnostic coronary angiography performed within 48 hours of presentation followed by revascularization as dictated by the coronary anatomical findings during angiography) should be considered in patients with high-risk features (dynamic ECG changes, positive troponin, hemodynamic instability, postinfarct angina, heart failure) of NSTE-ACS, whereas the use of an early conservative strategy (e.g., selectively invasive or delayed invasive) is more appropriate for low-risk patients with atypical presentations, absence of significant ECG changes, normal cardiac biomarkers, normal left ventricular function, and/or a low likelihood of ACS (Table 7.1). Hospitalized patients should receive aspirin at a dose of 162–325 mg initially, followed by lower dose aspirin (<150 mg) once daily, beta-blockers (IV for ongoing pain; otherwise PO), and antithrombotic therapy (unfractionated heparin, enoxaparin, or fondaparinux). Clopidogrel and GP IIb/IIIa inhibitors each provide benefit and their use is described on pp. 181, 184. Clopidogrel is of benefit in ACS patients whether they undergo PCI or CABG during the index hospitalization; however, to minimize the risk of perioperative bleeding, clopidogrel should be withheld 5–7 days prior to CABG. Additional measures include nitroglycerin (sublingual tablet or spray) for ongoing pain, and morphine sulfate for pulmonary congestion, severe agitation, or ongoing pain despite nitrates. Verapamil, amlodipine, or diltiazem should be considered for ongoing or recurrent ischemia if beta-blockers are contraindicated and LV function is preserved and for ACS due to variant angina or cocaine use. Nitrates should be avoided in RV infarction and within 24 hours of sildenafil (Viagra) (increased risk of severe hypotension), immediate-release nifedipine should be avoided without a beta-blocker (increased risk of MI, recurrent angina, and death), and fibrinolytics should be avoided due to their lack of clinical benefit and possible detrimental effect. Patients with refractory ischemia, hemodynamic instability, or refractory arrhythmias despite medical therapy should be considered for IABP as a bridge to urgent PCI. Initial assessment should also exclude the presence of a life-threatening mimic of ACS: pulmonary embolism, aortic dissection, pneumothorax, esophageal rupture, or ischemia/rupture of an intra-abdominal organ.

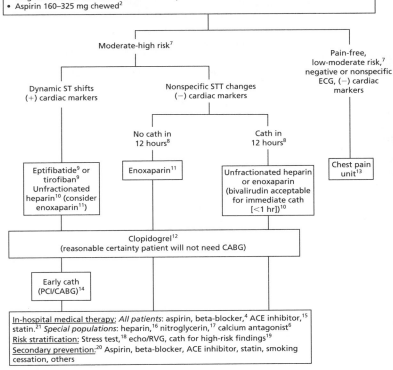

Figure 7.1. Management of NSTE-ACS

1. CK-MB every 6–8 hours × 3, cardiac troponins repeated at least once at 4–8 hours, complete blood count, platelet count, fibrinogen, lipid profile, electrolytes, BUN/creatinine, portable chest X-ray.

2. Buccal absorption of crushed or chewed nonenteric-coated aspirin produces the most rapid antiplatelet effects. Avoid enteric-coated preparations acutely due to delays in GI absorption and platelet inhibition. An aspirin suppository (325 mg) can be given to patients unable to take oral medications. For patients

Figure 7.1. Management of NSTE-ACS (cont'd)

who are allergic to aspirin, clopdiogrel 300 mg once at presentation, followed by 75 mg as a daily maintenance dose is recommend.

3. Up to three nitroglycerin tablets (0.4 mg) or three metered doses of nitroglycerin spray (0.4 mg) onto/ under tongue at 5-minute intervals. Avoid if systolic BP <90 mmHg, heart rate <50 bpm, suspected RV infarction. Avoid if sildenafil (Viagra) or vardenafil (Levitra) is used within 24 hours or if tadalafil (Cialis) is used within 48 hours.

4. Avoid beta-blocker acutely if systolic BP <90 mmHg, heart rate <50 bpm, severe heart failure, or history of significant bronchospasm. Given IV followed by PO to patients with ongoing pain or high-risk features. Can start PO in low-risk asymptomatic patients. See p. 178 for dosing and administration guidelines.

5. Morphine can be repeated in 2–8 mg increments every 5–15 minutes, as needed. Avoid in severe chronic lung disease (increased risk of respiratory depression). Hypoventilation can be reversed with naloxone (0.4–2.0 mg IV). Hypotension usually responds to leg elevation IV saline (200–300 cc if no pulmonary congestion). Bradycardia, nausea, and vomiting often improve with atropine (0.5–l.0 mg IV).

6. Diltiazem 120–320 mg/d (PO) or verapamil 120–480 mg/d (PO) in single or divided doses depending on the preparation. Also consider for non-Q-wave MI without pulmonary congestion, started on day 2–5 and continued up to 1 year.

7. See Table 6.2 (p. 65) for description of risk categories.

8. Early diagnostic angiography with anatomy-driven revascularization should be considered for patients with ongoing/recurrent pain, heart failure, hemodynamic instability, mitral regurgitation, or LV dysfunction. For immediate cath (<1 hour), unfractionated heparin, enoxaparin, or bivalirudin can be used as anticoagulants of choice. (The use of fondaparinux in this setting is generally not recommended. If it is used, additional anticoagulant support during PCI is recommended due to concern of higher incidence of catheter-related thrombosis.)

9. See Table 9.3 (p. 93) for dosing/administration guidelines for eptifibatide and tirofiban.

10. As medical therapy in conjunction with a GP IIb/IIIa inhibitor, UFH is given as 60–70 U/kg IV bolus (max. 5000 U) plus 12–15 U/kg/min (max. 1000 U/hr), adjusted to maintain aPTT at 1.5–2.5 times control (50–75 seconds). The SYNERGY trial randomized 10,027 high-risk ACS patients (two of the following: age >60, positive cardiac markers, transient ST elevation or ST depression) undergoing early cath/PCI to enoxaparin or UFH. There was no difference in the primary endpoint (death or MI) at 30 days, but TIMI major bleeding was increased in the enoxaparin group (see Table 9.7, p. 99).

11. See p. 101 for enoxaparin dosing.

12. See discussion of clopidogrel for non-ST-elevation ACS (p. 181).

13. For select patients with nondiagnostic or normal ECGs in whom the diagnosis of ACS is in doubt, one approach is to follow these patients in the emergency department for 8–12 hours and consider discharge to home if repeat serum cardiac markers are negative, serial ECGs remain stable, 2D echo (or possibly stress test) is normal, and there is no further evidence of ischemia. A stress test should be obtained within 48–72 hours if not performed in the emergency department prior to discharge.

14. Stent plus abciximab or eptifibatide (see Table 9.3, p. 93, for dosing regimens and use of adjunctive heparin/enoxaparin). Consider triage to CABG instead of PCI for significant left main disease, three-vessel disease with treated diabetes or LV dysfunction, or two-vessel disease with proximal LAD involvement and either LV dysfunction or ischemia on stress testing. Prior to CABG, discontinue clopidogrel × 5–7 days and GP IIb/IIIa inhibitors × several hours, and switch from enoxaparin to unfractionated heparin.

15. Start oral ACE inhibitor at low dose as soon as patient is stabilized from MI (after reperfusion and once blood pressure has stabilized; usually no sooner than 6 hours). Titrate upward over 1–4 days, as tolerated. See p. 174 for dosing and administration guidelines. Continue indefinitely if ejection fraction is reduced. For uncomplicated MI without LV dysfunction, discontinue after 4–6 weeks or consider long-term therapy for secondary prevention.

16. If anticoagulants are prescribed for several days due to higher risks of thromboembolism (e.g., large anterior MI, LV thrombus, atrial fibrillation, prior embolism), consider using enoxaparin or fondaparinux to decrease the likelihood of developing heparin-induced thrombocytopenia (HIT) with prolonged UFH treatment.

Figure 7.1. Management of NSTE-ACS (cont'd)

17. IV nitroglycerin should be continued × 24–48 hours for large anterior MI, heart failure, hypertension, or recurrent ischemia.

18. Predischarge stress testing is performed in low- and intermediate-risk patients without rest pain or heart failure after a minimum of 12–24 hours and 2–3 days (e.g., initial conservative or selectively invasive strategy), respectively. If baseline ECG abnormality precludes assessment of ST-segment shifts (e.g., LBBB, LVH with repolarization changes, female gender), an exercise test with radionuclide imaging is recommended. Patients unable to exercise should undergo a pharmacological stress test.

19. High-risk findings include any of the following: second troponin positive at 4–8 hours; repeat ECG shows ischemic ST-T changes; recurrent rest angina; recurrent exertional angina with heart failure or mitral regurgitation; LVEF <0.40; hemodynamic instability; sustained ventricular tachycardia; prior PCI within 6 months; prior CABG; or high-risk noninvasive test result (>3% annual mortality): rest or exercise LVEF <0.35; treadmill score ≤ −11; single large stress-induced perfusion defect or multiple moderate perfusion defects; large fixed perfusion defect or moderate stress-induced perfusion defect with LV dilatation or thallium uptake in lung; echo wall motion abnormality > two segments with low-dose dobutamine (<10 mcg/kg/min) or at a low heart rate (<120 bpm); or extensive ischemia on stress echo.

20. Secondary prevention measures include aspirin, beta-blocker, ACE inhibitor, statin, exercise, smoking cessation, weight control, Mediterranean or DASH diet. Consider gemfibrozil for low HDL cholesterol and fish oil (omega-3) supplement. Control hypertension (blood pressure ≤130/85 mmHg), diabetes mellitus (HgbAlc <7%), and dyslipidemia (LDL cholesterol ≤100 mg/dL; HDL-cholesterol >40 mg/dL; triglyceride ≤150 mg/dL). Provide instructions to patient and family on the use of nitrates for recurrent pain, when to return to the emergency room, the purpose and dose of each discharge medication, and the importance of compliance.

21. In-hospital initiation (within 10 days and after patient is stable) of intensive LDL-lowering drug therapy. See discussion on pp. 104–106.

EARLY MANAGEMENT OF NSTE-ACS BASED ON RISK CATEGORY

A. **High-Risk Patients.** These patients are best treated with early (<12–48 hours) catheterization followed by PCI (in conjunction with a GP IIb/IIIa inhibitor and antithrombin therapy) or CABG based on anatomy. Clinical trials have shown benefit for abciximab, eptifibatide, and tirofiban. In TARGET, the only head-to-head comparison of GP IIb/IIIa inhibitors to date, abciximab was superior to tirofiban at reducing the 30-day composite endpoint of death, MI, or urgent target vessel revascularization in ACS patients undergoing PCI (6.3% vs. 9.3%, p = 0.002). All high-risk patients without contraindications should also receive aspirin, clopidogrel, and a beta-blocker. Clopidogrel is of benefit in ACS patients treated by medical therapy alone or revascularization (PCI or CABG); however, to minimize the risk of perioperative bleeding, clopidogrel should be withheld 5–7 days prior to CABG. Because it is difficult to know if a patient will require CABG until angiography has been performed, and because many practices currently use early (<24 hours) angiography in such patients, some advocate withholding clopidogrel until the coronary anatomy is defined (see p. 181). Despite the established benefits for an early invasive approach, data from the CRUSADE quality improvement initiative indicate that high-risk patients are least likely to be transferred to an interventional center (from community hospitals without revascularization facilities) and are treated less aggressively during the acute phase of hospitalization than lower-risk patients.

B. Intermediate-Risk Patients. Patients with prior PCI or CABG should be treated the same as high-risk patients. Other intermediate-risk patients can be managed by the early invasive or early conservative approach to revascularization (see Table 7.1). Early conservative management consists of dual antiplatelet therapy with aspirin and clopidogrel plus anticoagulant therapy, followed by late angiography and revascularization for any of the following: elevated cardiac markers or ischemic ECG changes on repeat testing, recurrent rest angina, exertional angina with heart failure or mitral regurgitation, LV dysfunction (EF <0.40), high-risk noninvasive stress test result, hemodynamic instability, or sustained VT. High-risk (>3% annual mortality) findings on noninvasive testing include rest or exercise LVEF <0.35, treadmill score ≤ −11, single large or multiple moderate stress-induced perfusion defects, fixed perfusion defect with LV dilatation or thallium uptake in lung, and stress echo demonstrating extensive ischemia or echo wall motion abnormality in ≥ two myocardial segments with low-dose dobutamine (<10 mcg/kg/min) or at low heart rate (<120 bpm). All intermediate-risk patients without contraindications should receive aspirin, clopidogrel, and a beta-blocker. Clopidogrel is of benefit in ACS patients treated by medical therapy alone or revascularization (PCI or CABG); however, to minimize the risk of perioperative bleeding, clopidogrel should be withheld for 5–7 days prior to CABG.

C. Low-Risk Patients. Patients with new-onset or progressive angina without prolonged (>20 min) chest pain or other intermediate- or high-risk features should be triaged to PCI for the same indications as intermediate-risk patients. For asymptomatic, low-risk patients without ST-T changes or elevated cardiac troponins, one approach is to follow these patients in the emergency department for 8–12 hours and consider discharge to home if repeat serum cardiac troponins are negative, serial ECGs remain stable, 2D echo (or possibly stress test) is normal, and there is no further evidence of ischemia. Discharged patients are managed on an outpatient basis similar to patients with chronic stable angina; a stress test is recommended within 72 hours if not performed during observation in the emergency department.

Table 7.1. Approach to Revascularization for NSTE-ACS

Risk Category*	Approach**
High-risk	Early invasive approach.
Intermediate-risk	Early invasive or early conservative (selectively invasive) approach.
Low-risk	Early conservative approach or manage as outpatient.†

* See Table 6.2, p. 65, for description of risk categories.

** Early invasive approach: Early (within 48 hours) angiography and revascularization (PCI or CABG). Early conservative approach: angiography and revascularization for recurrent ischemia, LV dysfunction (EF <0.40), or high-risk finding on stress test.

† Low-risk patients with normal troponin levels on repeat testing, stable ECGs, no further ischemia, and a normal echocardiogram or stress test during observation in the emergency department may be considered for outpatient management similar to patients with chronic stable angina. Stress testing is recommended within 48–72 hours if not performed in the emergency department prior to discharge.

HOSPITAL MANAGEMENT

Aspirin, clopidogrel, and beta-blockers are continued throughout hospitalization. For patients initially triaged to PCI, a GP IIb/IIIa inhibitor and heparin are given before and during PCI. After PCI, heparin should be stopped, and the GP IIb/IIIa inhibitor infusion should be continued per labeled recommendations for 12–18 hours (Table 9.3, p. 93). For patients triaged to early conservative management, the benefit of eptifibatide or tirofiban in this setting is less certain and has a class IIb recommendation from the American College of Cardiology/American Heart Association guidelines, and abciximab should not be administered unless the patient is definitely planned to undergo PCI. The use of anticoagulants, such as UFH, enoxaparin, or fondaparinux is continued for 2–5 days or until hospital discharge for NSTE-ACS patients treated with an early conservative management strategy. Anticoagulant selection for patients with NSTE-ACS managed with an early invasive strategy include UFH, enoxaparin, fondaparinux, or bivalirudin. The recommendations from the ACC/AHA guidelines regarding the choice of anticoagulant and the level of evidence for each of the anticoagulants based on management strategy (early conservative vs. early invasive) are provided (Table 7.2). LDL-lowering drug therapy should be started in-hospital (within 10 days and after the patient is stable) and continued long term to reduce mortality and major cardiovascular events. Patients with hypertension, LV dysfunction, congestive heart failure, or diabetes mellitus should be treated with an ACE inhibitor or an angiotension receptor blocker during the hospitalization and upon discharge. Analgesics and anxiolytics are prescribed as needed, stool softeners are given to all patients, and IV nitroglycerin, prolonged heparin therapy, and calcium antagonists are considered for special patient populations (Table 3.4, p. 32). Vital signs should be assessed every 30 minutes until stable, then every 4 hours, and pulse oximetry is usually monitored for at least 1 day. Frequent assessment for mechanical, ischemic, and electrical complications (e.g., heart failure, acute mitral regurgitation, VSD, reinfarction, arrhythmias, heart block) is mandatory. Assessment of LV function with echocardiography, radionuclide ventriculography, or left ventriculography during angiography is recommended for all patients. Patients treated with an early conservative management strategy should undergo noninvasive stress testing to evaluate for inducible ischemia.

POST-DISCHARGE MEASURES

Therapeutic lifestyle changes and other secondary prevention measures are the same as for STEMI. Emphasis is placed on implementation of secondary prevention measures, including cardiac rehabilitation; lifestyle modification (Mediterranean diet, smoking cessation, weight control, exercise, stress management); treatment of hypertension (BP $\leq$130/85 mmHg), dyslipidemia (LDL cholesterol <70 mg/dL based on PROVE-IT, HDL cholesterol >40 mg/dL, triglyceride <150 mg/dL), and diabetes (Hgb Alc <7%); and use of aspirin, beta-blockers, statins, and ACE inhibitors (Table 3.5, p. 33).

Table 7.2. ACC/AHA Guidelines for Anticoagulants in NSTE-ACS Based on Management Strategy

Management Strategy	Anticoagulants	Recommendation	Level of Evidence
Early Conservative	UFH	Class I	A
	Enoxaparin	Class I	A
	Fondaparinux	Class I	B
Early Invasive	UFH	Class I	A
	Enoxaparin	Class I	A
	Fondaparinux	Class I	B
	Bivalirudin	Class I	B

Source: Adapted from Anderson JL, Adams CD, Antman EM, et al. ACC/AHA 2007 guidelines for the management of patients with unstable angina/non-ST-elevation myocardial infarction: a report of the American College of Cardiology/American Heart Association Task Force on Practice Guidelines (Writing Committee to Revise the 2002 Guidelines for the Management of Patients with Unstable Angina/Non-ST-Elevation Myocardial Infarction) developed in collaboration with the American College of Emergency Physicians, the Society for Cardiovascular Angiography and Interventions, and the Society of Thoracic Surgeons endorsed by the American Association of Cardiovascular and Pulmonary Rehabilitation and the Society for Academic Emergency Medicine. *J Am Coll Cardiol* Aug 14 2007; 50(7):e1–e157.

Chapter 8

Interventional Management of Non-ST-Elevation ACS (NSTE-ACS)

EARLY INVASIVE VS. EARLY CONSERVATIVE APPROACH TO REVASCULARIZATION

Four randomized trials of NSTE-ACS have compared early invasive management (early angiography within 48–72 hours with provisional revascularization) to early conservative management (angiography and revascularization reserved for patients with recurrent ischemia despite medical therapy or those with inducible ischemia on non-invasive stress testing) (Table 8.1).

A. Early Trials (TIMI-3B, VANQWISH). These trials showed no difference (TIMI-3B) or increased risk (VANQWISH) of death or MI with early invasive management. However, in TIMI-3B, Percutaneous transluminal coronary angioplasty (PTCA) resulted in earlier discharge, fewer readmissions, and less need for antianginal medication. Furthermore, 40% of the patients randomized to conservative management eventually required revascularization. In VANQWISH, the higher rate of in-hospital death or MI was primarily due to the high (10.4%) surgical mortality rate in the invasive group. There were also marked delays (8 days) prior to revascularization, low (21%) rates of PTCA or CABG in the invasive group, and patients at "very high risk" (e.g., those most likely to benefit the most from revascularization) were excluded from VANQWISH. Importantly, these trials were performed prior to the availability of coronary stents and GP IIb/IIIa inhibitors, limiting their relevance to current practice.

B. FRISC-2. In this trial, 2457 patients over 75 years old with NSTE-ACS and no prior CABG were randomized to an early invasive or early conservative strategy. If possible, patients were also treated with low molecular-weight heparin (dalteparin) for 4–5 days prior to angiography. Stents were used in 61% of cases. At 1 and 2 years, patients randomized to the early invasive strategy had a lower incidence of death or MI and less need for revascularization procedures.

Table 8.1. Early Invasive vs. Early Conservative Approach to NSTE-ACS*

Trial	N	Outcomes	Comments
		Invasive Vs. Conservative	
ISAR-COOL	410	Large MI or death at 30 days (5.9% vs. 11.6%, p = 0.04).	All patients were treated with intensive antithrombotic therapy (aspirin, clopidogrel, tirofiban, heparin), then randomized to cath/PCI at <6 hours or 3–5 days.

Table 8.1. Early Invasive Vs. Early Conservative Approach to NSTE-ACS* (cont'd)

Trial	N	Outcomes Invasive Vs. Conservative	Comments
RITA-3	1810	Death, MI, or refractory angina at 4 months (9.6% vs. 14.5%, p = 0.001), mainly due to a halving of refractory angina. No difference in death or MI between groups.	Angiography was performed within 48 hours. Enoxaparin was the antithrombin in both groups. Discretionary use of GP IIb/IIIa inhibitors. Invasive approach resulted in less angina and fewer antianginal meds at follow-up.
FRISC II	2457	1-year death (2.2% vs. 3.9%, p = 0.016), MI (8.6% vs. 11.6%, p = 0.015), death or MI (10.4% vs. 14.1%, p = 0.005); 2-year death (3.7% vs. 5.4%, p = 0.038), MI (9.2% vs. 12.7%, p = 0.005), death or MI (12.1% vs. 16.3%, p = 0.003).	In ACS patients treated with dalteparin (average. 6 days prior to angiography), the invasive approach demonstrated clear benefit at 6 months, 1 year, and 2 years. Most PCI patients underwent coronary stenting.
TACTICS-TIMI 18	2220	6-month death, MI, or readmission for ACS (15.9% vs. 19.4%, p = 0.025); 6-month death or MI (7.3% vs. 9.5%, p <0.05). Similar benefit in men and women.	In ACS patients treated with tirofiban (average. 22 hours prior to angiography), the early invasive approach was superior to the early conservative approach. Most PCI patients underwent coronary stenting.
VANQWISH	920	Hospital death (4.5% vs. 1.3%, p = 0.007), death or MI (7.8% vs. 3.3%, p = 0.004); 1-year death (12.6% vs. 7.9%, p = 0.025), death or MI (24% vs. 18.6%, p = 0.05).	High mortality rate in the invasive group was due to unusually high (10.4%) 30-day mortality after CABG. Most PCI patients underwent PTCA.
TIMI-3B	1473	Hospital death (2.4% vs. 2.5%, p = NS), MI (5.1% vs. 5.7%, p = NS), LOS (10.2 days vs. 10.9 days, p = 0.01); 6-week death (2.5% vs. 2.4%, p = NS), MI (5.7% vs. 5.1%, p = NS).	At 6 weeks, the invasive approach resulted in less readmission (7.8% vs. 14.1%, p = 0.001) and less need for >2 antianginals (44% vs. 52%, p = 0.02). Invasive group also had a shorter LOS. Most PCI patients underwent PTCA.

ACS = acute coronary syndrome, LOS = length of stay, MI = myocardial infarction, PCI = percutaneous coronary intervention, PTCA = percutaneous transluminal coronary (balloon) angioplasty, TVR = target vessel revascularization.

* Early invasive approach = routine angiography and revascularization as appropriate; early conservative approach = angiography and revascularization for recurrent ischemia or high-risk finding on stress test.

C. TACTICS-TIMI 18. In this more contemporary trial, 2220 patients with NSTE-ACS treated with aspirin, heparin, beta-blockers, and tirofiban on admission to the hospital were randomized to an early invasive strategy (routine catheterization within 48 hours followed by revascularization as appropriate) or an early conservative strategy (catheterization for recurrent ischemia or abnormal stress test). Stents were used in >80% of cases. The primary endpoint of death, MI, or rehospitalization for ACS at 6 months was reduced by 18% in the invasive group (15.9% vs. 19.4%, p = 0.025), with the greatest benefit among high- and intermediate-risk patients. For patients with elevated troponin levels, early invasive management resulted in a 10% absolute reduction and a 39% relative reduction in the primary endpoint at 6 months (p <0.001). In contrast, there was no advantage to early PCI in low-risk patients with normal cardiac troponins. The 4.7% rate of death or nonfatal MI at 30 days in the early invasive group is the lowest event rate reported in any ACS trial. Preprocedural (upstream) use of tirofiban (average 22 hours before PCI) appeared to prevent the increased risk of acute MI observed prior to PCI in FRISC-2 and other trials.

D. Other Trials. In ISAR-COOL, 410 patients with NSTE-ACS were treated with aspirin, clopidogrel (600-mg loading dose), unfractionated heparin, and tirofiban and then randomized to early (<6 hours) vs. late (3–5 days) angiography/PCI. Compared to deferred intervention for intensive antithrombotic pretreatment, early revascularization reduced the risk of large MI or death at 30 days by 51% (5.9% vs. 11.6%, p = 0.04).

In the Invasive Vs. Conservative Treatment in Unstable Coronary Syndromes (ICTUS) trial, 1200 patients with non-ST-segment ACS (chest pain, positive cardiac troponin T, and either ischemic ECG changes or history of coronary artery disease) were randomized to an initial invasive strategy vs. an initial conservative (selectively invasive) strategy. Both groups received recommended non-ST-segment ACS therapies including enoxaparin and statins. There was higher use of clopidogrel in the initial invasive strategy group. Results at 1 year demonstrated that the primary combined endpoint (death, MI, or rehospitalization for angina) occurred in 22.7% of the group assigned to early invasive and 21.2% of the group assigned to selectively invasive (RR 1.07; 95% CI 0.87, 1.33; p = 0.33). There were more nonfatal MIs, fewer rehospitalizations, and less angina in the group undergoing an initial invasive strategy. Furthermore, after a 4-year follow-up of the ICTUS cohort, there was still no difference in mortality between the two treatment arms but more frequent MIs in the invasively managed group.

STENTS VS. PTCA

In more than 7000 patients with unstable angina treated with stents or PTCA, stents resulted in fewer in-hospital ischemic complications, including less death (1.5% vs. 2.6%, p = 0.003), recurrent angina (23.5% vs. 47.4%, p <0.00001), Q-wave MI (0.4% vs. 1.9%, p <0.00001), repeat PTCA (13.8% vs. 30.6%, p <0.00001), and CABG (6.5% vs. 19.6%, p <0.00001), but there was no difference in mortality at 1 year. Further benefit on restenosis (but probably not death or MI) is likely to be achieved with drug-eluting stents (DES) which, in early trials, have led to 50% to 90% reductions in clinical and angiographic restenosis compared to standard stents (see Table 4.3). There have been concerns regarding delayed endothelialization with DES and greater risks of stent thrombosis and myocardial infarction compared to bare metal stents (BMS). In BASKET-LATE, 746 patients treated with BMS and DES were followed for 1 year after clopidogrel discontinuation for clinical outcomes. There were more clinical events (cardiac death or MI) in the DES group compared to the BMS group after clopidogrel was discontinued, including higher rates of late stent thrombosis and target vessel MI in the DES group. In a retrospective study, long-term outcomes in higher risk "real-world" patients receiving DES compared to BMS was evaluated using analytic methods for propensity scoring and weighted estimators to adjust for differences in treatment groups. These findings demonstrated that there were no significant differences in death or MI between groups but fewer target vessel revascularization procedures in the DES patients. The impact of clopidogrel use in patients who previously received an intracoronary stent on 2-year outcomes was further evaluated in a more recent study that demonstrated lower rates of death and MI in patients who received a DES and were taking clopidogrel but no significant reductions in death or death and MI among those who received a BMS, regardless of clopidogrel status. Current guidelines support at least 1 year of dual antiplatelet therapy in patients after receiving DES, but the optimal duration of clopidogrel treatment in NSTE-ACS patients having received an intracoronary stent requires an appropriately powered randomized trial with long-term follow-up.

GP IIB/IIIA INHIBITORS AND PCI

Data support the routine use of abciximab, eptifibatide, or tirofiban in patients with NSTE-ACS being treated with PCI, particularly those with elevated cardiac troponin levels or dynamic ST-segment changes. As adjuncts to aspirin, heparin, and beta-blockers, GP IIb/IIIa inhibitors reduce the risk of major adverse cardiac events after PCI by 30% to 40% (Tables 9.2 and 9.3). Only abciximab has shown long-term (>1 year) mortality benefit in stent patients. Eptifibatide reduced the rate of death or MI at 1 year in ESPRIT, and while the point estimate for mortality benefit with eptifibatide was similar to that observed with abciximab, the study was not designed to have adequate power to definitively establish the effect on mortality. In TARGET, the only head-to-head comparison of GP IIb/IIIa inhibitors as adjuncts to PCI, abciximab reduced the risk of MI at 30 days (5.8% vs. 8.5%, p = 0.004) and 6 months (7.2% vs. 8.8%, p = 0.013) in ACS patients compared to tirofiban, but 6-month mortality rates were the same in both groups (1.39%). Results from PURSUIT (eptifibatide), PRISM-PLUS (tirofiban), and CAPTURE (abciximab) suggest that upstream (preinterventional) administration of GP IIb/IIIa inhibitors can reduce the risk of acute MI prior to PCI by up to 70% (Table 8.2).

The optimal timing of GP IIb/IIIa inhibitors was recently evaluated in the EARLY ACS trial. The study compared early (≥12 hours before catheterization), routine administration of eptifibatide to delayed, provisional administration in 9492 patients with non-ST-segment ACS assigned to an invasive strategy for the primary efficacy endpoint (death, MI, recurrent ischemia requiring urgent revascularization, or thrombotic complication at PCI) at 96 hours. The results demonstrated no significant differences on the occurrence of the primary endpoint between early and delayed eptifibatide administration (9.3% vs. 10.0%, respectively; odds ratio 0.92; 95% CI 0.8 to 1.06; p = 0.23). There were no differences in the rate of death or MI at 30 days between the two groups, but patients in the early eptifibatide group had higher rates of bleeding and more transfusions than patients in the delayed eptifibatide group. Therefore, routine administration of eptifibatide shortly after presentation with non-ST-segment ACS was not found to be beneficial and was associated with more bleeding. Certain patient groups in EARLY ACS may have selectively benefited from early administration of eptifibatide, but that will be largely determined through secondary analyses.

CORONARY ARTERY BYPASS GRAFTING

Coronary artery bypass grafting (CABG) is the preferred method of revascularization for patients with ACS and either significant left main obstruction or LV dysfunction (or possibly treated diabetes) plus three-vessel disease or two-vessel disease with proximal LAD involvement. Because the risks of perioperative death (4%) and acute MI (10%) are high when CABG is performed on an urgent basis for NSTE-ACS patients, efforts should be made to stabilize patients pharmacologically and, if needed, with IABP counterpulsation prior to surgical revascularization.

RECOMMENDATIONS

The current weight of evidence favors early (within 48 hours) angiography with revascularization (including GP IIb/IIIa inhibitors for patients undergoing PCI) in conjunction with aspirin, clopidogrel, heparin, and beta-blockers. An initial conservative (selectively invasive) strategy is recommended in low-to-intermediate risk patients with NSTE-ACS, although studies have also demonstrated that troponin-positive patients may undergo this strategy without having worse clinical outcomes. A discussion with the patient regarding benefits and risks of both management strategies is paramount to providing good patient care. Technical considerations are similar to PCI for STEMI; stenting is usually performed on the culprit vessel to achieve a residual stenosis <30% and TIMI-3 flow. Patients should be started on evidence-based secondary prevention strategies while they are hospitalized. Patients failing an initial conservative strategy either due to recurrent symptoms or clinical events should be considered for angiography with revascularization.

Table 8.2. GP IIb/IIIa Inhibitors and Acute MI in Patients Awaiting PCI for NSTE-ACS

| Trial | GP IIb/IIIa Inhibitor | Incidence of MI Prior to PCI (%) | | |
		GP IIb/IIIa Inhibitor	Control	p-Value
PURSUIT	Eptifibatide	1.8	5.5	0.001
PRISM-PLUS	Tirofiban	0.8	2.4	0.01
CAPTURE	Abciximab	0.6	2.1	0.29

Chapter 9

Antiplatelet, Antithrombin, and Lipid Lowering Therapy for Non-ST-Elevation ACS (NSTE-ACS)

ASPIRIN

A. **Overview.** Aspirin is a salicylic acid derivative that exerts its antiplatelet effects by blocking the formation of thromboxane A_2 through irreversible acetylation of platelet cyclooxygenase. This effect is transient in nucleated cells but is permanent for the 10-day lifespan of anucleate platelets. Aspirin reduces the risk of death, MI, or stroke by 29% at 1 month following acute MI and by 36% at 6 months following unstable angina. Aspirin also reduces the risk of abrupt coronary occlusion after PCI by 50% to 75% and helps maintain saphenous vein graft patency after CABG. However, aspirin increases the risk of bleeding, has no impact on restenosis after PCI, and does not prevent platelet adhesion or platelet aggregation in response to thrombin, catecholamines, ADP, serotonin, or shear-stress. Up to 10% of patients with coronary artery disease are aspirin-resistant, and the antiplatelet effects of aspirin may diminish over time.

B. **Dose.** All patients should immediately receive two to four chewable nonenteric-coated baby aspirins (81 mg each) because buccal absorption of chewed aspirin is the fastest route for platelet inhibition. The initial dose (150 mg–325 mg) should be followed by low dose (<150 mg) daily thereafter. Rectal suppositories (325 mg) can be used for patients unable to take oral medications. Enteric-coated preparations should be avoided acutely due to delays in GI absorption and antiplatelet effects. In a pooled analysis of GUSTO IIb and PURSUIT, there was no difference in death at 6 months in patients receiving low-dose aspirin (<150 mg/d) vs. higher-dose aspirin (>150 mg/d), although there was a tendency for fewer MIs and more strokes in the higher-dose group. In CURE, bleeding risk increased with increasing aspirin doses, without increased benefit, suggesting an optimal aspirin dose of 75–100 mg/d, with or without clopidogrel.

CLOPIDOGREL

A. **Overview.** Clopidogrel is an inhibitor of adenosine diphosphate (ADP)-induced platelet activation and subsequent aggregation, acting by irreversible binding to the platelet $P2Y_{12}$ receptor and subsequently by ADP-mediated activation of the platelet GP IIb/IIIa receptor complex (Figure 9.1). Clopidogrel irreversibly modifies the platelet ADP receptor, so that platelets exposed to clopidogrel are affected for the remainder of their lifespan. Compared to ticlopidine, another thienopyridine derivative, clopidogrel has a longer duration of action, faster onset of action, and is better tolerated with fewer adverse hematologic effects.

B. Use in NSTE-ACS

   1. **Primary Medical Therapy.** The role for dual-antiplatelet therapy with aspirin and clopidogrel was evaluated in the CURE trial. In this study, 12,562 patients with unstable angina or NSTE-ACS were treated with aspirin (75–325 mg PO q24h) and randomized to clopidogrel (300 mg loading dose followed by 75 mg/day) or placebo for 3–12 months (average 9 months). Patients treated with GP IIb/IIIa inhibitors within 3 days or revascularization within 3 months were excluded from this study as were patients scheduled for the aggressive interventional approach to ACS. As shown in Table 9.1, clopidogrel resulted in a highly significant 20% reduction in the primary composite endpoint of cardiovascular death, MI, or stroke (9.3% vs.11.5%, p <0.001). Benefits were evident for patients treated by medical therapy alone or revascularization (PCI or CABG). There was a 1% absolute increase in major bleeding complications with clopidogrel, but these cases were effectively managed by blood transfusions, and there was no increase in fatal bleeding. To minimize the risk of perioperative bleeding, clopidogrel should be discontinued 5–7 days before elective CABG. In CURE, bleeding risk increased with increasing aspirin doses, without increasing benefit, suggesting an optimal aspirin dose of 75–100 mg/d, with or without clopidogrel, although this conclusion is subject to uncertainty because it is a nonrandomized comparison. Unlike GP IIb/IIIa inhibitors, which predominantly benefit patients with elevated troponins, clopidogrel improves cardiovascular outcomes in patients regardless of troponin status. When clopidogrel is discontinued after 30 days of treatment, markers of heightened platelet activity increase despite continued aspirin use. Based on CURE, clopidogrel should be added to aspirin as soon as possible on admission and continued for at least 9 to 12 months for NSTE-ACS patients in whom a noninterventional approach is planned.

   2. **Adjunct to PCI.** In CURE, 2658 of the 12,562 patients underwent PCI. Patients received study drug (clopidogrel or placebo) for a median of 10 days prior to PCI, then open-label clopidogrel for 2–4 weeks after PCI, then resumption of study drug for a mean of 8 months. Clopidogrel resulted in an overall (before and after PCI) reduction in cardiovascular death or MI by 31% (8.8% vs. 12.6%, p = 0.002). Although not a prespecified endpoint, clopidogrel did not increase the risk of major or life-threatening bleeding in patients receiving GP IIb/IIIa inhibitors. Preliminary cost analysis indicates that chronic use of clopidogrel after ACS falls within the range of societal standards with regard to cost effectiveness. Based on PCI-CURE, clopidogrel should be added to aspirin for at least 9 months in PCI patients not at high risk of bleeding. Clopidogrel should be withheld 5–7 days prior to CABG.

Table 9.1. Dual Antiplatelet Therapy for NSTE-ACS: Results of the CURE Trial

Endpoint (average 9 months)	Aspirin (n = 6303)	Aspirin + Clopidogrel (n = 6259)	Risk Ratio	p-Value
CV death, MI, or stroke (%)*	11.5	9.3	0.80	<0.001
CV death, MI, stroke, orrefractory ischemia (%)	19.0	16.7	0.88	0.0004
Major bleeding (%)	2.7	3.6	1.34	0.003
Minor bleeding (%)	8.6	15.3	1.78	<0.001

ACS = acute coronary syndromes; CURE = clopidogrel in unstable angina to prevent recurrent events; CV = cardiovascular; MI = myocardial infarction.

* Primary endpoint.

Source: Adapted from Yusuf S, Zhao F, Mehta SR, et al. Effects of clopidogrel in addition to asprin in patients with acute coronary syndromes without ST-segment elevation. *N Engl J Med* 2001;345:494–502.

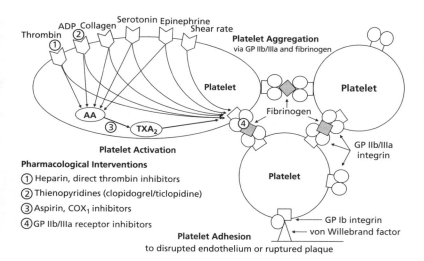

Figure 9.1. Mechanism of Antiplatelet Therapy

Adapted from: Peterson M, Dangas G, Fuster V, in: The Manual of Interventional Cardiology, 3rd ed. Safian R, Freed M (eds), Physician's Press, Royal Oak, MI.

3. **Unresolved issues.** Additional studies are required to assess the safety and efficacy of triple-antiplatelet therapy with aspirin, clopidogrel, and GP IIb/IIIa inhibitors for primary medical therapy of ACS. Because of this unresolved issue, one of three strategies is reasonable: (1) Initiate a GP IIb/IIIa inhibitor (small molecule eptifibatide or tirofiban) in high-risk patients and reserve clopidogrel until the coronary anatomy is visualized and a decision is made to proceed with PCI, (This approach is often used to avoid delays with the timing of CABG for patients who are found to have multivessel disease on angiography. Use of immediate clopidogrel would be reserved for patients not eligible for a GP IIb/IIIa inhibitor; i.e., patients with significant renal dysfunction.); (2) Initiate both clopidogrel and a GP IIb/IIIa inhibitor in high-risk patients and clopidogrel alone in low-risk patients; and (3) Initiate clopidogrel in all patients and withhold the GP IIb/IIIa inhibitor until the anatomy is visualized and a decision is made to proceed with PCI. Based on the preponderance of data, including the concerns raised by worse outcomes in the setting of major bleeding and transfusion requirements, an acceptable approach is to use of either small-molecule GP IIb/IIIa inhibitor or clopidogrel before angiography based of variables such as renal dysfunction and likelihood of requiring cardiac surgery (e.g., whether coronary anatomy has previously been determined) and reserving both therapies for patients with ongoing chest discomfort or dynamic ECG changes as well as expected long delays to angiography. Clopidogrel should be continued for at least 9 months following ACS and possibly long term (studies are underway). The optimal loading dose of clopidogrel (600 mg vs. 300 mg) prior to PCI and evaluation of clopidogrel responsiveness based on platelet function testing and the association with clinical outcomes, are being investigated.

C. **Other Uses for Clopidogrel**
   1. **Coronary stenting.** Numerous randomized trials have confirmed the superiority of dual-antiplatelet therapy compared with aspirin alone or aspirin plus warfarin at reducing ischemic events after coronary stenting. In the randomized CLASSICS trial of 1020 patients undergoing elective stenting, clopidogrel was better tolerated than ticlopidine, and in an analysis of eight randomized trials or registries, clopidogrel resulted in fewer major adverse cardiac events than ticlopidine. In CREDO, 2116 patients undergoing elective PCI were randomized to long-term (1-year) therapy with aspirin plus clopidogrel vs. short-term (4-week) therapy with aspirin plus clopidogrel followed by aspirin alone. At 1 year, long-term dual-antiplatelet therapy resulted in a 26.9% relative reduction in the combined endpoint of death, MI, or stroke (p = 0.02). In ISAR-REACT, 2195 low to moderate, risk patients undergoing elective PCI were randomized to clopidogrel alone (600-mg loading dose at least 2 hours before PCI followed by 75 mg/d) or clopidogrel plus abciximab. At 30 days, the addition of abciximab did not provide any further benefit regarding death, MI, or urgent revascularization.

   2. **Secondary prevention.** Clopidogrel proved somewhat more effective than aspirin for secondary prevention in CAPRIE, in which 19,185 patients with MI within 35 days, ischemic stroke within 6 months, or symptomatic peripheral arterial disease were

randomized to clopidogrel (75 mg/d) or aspirin (325 mg/d) for 1–3 years. At 1.6 years, clopidogrel reduced the composite endpoint of new ischemic stroke, new MI, or other vascular death by 8.7% relative to aspirin (5.32% vs. 5.83%, p = 0.043). Benefit was greatest in patients with peripheral arterial disease. Aspirin resulted in slightly more gastrointestinal bleeding compared with clopidogrel, and there was no difference in the incidence of severe neutropenia (0.1%).

The CHARISMA trial evaluated clopidogrel and aspirin compared with aspirin alone for reduction in cardiovascular outcomes over a median of 28 months in 15,603 patients with known cardiovascular disease or multiple cardiovascular risk factors. The study's primary endpoint did not demonstrate superiority of dual-antiplatelet therapy for the reduction of MI, stroke, or cardiovascular death in the study population (6.8% for clopidogrel plus aspirin vs. 7.3% for placebo plus aspirin, p = 0.22). In the pre-specified cohort of patients with known atherothrombosis ("symptomatic" group), there was a reduction in the primary endpoint with clopidogrel plus aspirin compared with aspirin alone. Of note, there was an observation of higher cardiovascular death in the clopidogrel plus aspirin arm compared with the aspirin alone arm among the cohort with multiple risk factors ("asymptomatic" group), raising concern about the use of dual-antiplatelet therapy in patients without established vascular disease. When comparing ischemic events to bleeding events, clopidogrel plus aspirin was associated with the reduction of 94 ischemic events at a cost of 93 bleeding (moderate or severe) events. In the study population tested, there is insufficient evidence from CHARISMA for the broad use of dual-antiplatelet therapy.

D. Safety Profile. The safety profile of clopidogrel is similar to that of low-dose aspirin, with a rare incidence of thrombotic thrombocytopenic purpura (TTP). The most frequent side effects include diarrhea, rash, and pruritus. Clopidogrel is not associated with an increased risk of neutropenia, so routine hematologic monitoring is not necessary for patients on chronic therapy. One report documented 11 cases of TTP among 3 million patients exposed to clopidogrel, although the incidence of TTP is substantially lower than that associated with ticlopidine. Due to an increased risk of perioperative bleeding, clopidogrel should be discontinued for 5–7 days prior to CABG. Clopidogrel is metabolized in the liver into an active metabolite that then irreversibly binds to the platelet $P2Y_{12}$ receptor, but has little impact on hepatic enzyme induction or drug metabolism. The antiplatelet/clinical effects of clopidogrel are not adversely affected by concomitant use of atorvastatin, based on platelet aggregometry data (INTERACTION study) and clinical trials (CREDO and others).

PRASUGREL

A. Overview. Prasugrel is a novel thienopyrdine ADP receptor antagonist that irreversibly inhibits platelet activation and aggregation mediated by the platelet $P2Y_{12}$ receptor. Compared with clopidogrel, prasugrel has been shown to demonstrate a faster onset of action, higher levels of platelet inhibition, and less response variability. Not unlike clopidogrel, prasugrel is a prodrug that requires metabolic conversion by carboxylesterases and multiple cytochrome P450 enzymes but the chemical pathways by which the prodrugs are converted to the active forms are different, with prasugrel undergoing a more efficient conversion such that more active metabolite is available to bind with platelets. Greater potency and bioavailability of prasugrel compared with clopidogrel on inhibition of ADP mediated platelet activation and aggregation has also been associated with a greater risk of bleeding, particularly notable among the elderly (e.g., $\geq$75 years of age), patients with prior transient ischemic attack (TIA) or stroke, and those with low body weight (<60 kg). Prasugrel has been FDA approved for the treatment of moderate to high risk ACS patients who are managed with PCI.

B. **Use in Moderate-to-High Risk ACS Patients Managed with PCI**
   1. **Adjunct to PCI.** The approval of prasugrel by the FDA was based on the results from the TRITON-TIMI 38 study which evaluated prasugrel vs. clopidogrel in moderate to high risk ACS patients undergoing PCI for their index event for clinical outcomes up to 15 months. In TRITON-TIMI 38, 13,608 patients across the spectrum of ACS were randomized to clopidogrel (300mg loading dose followed by 75mg daily maintenance dose) or prasugrel (60mg loading dose followed by 10mg daily maintenance dose) prior to scheduled PCI. Prasugrel, like clopidogrel, is a prodrug, but has a single oxidation step for activation, resulting in greater availability of the drug for $P2Y_{12}$ inhibition and less variablity among subjects. In TRITON, the primary composite endpoint (cardiovascular death, nonfatal MI, or nonfatal stroke) was significantly lower in the prasugrel arm compared with clopidogrel treated patients (9.9% vs. 12.1%; p <0.001). Target-vessel revascularization and stent thrombosis rates were also significantly lower in prasugrel treated patients. However, higher rates of major bleeding, including life-threatening and fatal bleeding, were observed in the prasugrel group. Patients with prior TIA or stroke, older age ($\geq$75 years), and lower body weight (<60 kg) were at the highest risk for bleeding complications in the TRITON study and less likely to have net clinical benefit from prasugrel. The higher risk of bleeding, particularly among certain subgroups, will be reflected in the labeling of prasugrel. Patients with prior cerebrovascular disease should not be treated with pragurel based on the results from TRITON. Although lower maintenance doses of prasugrel may offset the bleeding risk, doses lower than 10 mg per day of prasugrel have not been studied in large clinical outcome trials and thus neither efficacy nor safety data for such a strategy are known. A higher incident of gastrointestinal malignancies observed in the prasugrel group compared with the clopidogrel group from TRITON also remains an unanswered observation from the trial.

OTHER $P2Y_{12}$ INHIBITORS

Given that ACS patients remain at high risk for early and long-term cardiovascular events, several clincial studies have evaluated or are currently evaluating newer agents for $P2Y_{12}$ inhibition. The CHAMPION trial, a phase III trial, is comparing cangrelor, an injectable inhibitor of P2Y$_{12}$ with a short half-life, to clopidogrel in PCI-treated patients for the primary outcome of all-cause mortality, MI, and ischemia-driven revascularization. The pharmacokinetic substudy of CHAMPION will also provide a rich data set on cangrelor in PCI-treated patients. The PLATO-ACS trial is a large, phase III study evaluating ticagrelor, a oral direct-acting P2Y$_{12}$ inhibitor of which, similar to cangrelor, does not require metabolic conversion to form an active compound. Ticagrelor has been tested against clopidogrel as the active comparator in STEMI and NSTE-ACS patients in this large, double-blind, active-contol study on the occurrence of the primary outcome of death, nonfatal MI, or nonfatal stroke. The results from the PLATO-ACS trial should offer a better understanding of the relationship between P2Y$_{12}$ inhibition and clinical outcomes. The INNOVATE PCI trial is ongoing and is comparing the novel oral and IV direct-acting P2Y$_{12}$ inhibitor elinogrel to clopidogrel in patients undergoing nonurgent PCI. Because this is a phase II dose-finding study, information obtained regarding efficacy, safety, and tolerability among the dosing strata for elinogrel are the primary objectives of the trial.

PLATELET GLYCOPROTEIN (GP) IIB/IIIA RECEPTOR ANTAGONISTS

A. **Overview.** Activation of the platelet GP IIb/IIIa receptor complex is a critical event in the pathogenesis of arterial thrombosis and ACS. GP IIb/IIIa receptor antagonists represent a major breakthrough as adjuncts to PCI and in the medical management of high-risk patients.

B. **Mechanism of Action.** GP IIb/IIIa inhibitors prevent platelets from binding to fibrinogen via the GP IIb/IIIa receptor, the final obligatory pathway for platelet aggregation (Figure 9.2). GP IIb/IIIa inhibitors are the most potent antiplatelet agents available, blocking platelet aggregation in response to all platelet agonists (e.g., collagen, thrombin, ADP, epinephrine, thromboxane A$_2$). They do not, however, prevent platelet adhesion or the formation of thrombin, fibrin, or coagulation factors.

C. **Impact on Prognosis.** In more than 48,000 patients enrolled in 14 large-scale, randomized, placebo-controlled trials, GP IIb/IIIa inhibitors resulted in significant reductions in the relative risk of death or MI at 30 days when used as an adjunct to PCI (36% reduction) or as primary medical therapy for ACS (9% reduction) (Table 9.2). In a meta-analysis of 19 randomized trials of GP IIb/IIIa inhibitors vs. a placebo as adjuncts to PCI for elective indications or acute MI, GP IIb/IIIa inhibitors significantly reduced death by 31% at 30 days and 21% at 6 months. Early and late MI, and a composite outcome of death, MI, or revascularization were also reduced by GP IIb/IIIa inhibitors (p <0.001) (Table 9.3). The relative risk reduction was similar in patients with or without acute MI, in trials continuing or discontinuing heparin post-PCI, and in trials using stents or other PCI devices as the primaiy procedure. There was no excess in major bleeding when heparin was discontinued immediately after the procedure. Higher-risk patients derive the most benefit, especially those with elevated cardiac troponin levels.

D. Types of Inhibitors (Table 9.4). Two intravenous GP IIb/IIIa inhibitors (eptifibatide, tirofiban) have been approved for use in ACS; abciximab should be used in ACS only when PCI is clearly planned. Compared with competitive inhibitors (eptifibatide, tirofiban), noncompetitive inhibitors (abciximab) have longer biological half-lives, higher dissociation constants (resulting in more permanent binding), and more cross-reactivity with other cell-surface receptors. Adjunctive antiplatelet and antithrombin therapy is described in Table 9.5.

   1. Abciximab (ReoPro). Abciximab is the Fab fragment of the chimeric monoclonal antibody 7E3. In addition to GP IIb/IIIa inhibition, abciximab blocks the vitronectin receptor ($\alpha_v\beta_3$) on smooth-muscle and endothelial cells and the MAC-1 receptor on leukocytes. Abciximab also inhibits clot retraction, factor XIII and PAI-I, displaces fibrinogen, and prolongs the ACT, which may result in antiproliferative, anti-inflammatory, anticoagulant, and thrombolytic effects.

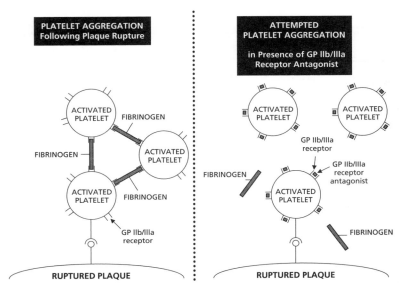

Figure 9.2. GP IIb/IIIa Receptor Antagonists and ACS

GP IIb/IIIa receptor antagonists are the most potent platelet inhibitors available and exert their antiplatelet effects by blocking the binding of fibrinogen to the GP IIb/IIIa receptor on the platelet surface, the final common pathway of platelet aggregation. Abciximab is a monoclonal antibody and noncompetitive inhibitor that binds 1:1 to the GP IIb/IIIa receptor molecule to induce a conformational change that renders the fibrinogen-binding site of the receptor inactive. Eptifibatide and tirofiban are small-molecule competitive inhibitors of the RGD tripeptide-binding domain of the GP IIb/IIIa receptor.

Table 9.2. GP IIb/IIIa Inhibitor Trials: 30-Day Death or MI

Study	GP IIb/IIIa Inhibitor	N	Death or MI at 30 Days (%)	
			Placebo	GP IIb/IIIa
Percutaneous Coronary Intervention (ACS or Elective Indication)				
EPIC	Abciximab	2099	9.6	6.6
EPILOG	Abciximab	2792	9.1	4.0
EPISTENT	Abciximab	2399	10.2	5.2
RAPPORT	Abciximab	483	5.8	4.6
CAPTURE	Abciximab	1265	9.0	4.8
IMPACT II	Eptifibatide	4010	8.4	7.1
ESPRIT	Eptifibatide	2064	10.2	6.4
RESTORE	Tirofiban	2141	6.3	5.1
Total		**17,253**	**8.9**	**5.7**
Medical Therapy for NSTE-ACS (Patients Not Scheduled for PCI)				
PARAGON A	Lamifiban	2282	11.7	11.3
PARAGON B	Lamifiban	5225	11.4	10.6
PRISM	Tirofiban	3231	7.1	5.8
PRISM-PLUS	Tirofiban	1570	12.0	8.7*
PURSUIT	Eptifibatide	10,948	15.7	13.4*
GUSTO-IV ACS	Abciximab	7800	8.0	8.2*
Total		**31,402**	**11.8**	**10.8**
All Studies		**48,655**	**10.8**	**9.0**

Fourteen large-scale, randomized, placebo-controlled trials of GP IIb/IIIa inhibitors. At 30 days, GP IIb/IIIa inhibitors reduced the composite endpoint of death or MI by 36% in PCI trials ($p < 0.001$), by 9% in trials of medical therapy for non-ST-elevation ACS ($p = 0.015$), and by 17% for all trials. Risk reduction was greatest for troponin-positive patients.

* Best dosage regimen selected for analysis.

Sources: Adapted from *Lancet* 2002;359:189–198; Clev Clinic J Med 2000;67:131.

2. **Eptifibatide (Integrilin).** Eptifibatide is a synthetic cyclic K-G-D (lysine-glycine-aspartic acid) heptapeptide. In contrast to abciximab, eptifibatide is a competitive antagonist of the GP IIb/IIIa receptor, has a short half-life (2.5 hours), and does not cross-react with the vitronectin receptor. Platelet function returns to baseline within 4–8 hours after drug discontinuation.

3. **Tirofiban (Aggrastat).** Tirofiban is a synthetic small-molecule nonpeptide mimetic of the R-G-D (arg-gly-asp) sequence of fibrinogen. Like eptifibatide, tirofiban is a competitive antagonist of the GP IIb/IIIa receptor, is rapidly reversible and highly selective, and does not cross-react with the vitronectin receptor.

E. **Indications in NSTE-ACS.** GP IIb/IIIa inhibitors are indicated as adjuncts to PCI and as initial medical therapy for high-risk patients (e.g., elevated troponin or CK-MB levels, ST-segment depression or dynamic ST-segment shifts, prolonged refractory chest pain, hemodynamic instability) planned for early invasive management.

Table 9.3. Meta-Analysis of GP IIb/IIIa Inhibitor Trials as Adjuncts to PCI for Acute MI or Elective Indication: 30-Day and 6-Month Outcomes

Outcome	GP IIb/IIIa Inhibitor	Placebo	RR (95% CI)*	RRR (%)
Death (%)*				
30 days	0.9	1.37	0.69 (0.53–0.90)	31
6 months	1.98	2.53	0.79 (0.64–0.97)	21
MI (%)				
30 days	4.6	6.9	0.63 (0.56–0.70)	37
6 months	5.7	8.1	0.67 (0.60–0.76)	33
Composite†				
30 days	7.9	11.6	0.65 (0.59–0.72)	35
6 months	21.4	24.0	0.85 (0.80–0.90)	15

CI = confidence intervals; RR = relative risk; RRR = relative risk reduction.

* RR (95% CI) for GP IIb/IIIa inhibitors in acute MI population: At 30 days 0.69 (0.45–1.05); at 6 months 0.76 (0.55–1.05).

† Death, MI, or revascularization.

Source: Adapted from Karvouni E, Katritsis DG, Ioannidis JPA. Intravenous glycoprotein IIb/IIIa receptor antagonists reduce mortality after percutaneous coronary interventions. *J AM Coll Cardiol* 2003;41:26–32.

Table 9.4. GP IIb/IIIa Inhibitors for NSTE-ACS

	Abciximab (ReoPro)	Eptifibatide (Integrilin)	Tirofiban (Aggrastat)
Description	Monoclonal antibody; noncompetitive inhibitor.	Peptide; competitive inhibitor.	Nonpeptide; competitive inhibitor.
Duration of effect	24–48 hours after infusion.	4–8 hours after infusion.	4–8 hours after infusion.
GP IIb/IIIa specificity	Cross-reacts with other receptors.	Highly specific.	Highly specific.
GP IIb/IIIa binding	Permanent.	Reversible.	Reversible.
Dose *Upstream Use Before Angiography*	Not approved.	**PURSUIT dose:** 180 mcg/kg IV bolus plus 2.0 mcg/kg/min IV infusion for up to 72–96 hours.* For arrival to the cath lab >2 hours after initiating therapy, no additional bolus is required; otherwise, a second bolus of 180 mcg/kg is given. For CrCl <50 mL/min, the infusion rate is reduced to 1.0 mcg/kg/min.	**PRISM-PLUS dose:** 0.4 mcg/kg/min IV loading infusion × 30 min plus 0.1 mcg/kg/min IV infusion for up to 48–96 hours. For CrCl <30 cc/min, the infusion rate is reduced by 50%.
Adjunct to PCI	0.25 mg/kg IV bolus at the time of PCI plus 0.125 mcg/kg/min (max. 10 mcg/min) IV infusion x 12 hours. For patients with unstable angina scheduled for PCI within 24 hours, bolus plus infusion abciximab (PCI dose) can be started up to 24 hours prior to PCI and continued until 1 hour after the procedure.	**ESPRIT dose:** 2 × 180 mcg/kg IV boluses, 10 minutes apart, at time of PCI plus 2 mcg/kg/min IV infusion × 18–24 hours.*	**RESTORE/TACTICS dose:** 10 mcg/kg IV bolus over 3 minutes immediately prior to PCI plus 0.15 mcg/kg/min IV infusion × 18–24 hours. For CrCl <30 cc/min, the infusion rate is reduced by 50%.

CrCl = creatinine clearance, PCI = percutaneous coronary intervention, UFH = unfractionated heparin.

* For estimated CrCl <50 mL/min, reduce infusion to 1 mcg/kg/min. Estimated CrCl = [(140 − age)/Cr] × [wt. kg/72] × [0.85 if female].

Table 9.5. Adjunctive Antithrombin and Antiplatelet Therapy for GP IIb/IIIa Inhibitors for NSTE-ACS

Therapy	Dose
Heparin (unfractionated)	• As medical therapy in conjunction with a GP IIb/IIIa inhibitor: 60–70 U/kg IV bolus (max. 5000 U) plus 12–15 U/kg/min IV infusion (max. 1000 U/hr), adjusted to maintain aPTT at 1.5–2.5 times control (50–75 seconds). • As adjunct to PCI in conjunction with a GP IIb/IIIa inhibitor: 60 U/kg IV bolus to achieve intraprocedural ACT of 200–250 seconds. Higher heparin doses and target ACTs have been used with eptifibatide and tirofiban. No additional heparin is given after PCI.
Enoxaparin (as alternative to UFH)*	• As primary medical therapy in conjunction with a GP IIb/IIIa inhibitor: 1 mg/kg SQ q12h × 2–8 days. • As an adjunct to PCI in conjunction with a GP IIb/IIIa inhibitor: 0.75 mg/kg IV bolus. If the patient has been treated with SQ enoxaparin and the last SQ dose was <8 hours, no additional enoxaparin is required; if the last SQ dose was >8 hours, an additional 0.3 mg/kg IV should be given just before PCI.
Aspirin/clopidogrel	325 mg started at least 1 day prior to PCI followed by 75–325 mg PO q24h long term; for urgent PCI, give four chewable nonenteric-coated baby aspirins (325 mg total). For stent procedures, add clopidogrel 300 mg PO load followed by 75 mg PO q24h for at least 1 month and possibly for up to 9 months.

ACT = activated clotting time, ACS = acute coronary syndromes, PCI = percutaneous coronary intervention, UFH = unfractionated heparin.

* As an alternative to UFH, enoxaparin may be easier to administer and associated with better clinical outcomes (ASSENT-3, p. 57), but further testing will be needed before it is adopted widely.

F. **Safety Concerns.** A number of safety concerns have been raised about the use of GP IIb/IIIa inhibitors in general and about abciximab in particular, including bleeding complications, the potential requirement for emergency CABG, severe thrombocytopenia, and potential drug interactions. Virtually all of these considerations are readily prevented or treated and do not preclude the use of these agents.

1. **Bleeding.** In contrast to earlier abciximab trials using standard-dose heparin to maintain high activated clotting time (ACT) levels, trials using low-dose heparin, early sheath removal, and target ACT levels of 200–250 seconds (EPILOG, CAPTURE, EPISTENT) reported no difference in major or minor bleeding for patients treated with abciximab vs. a placebo. These studies indicate that the risk of bleeding associated with abciximab can be minimized by low-dose heparin, early sheath removal, avoidance of venous sheaths, and fastidious postprocedure groin care. No GP IIb/IIIa inhibitor has been associated with an increased risk of intracranial hemorrhage.

2. **Thrombocytopenia.** The incidence of thrombocytopenia appears to be higher with abciximab than with eptifibatide or tirofiban. In abciximab trials, the incidence of

mild thrombocytopenia (<100,000/mm³) was 2.6% to 5.6% and severe thrombocytopenia (<50,000/mm³) was 0.9% to 1.6%; platelet transfusions were needed in 1.6% to 5.5%. Unlike heparin-induced thrombocytopenia, abciximab-associated thrombocytopenia responds promptly to platelet transfusions (although severe thrombocytopenia after abciximab retreatment may not respond as effectively).

3. **Emergency CABG.** The risk of bleeding during emergency CABG is increased in patients receiving abciximab plus heparin. The hemostatic defect caused by abciximab is largely reversible with platelet transfusions, but the benefit is not immediate or complete. Key factors in reducing the risk of bleeding during emergency CABG include careful titration of heparin dose and liberal use of platelet transfusions, especially after coming off cardiopulmonary bypass. In contrast to abciximab, antiplatelet effects with eptifibatide or tirofiban usually resolve in 4–8 hours and platelet transfusions are ineffective. GP IIb/IIIa inhibitors should be discontinued prior to emergency CABG.

G. **Unresolved Issues.** Ongoing or planned trials will help determine the optimal GP IIb/IIIa inhibitor for NSTE-ACS, including dose, duration, timing, and adjunctive use of antithrombin therapy (unfractionated heparin, low molecular-weight heparin, direct thrombin inhibitors) and other antiplatelet agents (aspirin, clopidogrel).

LOW MOLECULAR-WEIGHT HEPARIN (LMWH)

A. **Overview.** LMWHs are homogeneous glycosaminoglycans with a mean molecular weight of 4000–6000 formed by controlled enzymatic or chemical depolymerization of unfractionated heparin (UFH). Enoxaparin has shown benefit over UFH for non-ST-elevation ACS in two randomized trials.

B. **LMWH vs. Unfractionated Heparin** (Table 9.6)
   1. **Mechanism of action.** LMWH and UFH inhibit clotting factors IIa (thrombin activity) and Xa (thrombin generation). LMWHs have more anti-Xa activity and less anti-IIa activity than UFH, and their anticoagulant effect, which is mediated primarily by inhibition of thrombin generation, is not fully reflected in the aPTT (Figure 9.3).

   2. **Ease of use, reliability of anticoagulation, and risk of thrombocytopenia.** LMWHs have several advantages over UFH, including better inhibition of thrombin generation (higher anti-Xa–to–anti-IIa ratio), lack of need to monitor aPTT (due to enhanced bioavailability and a more reliable anticoagulant effect), ease of administration (reliable anticoagulation via subcutaneous route), lack of inhibition by platelet factor IV, and a lower risk of heparin-induced thrombocytopenia. In clinical trials, LMWHs were associated with more minor bleeding than UFH, but there was no increase in major bleeding complications. Protamine is less effective at reversing the anticoagulant effects of LMWHs than UFH.

Table 9.6. Comparison of Low Molecular-Weight Heparin (LMWH) to Unfractionated Heparin (UFH)

	UFH	LMWH
Composition	Heterogeneous mixture of polysaccharides; molecular weight 3,000–30,000.	Homogeneous glycosaminogycans; molecular weight 4,000–6,000.
Mechanism of anticoagulation	Activates antithrombin; equivalent activity against factor IIa (thrombin) and factor Xa.	Less activation of antithrombin; greater activity against factor Xa than factor IIa (thrombin); releases TFPI from endothelium.
Pharmacokinetics	Variable binding to plasma proteins, endothelial cells, and macrophages results in unpredictable anticoagulant effects and short half-life.	Minimal binding to plasma proteins, endothelial cells, and macrophages results in predictable anticoagulation and longer half-life.
Laboratory monitoring	Essential because of unpredictable anticoagulant effects; monitor aPTT or ACT.	Unnecessary except in renal failure or body weight <45 kg or >80 kg; monitor antifactor Xa levels.
Clinical uses	ACS; venous thrombosis; ischemic stroke. Routinely used during PCI. Preferred over LMWH for anticoagulation during CABG.	At least as effective as UFH for NSTE-ACS (enoxaparin may be better than UFH); venous thrombosis; ischemic stroke. At least as safe and effective as UFH during PCI with or without GP IIb/IIIa inhibitors.
Neutralization	Protamine neutralizes antithrombin activity.	Protamine neutralizes antithrombin activity but only partially reverses antifactor Xa activity.
HIT-2	Should not be used in patients with a history of HIT-2.	Should not be used in patients with a history of HIT-2.
Cost	Inexpensive.	More expensive than unfractionated heparin, but costs are offset by lack of need for monitoring and fewer adverse events (enoxaparin).

ACS = acute coronary syndrome, CABG = coronary artery bypass graft surgery, HIT-2 = heparin-induced thrombocytopenia, TFPI = tissue factor pathway inhibitor.

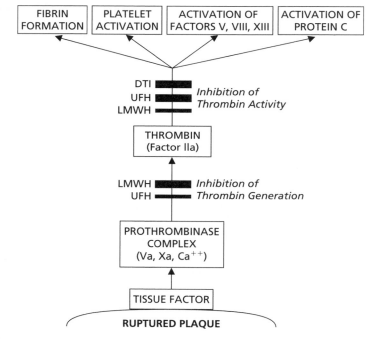

Figure 9.3. Antithrombin Therapy and ACS

Various antithrombonins are used in clinical practice. Low-molecular weight heparins (LMWH) and unfractioned heparin (UFH) bind factors Xa and IIa (thrombin) to reduce thrombin generation and thrombin activity, respectively. Direct thrombin inhibitors (DTI) (e.g., hirubin) reduce thrombin activity only. LMWHs have greater anti-Xa activity than UFH, resulting in greater inhibition of thrombin generation. Standard weight-adjusted dosing of LMWH produces a predictable level of anticoagulation, which is not fully reflected in the activated partial thromboplastin time (aPTT). Neither UFH nor LMWH bind clot-bound thrombin, in contrast to direct thrombin inhibitors. Since thrombin itself is a potent platelet activator, antithrombin agents also decrease platelet activation.

3. **Clinical Trials of LMWH for NSTE-ACS**
   a. **Primary medical therapy (patients not scheduled for PCI).** Four major randomized trials compared LMWH to UFH as primary medical therapy for NSTE-ACS (Table 9.7). A meta-analysis of two enoxaparin trials (ESSENCE, TIMI 11b) included a total of 7081 patients and showed a significant (20%) reduction in the composite endpoint of death or MI at 8 days (4.1% vs. 5.3%, p = 0.02)

and at 6 weeks (7.1% vs. 8.6%, p = 0.02) in favor of enoxaparin, without an increase in major bleeding complications. (There is an increased risk of recurrent ischemic events in the 24 hours following discontinuation of enoxaparin or UFH; close monitoring is recommended for high-risk patients.) At 1 year, enoxaparin reduced the risk of death, MI, or urgent revascularization compared to UFH by 12% (23.3% vs. 25.8%, p = 0.008). In contrast, dalteparin (FRIC) and nadroparin (PRAXIS) had no impact on clinical outcome, suggesting important differences between LMWHs.

b. **Adjunct to PCI.** Because ACT and aPTT levels do not accurately reflect the degree of anticoagulation with LMWHs, UFH is preferred by most interventional cardiologists during PCI. However, recent observational studies (NICE-1, NICE-3, NICE-4) and randomized trials (ACUTE II, CRUISE, INTERACT, SYNERGY) have addressed this question. Among 746 high-risk patients with non-ST-elevation ACS treated with eptifibatide and randomized to enoxaparin or UFH in the INTERACT trial, enoxaparin resulted in fewer major bleeding episodes at 96 hours (1.8% vs. 4.6%, p = 0.03) and less death or MI at 30 days (5% vs. 9%, p = 0.031). The SYNERGY trial randomized 10,027 high-risk patients with non-ST-elevation ACS—defined as having two of the following three criteria: age >60 years, transient ST elevation or ST depression, or positive cardiac markers— to enoxaparin or UFH. The combined primary endpoint rate (death or MI) at 30 days was similar in the enoxaparin and UFH arms (14% vs. 14.5%). Enoxaparin was associated with a small, statistically significant increase in TIMI major bleeds (9.1% vs. 7.6%, p = 0.008). Collectively, these data indicate that enoxaparin is a safe and effective alternative to UFH for procedural anticoagulation (with or without GP IIb/IIIa inhibitors) with similar rates of ischemic events and major bleeding complications.

Table 9.7. Clinical Trials of Low Molecular-Weight Heparin vs. Unfractionated Heparin for NSTE-ACS (cont'd)

Trial	LMWH	Design	Results (LMWH vs. UFH)
SYNERGY	Enoxaparin	10,027 high-risk ACS patients undergoing early cath/PCI randomized to enoxaparin or UFH. High-risk defined as two of the following: age >60 years, positive cardiac markers, transient ST elevation or ST depression.	No difference in death or MI at 30 days (14% vs. 14.5%). More TIMI major bleeding with enoxaparin (9.1% vs. 7.6%, p = 0.008) but no increase in blood transfusions. More bleeding complications in patients switched from one antithrombin to the other.

Table 9.7. Clinical Trials of Low Molecular-Weight Heparin vs. Unfractionated Heparin for NSTE-ACS (cont'd)

Trial	LMWH	Design	Results (LMWH vs. UFH)
A-to-Z	Enoxaparin	3987 high-risk ACS patients treated with tirofiban and randomized to enoxaparin or UFH for maximum of 12 hours (~60% underwent cardiac catheterization in first 30 days).	No difference in death, MI, or refractory ischemia (8.4% vs. 9.4%).
INTERACT	Enoxaparin	746 high-risk ACS patients treated with eptifibatide and randomized to enoxaparin or UFH (60% underwent early PCI).	Enoxaparin resulted in less death or MI at 30 days (5% vs. 9%, p = 0.031) and less major bleeding at 96 hours (1.8% vs. 4.6%, p = 0.03).
TIMI 11b	Enoxaparin	3910 patients randomized to enoxaparin (30 mg IV bolus followed by 1 mg/kg SQ q12h) or UFH (70 U/kg IV bolus followed by 15 U/kg/hr IV infusion to maintain aPTT 1.5–2.5 times control) × 3–5 days (median duration: enoxaparin 4.6 days; UFH 3 days). Outpatient phase with rerandomization of UFH patients to enoxaparin or placebo × 6 weeks.	Enoxaparin was superior to UFH at reducing death, MI, or urgent revascularization at 8 days (12.4% vs. 14.5%, p = 0.048) and at 43 days (17.3% vs. 19.6%, p = 0.048). No incremental benefit for outpatient enoxaparin. Minor bleeding was increased with enoxaparin, but not major bleeding.
ESSENCE	Enoxaparin	3171 patients randomized to enoxaparin (1 mg/kg SQ q12h) or UFH (5000 U IV bolus followed by an IV infusion to maintain aPTT at 55–86 sec.) × 2–8 days (median treatment 2.6 days).	Enoxaparin was superior to UFH at reducing death, MI, or recurrent angina at 14 days (19.8% vs. 23.3%, p = 0.019) and at 30 days (19.8% vs. 23.3%, p = 0.017).
FRAXIS	Nadroparin	3468 patients randomized to nadroparin (6 or 14 days) vs. UFH.	No difference in death, MI, or refractory angina at 14 days (6-day nadroparin 17.8% vs. 14-day nadroparin 20.0% vs. UFH 18.1%) or at 3 months (22.3% vs. 22.3% vs. 26.2%). Trend toward increased death or MI in nadroparin group at all time points.

Table 9.7. Clinical Trials of Low Molecular-Weight Heparin vs. Unfractionated Heparin for NSTE-ACS (cont'd)

Trial	LMWH	Design	Results (LMWH vs. UFH)
FRIC	Dalteparin	1482 patients randomized to dalteparin (120 IU/kg SQ q12h) or UFH × 6 days. At day 6 until day 45, second randomization to dalteparin (120 IU/kg SQ q24h) or placebo.	No difference in death, MI, or recurrent angina (14% vs. 12.9%) or in bleeding (1.1% vs. 1%) at 45 days. Trend toward increased early risk of death, MI, or recurrent angina in dalteparin group (9.3% vs. 7.7% at 6 days, p = 0.33).

aPTT = activated partial thromboplastin time, FV = intravenous, MI = myocardial infarction, SQ = subcutaneous, UFH = Unfractionated heparin.

C. Indications. Enoxaparin is indicated as a primary medical therapy for NSTE-ACS to reduce the risk of death, MI, or target-vessel revascularization. Contraindications include active major bleeding, thrombocytopenia with positive antiplatelet antibody tests, or hypersensitivity. Caution should be used in uncontrolled hypertension, diabetic retinopathy, serum creatinine <30 cc/min, and in conditions associated with an increased risk of bleeding. UFH is preferred over LMWH in patients scheduled for CABG within 24 hours because the anticoagulant effects of UFH are more reliably reversed with protamine.

D. Dose. *For primary medical therapy:* Enoxaparin 1 mg/kg SQ q12h × 2–8 days (median duration: ESSENCE 2.6 days; TIMI 11b 4.6 days) in patients with normal renal function, with modification of dosing interval to q24h if CrCl <30 mL/min.

As an adjunct to PCI:

    (1) If the patient has received prior enoxaparin: at the time of the procedure, give 1.0 mg/kg IV if no GP IIb/IIIa inhibitor; 0.75 mg/kg IV if a GP IIb/IIIa inhibitor is used.

    (2) If the patient has received prior enoxaparin (e.g., initial 30 mg IV loading dose or two doses of SQ enoxaparin with or without IV loading dose):
- Procedure <8 hours of last SQ dose: no additional enoxaparin.
- Procedure within 8–12 hours of the last SQ dose: give booster dose of 0.3 mg/kg IV in the catheterization laboratory.

    (3) If the patient has received no initial 30 mg IV dose and only one SQ dose: at the time of the procedure, give a booster dose of 0.3 mg/kg IV.

E. Monitoring. Platelet count (baseline, twice weekly), CBC, serum creatinine (baseline, change in renal function), and daily clinical evaluation for bleeding. The aPTT/ACT does not need to be monitored, because antithrombin activity is not fully reflected in these parameters.

F. Complications

   1. Bleeding. For significant bleeding warranting immediate reversal of anticoagulation, enoxaparin's anticoagulant effect can be partially reversed with protamine. Dosing is based on the time elapsed since the last enoxaparin dose:

   - Last enoxaparin dose ≤8 hours: protamine 1 mg for each 1 mg of enoxaparin as a slow IV infusion. A second dose of 0.5 mg for each 1 mg of enoxaparin may be needed if the aPTT 2–4 hours after the first dose is prolonged.

   - Last enoxaparin dose >8 hours but ≤12 hours: protamine 0.5 mg for each 1 mg of enoxaparin.

   - Last enoxaparin dose >12 hours: protamine may not be required.

   2. Thrombocytopenia. Enoxaparin should be discontinued if the platelet count drops below 100,000/mm^3 or ≥50% from baseline.

   3. Renal insufficiency. For CrCl ≥30 mL/minute, no specific dose adjustment is recommended (per manufacturer); monitor closely for bleeding. For CrCl <30 mL/minute in unstable angina/non-Q-wave MI (with aspirin), the dose is 1 mg/kg SQ q24h. Enoxaparin has not been approved by the FDA for use in dialysis patients. Serious bleeding complications have been reported with use in patients who are on dialysis or have severe renal failure. LMWH administration at fixed doses without monitoring has greater unpredictable anticoagulant effects in patients with chronic kidney disease. If used, dosages should be reduced and anti-Xa activity frequently monitored because accumulation may occur over days (enoxaparin elimination is primarily via the renal route). Many clinicians would not use enoxaparin in this population, especially without timely anti-Xa activity assay results.

G. Recommendations and Unresolved Issues. Enoxaparin is recommended in conjunction with aspirin, clopidogrel, and GP IIb/IIIa inhibitors (in higher-risk patients) for primary medical management of NSTE-ACS at a dose of 1 mg/kg SQ q12h × 2–8 days. UFH can also be used in this setting, but most data support the use of enoxaparin. Patients requiring PCI can be treated with either enoxaparin or UFH (maintain intraprocedural ACT at 300–500 seconds, or 200–250 seconds if a GP IIb/IIIa inhibitor is used). Findings from the SYNERGY trial demonstrated that enoxaparin was as safe as UFH in high-risk ACS patients undergoing PCI, with a trend toward less death and myocardial infarction. Enoxaparin was associated with a small increase in TIMI major bleeding but no increase in blood transfusions. Switching from one antithrombin to another was associated with more bleeding complications in SYNERGY and is not recommended.

Although still not widely used in the United States given concerns regarding catheter-thrombosis and a long duration of action, fondaparinux, a synthetic factor Xa inhibitor, was found to be noninferior to enoxaparin in ACS patients in OASIS-5. Fondaparinux was associated with a similar incidence of the primary outcome (death, MI, or refractory ischemia) at 9 days, but was associated with a significant reduction in major bleeding and 30-day mortality compared with enoxaparin. The available evidence suggests that fondaparinux may be an excellent anticoagulant in patients who are managed with an early conservative strategy for NSTE-ACS. Recommendations are to include supplemental antithrombotic therapy (UFH or enoxaparin) with anti-IIa activity in fondaparinux-treated patients in the setting of PCI.

DIRECT THROMBIN INHIBITORS

Direct thrombin inhibitors are classified as polypeptide inhibitors (hirudin, bivalirudin) or low molecular-weight inhibitors (argatroban). In contrast to UFH, hirudin and bivalirudin do not require antithrombin III for anticoagulant effect, form highly stable noncovalent complexes with circulating and clot-bound thrombin, and are not inhibited by platelet factor IV. In a recent meta-analysis of 11 randomized trials comparing direct thrombin inhibitors with UFH for primary medical therapy of ACS or as adjuncts to PCI, direct thrombin inhibitors were associated with less death or MI at 1 week (4.3% vs. 5.1%, p = 0.001) and at 30 days (7.4% vs. 8.2%, p = 0.02). Clinical benefit was observed for bivalent inhibitors (hirudin, bivalirudin) but not univalent inhibitors. The risk of major bleeding was increased with hirudin and decreased with bivalirudin. (In patients without ACS undergoing elective PCI, bivalirudin plus provisional GP IIb/IIIa blockade was a safe and effective alternative to UFH plus planned GP IIb/IIIa blockade for procedural anticoagulation in REPLACE-2.) Bivalirudin is approved for procedural anticoagulation in unstable angina, and lepirudin (Refludan), a recombinant hirudin, and argatroban (Acova) are approved for use in patients with heparin-induced thrombocytopenia who require IV anticoagulation. Lepirudin is administered as an initial bolus of 0.4 mg/kg (max. 44 mg) over 15–20 seconds followed by a continuous infusion of 0.15 mg/kg/hr (max. 16.5 mg/hr). The infusion rate should be reduced by 50%, 70%, and 85% for creatinine clearances of 45–60 mL/min, 30–44 mL/min, and 15–29 mL/min, respectively, and lepirudin should be avoided/discontinued if the creatinine clearance is <15 mL/min. Argatroban is administered as a constant infusion of 2 mcg/kg/min (0.5 mcg/kg/min for patients with moderate hepatic impairment). Monitoring is accomplished using the same aPTT guidelines as for UFH.

The ACUITY trial evaluated three different antithrombotic strategies: UFH or enoxaparin plus GP IIb/IIIa inhibition, bivalirudin plus GP IIb/IIIa inhibition, or bivalirudin alone on the incidence of ischemia, major bleeding, and the net clinical outcome (combination of composite ischemia or major bleeding) at 30-days in 13,819 patients with moderate to high-risk ACS assigned to an invasive strategy. GP IIb/IIIa use was allowed for thrombotic complications during PCI in the bivalirudin monotherapy group. Among the groups treated with a GP IIb/IIIa, the use of bivalirudin compared with heparin-based regimen was noninferior for ischemia, major bleeding, or the net clinical outcome at 30 days. Bivalirudin monotherapy compared with heparin-based regimens plus a GP IIb/IIIa was associated with a noninferior rate of composite ischemia but nearly two times the reduction in major bleeding (3.0% vs. 5.7%, p <0.001). Composite ischemia or mortality was no different at 1-year follow-up among the three treatment groups. The findings demonstrated that bivalirudin is noninferior to heparin-based regimens plus a GP IIb/IIIa inhibitor for invasively managed patients with non-ST-elevation ACS and that bivalirudin monotherapy was associated with reduced rates of major bleeding. The observation that high and similar use of clopidogrel among all three study groups must be emphasized and that ACS trials of antithrombotic strategies must also factor in major bleeding when designing primary endpoints given the association of bleeding complications with early and late mortality in ACS patients.

HMG COA-REDUCTASE INHIBITORS (STATINS)

Dyslipidemia is the most prevalent and important modifiable risk factor for atherosclerosis, affecting one in two U.S. adults. Proper treatment reduces the risk of acute MI and stroke by 25% to 80%, cardiovascular and all-cause mortality by 20% to 40%, and revascularization procedures by 22% to 30%. It has been estimated that for each 1% decrease in LDL cholesterol and each 1% increase in HDL cholesterol, the risk of cardiovascular events falls by 2% and 3%, respectively. Angiographic trials of statin therapy have consistently demonstrated less progression of existing plaque and a reduction in the development of new atherosclerotic lesions. Despite marked benefits of lipid therapy, dyslipidemia is grossly undertreated: 80% of patients with coronary artery disease do not meet the LDL cholesterol targets established by the National Cholesterol Education Program Adult Treatment Panel (NCEP ATP) III. Recent data suggest a role for in-hospital initiation of statins in ACS. In MIRACL, 3086 patients were randomized to atorvastatin 80 mg or a placebo 1–4 days after admission for ACS. At 16 weeks, atorvastatin reduced the risk of death, MI, resuscitated cardiac arrest, or unstable angina by 16% (14.8% vs. 17.4%, p = 0.048). Although the benefit was primarily due to a reduction in hospitalization for recurrent ischemia (as opposed to "hard" endpoints like death or MI), there was no apparent major harm associated with use of atorvastatin. A substudy from PRISM found that statin use for ≥30 days prior to the onset of ACS was associated with a 51% reduction in death or MI at 30 days, and that stopping statins in these patients was associated with a threefold increased risk of death or MI. Importantly, recent results from the PROVE IT trial indicate that compared to in-hospital initiation of standard statin therapy (LDL 95 mg/dL), more intensive statin therapy (LDL 62 mg/dL) provides greater protection against death or major cardiovascular events at 18–36 months following ACS. In this trial, 4162 patients hospitalized for ACS within 10 days were randomized to atorvastatin 80 mg/d (intensive therapy) or pravastatin 40 mg/d (standard therapy). At a mean follow-up of 24 months, atorvastatin reduced the primary endpoint (death, MI, unstable angina requiring hospitalization, revascularization 30 days after randomization, stroke) by 16% compared to pravastatin (22.4% vs. 26.3%, p = 0.005) (Table 9.8). Benefits were evident in as early as 30 days and continued throughout the study. Statins were also well tolerated and very safe: rates of elevated liver enzymes > three times normal were low (1.1% to 3.3%), statins were discontinued in only 2.7% to 3.3% of patients due to myalgias or elevated CK; and there were no cases of rhabdomyolysis.

Based on these compelling results, the NCEP ATP III issued a recent guideline update recommending more intensive statin therapy for ACS patients, with an optional LDL target <70 mg/dL, starting in-hospital (within 10 days and after the patient is stable) and continued long term to reduce the early and late risk of death or recurrent ischemia. LDL measurement within 24 hours of hospitalization can help guide therapy: For patients with baseline LDL levels <100–110 mg/dL, a standard dose of a statin is recommended to reduce LDL cholesterol by 30% to 40% (Table 9.9); for the many patients with higher baseline LDL levels who require ≥50% reductions in LDL, either a high dose of a statin or the standard dose of a statin plus ezetimibe is usually required to reduce LDL levels to <70 mg/dL (Table 9.10).

Table 9.8. Intensive LDL-Lowering with High-Dose Statin Therapy Improves Outcomes in ACS: Results of the PROVE IT Trial

Results at 2 years	Atorvastatin 80 mg/d (n = 2099)	Pravastatin 40 mg/d (n = 2063)	Risk Reduction	p-Value
Mean LDL	62 mg/dL	95 mg/dL	–	<0.001
Death, MI, unstable angina requiring hospitalization, revascularization 30 days after randomization, stroke*	22.4%	26.3%	16%	0.005
Death from CHD, MI, revascularization†	19.7%	22.3%	14%	0.029
Need for revascularization	16.3%	18.8%	14%	0.04
Recurrent unstable angina	3.8%	5.1%	29%	0.02
Death from any cause	2.2%	3.2%	28%	0.07
Death or MI	8.3%	10.0%	18%	0.06

* Primary endpoint; † Secondary endpoint.

Source: Adapted from Cannon CP, Braunwald E, McCabe CH, et al. Comparison of intensive and moderate lipid lowering with stains after acute coronary syndromes. *N Engl J Med* 2004;350.

Table 9.9. Doses of Statins Required to Attain an Approximate 30% to 40% Reduction in LDL Cholesterol Levels (Standard Dose)

Drug	Dose (mg/d)	LDL Reduction (%)
Rosuvastatin	5–10	39–45
Atorvastatin	10	39
Simvastatin	20–40	35–41
Pravastatin	40	34
Lovastatin	40	31
Fluvastatin	40–80	25–35

Source: Reprinted with permission © 2004 American Heart Association, Inc.

Table 9.10. Minimum Drug Doses Required to Attain ≥50% Reductions in LDL Cholesterol Levels

Drug	Dose (mg/d)	LDL Reduction (%)
Atorvastatin	80	51–54
Ezetimibe/Simvastatin	10/20	50–52
Rosuvastatin	20	52

Chapter 10
Special Patient Populations and Non-ST-Elevation ACS (NSTE-ACS)

The management of NSTE-ACS in women, diabetics, and post-CABG patients is similar to that of other ACS patients. Special considerations are required in the very elderly, and nitrates and calcium antagonists are particularly useful for ACS secondary to variant (Prinzmetal's) angina or cocaine use (Table 10.1).

Table 10.1. Treatment of ACS in Special Patient Populations

Group	Treatment	Comments
Women	Treated similar to men.	38% of women die in the year following MI compared to 25% of men, and women <65 years are twice as likely to die from acute MI as men. Six years post-MI, 35% of women vs. 18% of men will have had recurrent MI. Women are older at presentation, have greater comorbidity, are more likely to present with atypical symptoms, and derive less benefit from GP IIb/IIIa inhibitors as primary medical therapy. (Troponin-positive women given GP IIb/IIIa inhibitors derive benefit similar to troponin-positive men, but men are twice as likely to be troponin-positive than are women.) Hormone replacement therapy is not recommended for secondary prevention of cardiovascular events. Cardiovascular disease causes more than twice the number of deaths as cancer, but <10% of women perceive heart disease as their greatest threat.
Age >75 years	Intensity of management depends on overall general health and healthcare goals of the patient. Enoxaparin, clopidogrel, and GP IIb/IIIa inhibitors improve outcomes, but these medications must be properly dosed in older adults with particular attention to the patient's body weight and calculated creatinine clearance.	Elderly patients have greater comorbidity, more heart failure, worse outcomes, and are more likely to manifest atypical symptoms. Baroreceptor sensitivity and cerebral autoregulation are often impaired, resulting in exaggerated hypotensive responses to nitrates and other vasodilators, including orthostatic intolerance. However, benefits from evidence-based therapies, including revascularization, are similar, if not greater, among older adults. Age alone should not be the sole basis by which beneficial therapies are not provided to eligible patients.

Table 10.1. Treatment of ACS in Special Patient Populations (cont'd)

Group	Treatment	Comments
Diabetics	Treated similar to nondiabetics. Tight glucose control is recommended.	Diabetics have greater comorbidity, more extensive coronary disease, worse LV function, more silent ischemia, and worse prognosis after revascularization. The risk of death in the first year after MI is 50%, half of which occurs before reaching the hospital. In BARI, diabetics with multivessel disease had better long-term outcomes after CABG vs. PCI, but stents were not used in this study.
Prior CABG	Treated similar to patients without CABG. Low threshold for angiography.	Prior CABG patients have more extensive coronary disease, worse LV function, more prior MI, and worse prognosis after ACS. Saphenous vein graft (SVG) plaques are often highly friable, ulcerated, and thrombotic. PCI of acute SVG occlusions is associated with lower procedural success and higher early and late mortality compared to PCI of native vessel occlusions.
Chest pain after cocaine use	Nitrates and calcium antagonists for ST-elevation or depression with ischemic chest pain. Angiography for persistent ST-segment changes, and fibrinolytics (PCI) for intracoronary thrombus.	Cocaine use increases the risk for coronary spasm and intravascular thrombosis. Controversy exists regarding whether beta-blockers can be safely administered to NSTE-ACS who are cocaine-positive.
Variant (Prinzmetal's) angina	Nitrates, calcium antagonists, smoking cessation.	PCI is useful for obstructive CHD.

CABG = coronary artery bypass grafting, CHD = coronary heart disease, LV = left ventricular, MI = myocardial infarction, PCI = percutaneous coronary intervention.

SECTION 4

NON-MEDICAL THERAPY, MONITORING, RISK STRATIFICATION

Chapter 11

Non-Medical Therapy and Monitoring Techniques

This section describes non-medical therapies and monitoring techniques used for the management of ACS. When used in conjunction with medical therapy, proper application of these modalities can reduce infarct size; preserve LV function; minimize ischemic, mechanical, and electrical complications; and improve survival.

NON-MEDICAL THERAPY AND MONITORING TECHNIQUES FOR ACS

A. Transfer to a Facility Equipped for PCI and CABG

1. **Indications.** Lytic-ineligible patients with STEMI patients who can be rapidly transported for primary PCI with a total door-to-balloon time of <90 minutes; persistent ischemia after fibrinolytic therapy; recurrent chest pain; hemodynamic instability (heart failure, hypotension, shock); suspected mechanical defect (VSD, free-wall rupture, acute MR); recurrent VT or VF that is difficult to control; possibly for lytic-eligible patients with STEMI.

2. **Comments.** The decision to transfer by ambulance or helicopter depends upon distance and driving time (for driving times >90 minutes, helicopter transfer is recommended). During transfer, a paramedic or intensive care nurse should accompany the patient, and the ability to communicate by radio or phone with a physician is recommended. Arrhythmias, hypotension, and bleeding complications that develop during transfer can be treated effectively and are associated with low mortality rates.

B. Primary PCI

1. **Indications.** STEMI; high-risk NSTE-ACS, cardiogenic shock.

2. **Comments.** Compared to fibrinolytic therapy for STEMI, primary PCI is associated with less reinfarction and recurrent ischemia, fewer strokes in high-risk patients, shorter hospital stay, and improved survival (Chapter 3). Stents are superior to PTCA, and routine use of GP IIb/IIIa inhibitors is reasonable. For high-risk patients with NSTE-ACS (e.g., elevated cardiac troponins, dynamic ST-segment changes, ongoing ischemia), an early invasive strategy plus a GP IIb/IIIa inhibitor is superior to an early conservative strategy of PCI for recurrent ischemia only (Chapter 8). Early revascularization (PCI or CABG) improves survival in cardiogenic shock.

C. Immediate PCI After Successful Fibrinolysis (Patent Vessel)

1. **Indications.** Continued or recurrent ischemia, hemodynamic instability, or shock.

2. **Comments.** Routine immediate PCI should not be performed on asymptomatic patients after successful fibrinolytic therapy. Compared to a conservative strategy, routine PTCA resulted in higher rates of emergency CABG and blood transfusions, similar reocclusion rates, no improvement in LV function, and a trend toward increased mortality.

D. Rescue PCI for Failed Fibrinolysis (Occluded Vessel)

1. **Indications.** Ongoing chest pain; hemodynamic instability; persistent ST-elevation with ongoing chest pain 30–60 minutes after starting fibrinolytic therapy, especially for large anterior MI, prior MI or impaired ventricular function in noninfarct zone.

2. **Comments.** Rescue PCI may improve clinical outcome and regional function of the infarct zone in high-risk patients with anterior MI. Reocclusion rates are higher after rescue PCI than after primary PCI; therefore, stenting plus a GP IIb/IIIa inhibitor is recommended to reduce the risk of reocclusion. When assessing the response to fibrinolytic therapy, the ECG lead with maximal ST-elevation at baseline should be evaluated for >50% resolution (much more accurate and useful marker of persistent occlusion than persistent chest pain).

E. Delayed PCI (2–7 Days After Fibrinolysis)

1. **Indications.** Spontaneous or inducible ischemia; LVEF <40%; heart failure; serious ventricular arrhythmias; heart failure during acute episode even if LV function is preserved on subsequent testing.

2. **Comments.** Routine delayed PCI should not be performed on asymptomatic patients with patent vessels. Compared to a conservative strategy of PCI for recurrent ischemia, routine PCI resulted in higher rates of abrupt closure, reinfarction, and urgent CABG, no improvement in LV function, and a trend toward increased mortality (Chapter 5). Late revascularization is recommended for recurrent ischemia and should be considered for high-risk patients with prior MI, LV dysfunction, multivessel disease, or stenosis >90% supplying a moderate or large area of myocardium. Whether stable patients should undergo PCI of the infarct-related occluded artery after the period of myocardial salvage has passed was tested in the OAT trial. This study randomized 2166 patients with depressed LV function or proximal occlusion and who were at least 3 days, but not more than 28 days, post-MI to routine PCI or no PCI. Patients were followed over a mean period of 3 years. Both groups received background optimal medical therapy. The primary event rate of death, MI, or class IV heart failure was not significantly different between patients managed with PCI vs. those without PCI (17.2% vs. 15.6%, p = 0.20), and a trend toward increased nonfatal reinfarction among PCI-treated stable patients was observed.

F. CABG Surgery

1. **Indications.** Failed PCI with ongoing ischemia or hemodynamic instability; left main disease; three-vessel disease; two-vessel disease with proximal LAD obstruction and either LV dysfunction or treated diabetes; proximal three-vessel disease with a patent infarct vessel, especially if unsuitable for PCI. CABG can also be considered for patients with stable postinfarct angina with one- or two-vessel disease without significant proximal LAD obstruction but with a large area of viable myocardium and high-risk criteria on noninvasive testing (e.g., rest or exercise LVEF <0.35; treadmill score ≤ −11, single large stress-induced perfusion defect or multiple moderate perfusion defects, large fixed perfusion defect or moderate stress-induced perfusion defect with

LV dilatation or thallium uptake in lung, echo wall motion abnormality > two segments with low-dose dobutamine [<10 mcg/kg/min] or at a low heart rate [<120 bpm]; or extensive ischemia on stress echo). Additional surgical procedures are required for ruptured papillary muscle, VSD, LV pseudoaneurysm, and free-wall rupture.

2. **Comments.** Perioperative mortality rates for elective CABG 3–7 days after acute MI are similar to other elective indications. Mortality rates are high for acute MI complicated by failed fibrinolytic therapy (13% to 17%), acute mitral regurgitation (27% to 55%), or VSD (anterior MI 20%; posterior MI 70%). After fibrinolytic therapy, there is a 4% risk of reoperation for bleeding. Bypass Angioplasty Revascularization Investigation (BARI) reported better outcomes with CABG vs. PTCA for patients with multivessel disease and treated diabetes, but coronary stents and GP IIb/IIIa inhibitors were not tested in this trial. Compared to diabetics with prior PTCA, diabetics with prior CABG were more likely to survive spontaneous Q-wave MI. Aspirin should not be withheld prior to CABG, but clopidogrel should be withheld for 5–7 days to minimize the risk of perioperative bleeding.

G. Intra-Aortic Balloon Pump (IABP) Counterpulsation

1. **Indications.** Cardiogenic shock or severe hypotension not responding promptly to therapy; as a stabilizing bridge to surgical repair of ruptured chordae/papillary muscle or VSD; as a stabilizing bridge to revascularization for refractory postinfarct angina, significant left main disease, or critical three-vessel disease with LV dysfunction; persistent ischemia; or hypotension. Reasonable for management of refractory polymorphic VT to reduce myocardial ischemia. Use of the IABP can provide significant hemodynamic support with rare complications.

2. **Comments.** IABP improves coronary perfusion via augmentation of diastolic blood pressure and improves cardiac output and lowers filling pressures via afterload reduction of the left ventricle. Routine use of IABP after successful primary PCI has not been shown to improve outcome in low-intermediate risk or hemodynamically stable patients.

H. Temporary Pacemaker, Prophylactic (Table 11.1)

1. **Indications.** Mobitz II 2° AV block, new LBBB, RBBB with left anterior or left posterior fascicular block (LAFB/LPFB), 1° AV block with RBBB or LBBB, alternating LBBB and RBBB, or RBBB with alternating LAFB and LPFB.

2. **Comments.** Prophylactic pacing (usually for 48–72 hours) is recommended to prevent hemodynamic collapse in the event that conduction-delay progresses to complete heart block. Transcutaneous leads are preferred over transvenous leads because they can be applied quickly and used in standby mode for potentially unstable patients. Transcutaneous systems also avoid the risk of pneumothorax, cardiac perforation, and bleeding complications if anticoagulants/fibrinolytics are used. Nevertheless, a transvenous lead should be placed in patients who require more than brief transcutaneous pacing; are at high risk of progression to complete heart block; or develop asystole, complete heart block, or bradycardia with hypotension or recurrent sinus pauses >3 seconds unresponsive to atropine.

Table 11.1. Early Management of Atrioventricular and Intraventricular Conduction Disturbances During Acute MI

Intraventricular Conduction	Atrioventricular Conduction			
	Normal	1° AVB	Mobitz 1, 2° AV Block	Mobitz 2, 2° AV Block
Normal	O	O	TC	TC
Old or new LAFB or LPFB	O	TC*	TC	TC
Old BBB	O	TC	TC	TC
New BBB	TC	TC	TC	TV
Fascicular block + RBBB	TC	TC	TC	TV
Alternating RBBB + LBBB	TV	TV	TV	TV

BBB = bundle branch block, LAFB = left anterior fascicular block, LBBB = left bundle branch block, LPFB = left posterior fascicular block, RBBB = right bundle branch block.

This table indicates the highest level recommendation for each combination of atrioventricular and intraventricular conduction, as provided for in the 2004 ACC/AHA Guidelines for the Management of STEMI. All recommendations in this table are class I recommendations, except for transcutaneous pads/pacing for 1° AV block with old or new LAFB or LPFB (TC*), which is a class IIa recommendation for nonanterior MI. See the full-text of guidelines at www.acc.org/clinical/guidelines/stemi/index.pdf for other treatment options/considerations. Temporary pacing is not by itself an indication for permanent pacing.

Management Codes/Recommendations

O = observe: continued ECG monitoring, no further action planned.

TC = application of transcutaneous pads and standby transcutaneous pacing with no further progression to transvenous pacing imminently planned. If the patient becomes pacemaker-dependent due to a persistent conduction abnormality, temporary transvenous pacing is preferred over long-term transcutaneous pacing.

TV = temporary transvenous pacing; standby transcutaneous pacing until transvenous pacing initiated.

Reprinted from: Antman EM, Anbe DT, Armstrong PW, Bates ER, Green LA, Hand M, Hochman JS, Krumholz HM, Kushner FG, Lamas GA, Mullany CJ, Ornato JP, Pearle DL, Sloan MA, Smith SC Jr. ACC/AHA guidelines for the management of patients with ST-elevation myocardial infarction: a report of the American College of Cardiology/American Heart Association Task Force on Practice Guidelines (Committee to Revise the 1999 Guidelines for the Management of Patients With Acute Myocardial Infarction). *Circulation*. 2004;110;e82–e293.

I. **Temporary Pacemaker, Therapeutic (Transvenous Lead Required) (Table 11.1)**

   1. **Indications.** Asystole; 3° AV block; bradycardia with hypotension not responding to atropine; recurrent sinus pauses >3 seconds not responding to atropine.

   2. **Comments.** Patients with hemodynamic instability may require transcutaneous pacing until a transvenous lead can be placed. Given unacceptably high rates of failure with prolonged transcutaenous pacing, including patient discomfort with this method of chronotropic support, consideration for transvenous pacing should be made early. Temporary pacing may not be required for 3° AV block that occurs with inferior MI and resolves with atropine or after successful reperfusion. AV sequential pacing may be preferred over ventricular pacing to optimize AV synchrony

("atrial kick") and cardiac output in patients with severe LV dysfunction, LVH, or RV infarction. Frequent testing of pacing threshold is recommended; pacing energy is usually set at least three times threshold.

J. Permanent Pacemaker

1. **Indications.** Persistent 2° AV block in the His-Purkinje system accompanied by bilateral bundle branch block or complete heart block within or below the His-Purkinje system at any time during MI, bundle branch block with even transient infranodal 2° or 3° AV block (if site of block is uncertain, an EP study may be needed), or persistent, symptomatic 2° or 3° AV block. May be considered for persistent 2° or 3° AV block at the AV node. Permanent pacing is also recommended for persistent sinus node dysfunction, including mildly symptomatic sinus bradycardia, sinus pauses >3 seconds, or sinus bradycardia <40 bpm with hypotension or hemodynamic compromise resistant to atropine. (*Note*: Many cases of sinus node dysfunction resolve spontaneously after MI, requiring only temporary pacing.) Patients with indications for permanent pacing should also be evaluated for biventricular pacing and/or ICD implantation.

2. **Comments.** Temporary pacing after acute MI is not by itself an indication for permanent pacing. Most of the excess mortality associated with high-grade conduction disturbances is caused by heart failure and ventricular arrhythmias from extensive myocardial necrosis, not progressive heart block.

K. Implantable Cardioverter-Defibrillator (ICD) (see Figure 12.1, p. 122)

1. **Indications.** VF or hemodynamically significant sustained VT >48 hours from MI if not due to transient/reversible ischemia or reinfarction; STEMI at least 1 month prior with LVEF <30%; STEMI at least 1 month prior with LVEF 31% to 40%, electrical instability (e.g., nonsustained VT), or inducible VF or sustained VT on EP testing.

2. **Comments.** In MADIT, patients with prior MI, EF <36%, nonsustained VT, and inducible VT were randomized to ICD or best conventional therapy. At 4 years, the risk of death was reduced by 71% with prophylactic ICD (14% vs. 49%). In MUSTT, ICDs were better than EP-guided drug therapy at reducing arrhythmic death in patients with coronary artery disease, nonsustained VT, and inducible VT during EP testing. In DINAMIT, 674 high-risk patients with LV ejection fractions ≤35% between 6–40 days post-MI were randomized to optimal medical therapy plus ICD vs. medical therapy alone. At 2.5 years, ICDs reduced the risk of arrhythmic death by 58% (1.5% versus 3.5% per year, p = 0.009), which was offset by a 78% increase in nonarrhythmic death. In MADIT-2, 1232 patients with prior MI and severe LV dysfunction (EF ≤0.30) were randomized without EP testing to ICD or medical therapy. At 20 months, the risk of death was reduced by 31% with prophylactic ICD (14.2% vs. 19.8%, p = 0.016). In SCD-HeFT, 2521 patients with ischemic (48%) or nonischemic (52%) cardiomyopathy, class 2 or 3 heart failure, and LV ejection fraction ≤35% were randomized to ICD, amiodarone, or placebo. At 5 years, ICDs reduced

the risk of death by 23% (28.9% vs. 35.8%, p = 0.007). (Patients with class 3 heart failure treated with amiodarone experienced a 6% increase in mortality compared to placebo.) These data indicate significant survival benefit for ICD prophylaxis in patients with prior MI and LV dysfunction. Based on MADIT-2, there are 3–4 million potential ICD candidates now and 400,000 new candidates each year. Of note, patients should be screened for ICD therapy 1 month after MI or 3 months after CABG because previous studies treating patients with ICD therapy immediately after MI have not demonstrated a benefit.

L. Pulmonary Artery (PA) Catheterization

1. Indications. To differentiate cardiogenic shock from hypovolemic shock after failure of initial therapy with volume expansion or inotropic drugs; to guide management of cardiogenic shock, progressive hypotension, mechanical complications (VSD, papillary muscle rupture, cardiac tamponade); RV infarction with persistent hypotension or low cardiac output not responding to volume expansion and inotropes; and acute pulmonary edema not responding to diuretics, nitroglycerin, and inotropes.

2. Comments. PA catheterization allows determination of pulmonary capillary wedge pressure, cardiac output, and systemic vascular resistance. This information can be used to identify the etiology of hypotension (e.g., hypovolemia, RV infarction, low cardiac output, acute VSD) and guide therapy in a variety of settings. PaO_2 measurements in the superior vena cava, right atrium, right ventricle, and pulmonary artery can be used to diagnose VSD and assess the severity of left-to-right shunting. Information obtained from PA catheterization (Table 11.2) and echocardiography with Doppler should be integrated into the decision-making process for critically ill patients.

M. Intra-Arterial Pressure Monitoring

1. Indications. Severe hypotension (systolic BP <80 mmHg) or cardiogenic shock, use of IV vasopressors or inotropes (e.g., dopamine, dobutamine).

2. Comments. Monitoring via the radial artery is preferred, but the brachial or femoral artery can be used if needed. The intra-arterial catheter may remain in place at a single site up to 4 days as long as there is no evidence of thrombosis or infection, although in certain patients with difficult access it may be reasonable to leave the catheter in place longer.

Table 11.2. Pulmonary Artery Catheterization in ACS

Complication	Usual Hemodynamic Findings
RV infarction	↑ RAP; RAP/PCWP ratio >0.8; ↓ CO.
Cardiogenic shock	↓ BP; ↓ CO; ↑ PCWP; ↑ SVR.
Acute MR	↑ PCWP (prominent V-wave may be seen); CO usually ↓.
Acute VSD	≥8% oxygen step-up from RA to RV/PA. CO calculations are falsely elevated (reflecting left-to-right shunting with increased pulmonary blood flow).
Cardiac tamponade	↓ BP; paradoxical pulse; RAP ~ PCWP; ↓ CO; prominent X-descent may be seen on RA tracing. May need echo to distinguish from RV infarction.
Massive pulmonary embolism	↓ BP; ↓ CO; ↑ PA pressure and PVR; normal PCWP.

BP = blood pressure, CO = cardiac output, MR = mitral regurgitation, PA = pulmonary artery, PCWP = pulmonary capillary wedge pressure, PVR = pulmonary vascular resistance, RA = right atrium, RAP = right atrial pressure, RV = right ventricular, SVR = systemic vascular resistance, VSD = ventricular septal defect.

Source: Reprinted from Freed M, Grines C. In: *Essentials of Cardiovascular Medicine*, Physician's Press, Royal Oak, MI, 1994.

Chapter 12
Risk Stratification Post-MI

Predischarge risk stratification is indicated for all patients with ACS. If not performed early, cardiac catheterization is indicated to define coronary anatomy and assess LV function in patients with prior MI or CABG, known LV dysfunction, or a hospital course complicated by heart failure, hypotension, recurrent ischemia, failed fibrinolysis, suspected mechanical defect, or ventricular tachycardia or fibrillation >48 hours from MI. All other patients should undergo stress testing, followed by cardiac catheterization for inducible ischemia, especially at low workloads

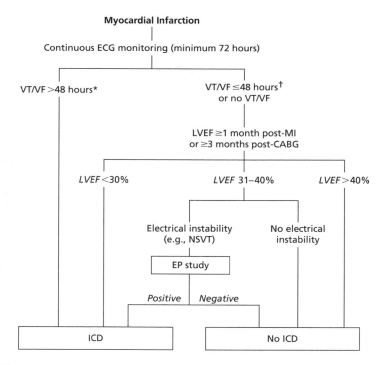

Figure 12.1. Screening and Evaluation of Arrhythmias Post-MI

CABG = coronary artery bypass grafting, EP = electrophysiology, ICD = implantable cardioverter-defibrillator, LVEF = left ventricular ejection fraction, NSVT = nonsustained ventricular tachycardia, VF = ventricular fibrillation, VT = ventricular tachycardia.

* If VT/VF due to transient ischemia or reinfaction, perform cardiac catheterization and revascularization. Then follow "no VT/VF" scheme to determine need for ICD therapy.

† Correct metabolics abnormalities; start beta-blockers; administer IV antiarrhythmic × 24 hours.

(<5 METS), or for other high-risk results (e.g., fixed perfusion defect with LV dilation or increased lung uptake of thallium, exercise-induced LV dysfunction or a drop in systolic blood pressure). All patients should have their left ventricular ejection fraction measured after MI. Guidelines for screening and evaluation of arrhythmias post-MI are proposed in Figure 12.1. This section describes modalities used for risk stratification following acute MI.

RISK STRATIFICATION MODALITIES

A. **Stress Test**
   1. **Indications.** (1) All patients who do not undergo coronary angiography; OR (2) In select patients to assess functional capacity and the effectiveness of antianginal therapy.

   2. **Comments.** No single approach to exercise testing is universally accepted. One approach is to perform a submaximal stress test (70% of predicted maximal heart rate or up to 120–130 bpm) prior to discharge followed by a symptom-limited (maximal) stress test at 4–6 weeks. Another approach is to perform a symptom-limited stress test prior to discharge, which will identify a higher percentage of patients with residual ischemia compared to a submaximal test (40% versus 23%). Patients with resting ECG changes that preclude assessment of ST-segment shifts (e.g., LBBB, LVH with repolarization abnormality, ST elevation, or depression at rest) should undergo stress testing with radionuclide imaging. Patients unable to exercise should undergo a pharmacological stress test. Predictors of future cardiac events in patients who have not undergone reperfusion therapy include the inability to exercise 6 minutes, chest pain, ST-depression, hypotensive response to exercise, reversible thallium defects, thallium uptake in lung, and ≥5% fall in exercise ejection fraction. Stress testing is not routinely recommended following successful PCI.

B. **Echocardiogram**
   1. **Indications.** Heart failure; anterior MI; pericarditis; new murmur; sustained hypotension; inferior MI with clinical instability and suspicion of RV infarction.

   2. **Comments.** Echocardiography can be used to assess LV function, evaluate the etiology of hypotension, and identify structural abnormalities post-MI (e.g., LV thrombus, aneurysm, pseudoaneurysm, pericardial effusion, RV infarction, ruptured papillary muscle). In conjunction with Doppler imaging, echocardiography can be used to identify acute mitral regurgitation and VSD. In conjunction with stress testing (exercise or dobutamine), echocardiography can be used to assess inducible ischemia and myocardial viability to determine the need for revascularization.

C. **Ambulatory (Holter) ECG Monitor**
   1. **Indications.** Not routinely indicated; obtain if patient is not on a computer-monitored telemetry system.

   2. Comments. Frequent VPCs or VT >48 hours from MI identifies patients at increased risk of death. Based upon findings from MUSTT, ICDs are beneficial for patients with nonsustained VT >96 hours after MI, LVEF ≤0.40, and inducible VT.

D. Electrophysiology (EP) Study

   1. Indications. Nonsustained monomorphic VT >96 hours from MI.

   2. Comments. The utility of programmed electrical stimulation in post-MI patients remains controversial, because poor specificity results in many false positive tests. In MUSTT there was no difference in outcome for patients with coronary artery disease and inducible VT treated by EP-guided medical therapy or no therapy; survival was greatest with ICD implantation.

E. Cardiac Catheterization Post-MI

   1. Indications. Recurrent ischemia (spontaneous or provoked by minimum exertion during recovery from MI); heart failure or hemodynamic instability; LV dysfunction (EF ≤0.40); clinical heart failure during acute MI but well-preserved LV function post-MI; new murmur with suspected mechanical defect; prior MI or CABG; VT >48 hours from MI; inability to exercise; ischemia, arrhythmia, or fall in blood pressure during exercise testing.

   2. Comments. Current guidelines recommendations endorse routine early cardiac catheterization for ACS patients with high-risk features to eliminate the need for multiple costly noninvasive tests that subsequently would indicate the need for catheterization in >60% of patients with acute MI. Patients undergoing routine coronary angiography and revascularization based on coronary anatomy have improved outcomes after hospital discharge. Poor prognostic factors on cardiac catheterization include occluded infarct vessel or suboptimal flow, multivessel or left main disease, LV dysfunction (EF <0.40), hypokinesis of noninfarct zone, and mechanical defects (acute mitral regurgitation, VSD).

SECTION 5

COMPLICATIONS OF ACUTE MI

The likelihood of developing a major complication in the days following acute myocardial infarction is related to the location of the infarct, the amount of myocardial necrosis, the degree of LV dysfunction, and the extent of residual coronary artery disease. Some complications are transient, easily managed, and relatively benign (e.g., bradycardia with inferior MI, pericarditis); other complications are associated with a significant risk of death and require emergency management (e.g., shock, ruptured papillary muscle, ventricular tachycardia). This section details the management of electrical, ischemic, and mechanical complications of acute MI.

Chapter 13

Arrhythmias and Conduction Disturbances in Acute Myocardial Infarction

SINUS TACHYCARDIA

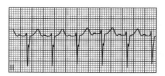

A. Overview. There are many potential causes of sinus tachycardia in the setting of ACS, including myocardial ischemia or infarction, heart failure, drug-induced (e.g., dobutamine, dopamine, vasodilators), pericarditis, atrial infarction, acute mitral regurgitation, and ventricular septal defect. Sinus tachycardia can also be a physiological response to pain, anxiety, fever, hypovolemia, hypoxemia, or hypotension. Sinus tachycardia is associated with larger infarctions and increased mortality risk and is one of the more ominous electrocardiographic findings after ACS.

B. ECG Characteristics. Sinus P-waves (upright in leads I, II, aVF) at a rate >100 per minute. P-wave amplitude often increases and the PR interval often shortens with increasing heart rates.

C. Treatment. The primary goal in the evaluation and treatment of sinus tachycardia is identification and correction of the underlying etiology (e.g., myocardial ischemia, pain, anxiety, hypovolemia, fever, heart failure). Drug therapy should not be used to slow reflex tachycardia caused by hypovolemia or compensatory tachycardia caused by heart failure.

SINUS BRADYCARDIA

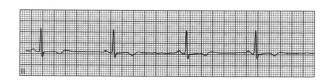

A. Overview. Sinus bradycardia occurs in up to one-third of patients with acute MI and is more common with inferior MI and following coronary reperfusion. In the setting of ACS, common causes include high vagal tone (Bezold-Jarisch reflex with inferior MI) and drugs (beta-blockers, verapamil, diltiazem, digitalis, Type IA/IB/IC antiarrhythmics, amiodarone, sotalol). Sinus bradycardia often occurs in conjunction with sinus arrest, sinoatrial exit block, AV junctional escape rhythm, and bradycardia alternating with tachycardia as a component of the sick sinus syndrome.

B. ECG Characteristics. Sinus P-waves (upright in leads I, II, and aVF) at a rate <60 per minute.

C. Treatment. No treatment is indicated for asymptomatic patients. Atropine should be considered for heart rates <40 bpm with associated hypotension, ischemia, or ventricular arrhythmias, at a dose of 0.6–1.0 mg IV; this may be repeated up to a total dose of 0.04 mg/kg. (Atropine can cause paradoxical slowing of heart rate at low [<0.5 mg] doses and myocardial ischemia at high doses.) Transcutaneous or transvenous (preferably atrial) temporary pacing is indicated for symptomatic bradycardia unresponsive to atropine. Dopamine 5–20 mcg/kg/min IV or epinephrine 2–10 mcg/min IV can be used acutely for refractory cases (as the patient is being prepared for temporary pacemaker insertion); however, in the setting of ACS, they may also promote ventricular arrhythmias. Permanent pacing is indicated for persistent, symptomatic sinus bradycardia.

SINUS PAUSE/ARREST

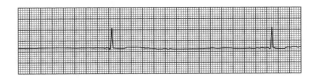

A. Overview. Sinus pauses and sinus arrest are due to transient failure of impulse formation at the sinoatrial (SA) node. They occur infrequently with acute MI but are more common with inferior MI and following coronary reperfusion.

B. ECG Characteristics. PP interval (pause) exceeds 1.6–2.0 seconds and is not a multiple of the basic sinus PP interval. Sinus pauses must be differentiated from sinus arrhythmia (phasic, gradual change in PP interval); Mobitz Type I second-degree sinoatrial exit block (progressive shortening of the PP interval until a P-wave fails to appear); Mobitz Type II second-degree sinoatrial block (PP pause is a multiple of the basic sinus PP interval); abrupt change in autonomic tone (e.g., vagal reaction); and "pseudo" sinus pauses from nonconducted atrial premature complexes (P-wave appears to be absent but is actually buried in the T-wave, as suggested by subtle deformity of the T-wave at the beginning of the pause). Complete failure of sinoatrial conduction (third-degree sinoatrial exit block) cannot be differentiated from a complete sinus arrest on surface ECG.

C. Treatment. Sinus pauses >3 seconds and frequent sinus pauses associated with hypotension, heart failure, or other low output symptoms should be treated the same as symptomatic sinus bradycardia (p. 128).

ATRIAL FLUTTER

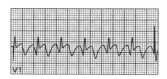

A. Overview. Atrial flutter is an uncommon arrhythmia during ACS and suggests associated atrial disease.

B. ECG Characteristics. Rapid, regular, atrial undulations (flutter or "F"-waves) usually at a rate of 240–340 per minute. Typical atrial flutter morphology is usually present, with inverted F-waves without an isoelectric baseline ("picket-fence" or "sawtooth" appearance) in leads II, III, and aVF, and small, positive deflections with a distinct isoelectric baseline in lead V_1. QRS complexes are usually normal but can be wide in the setting of underlying bundle branch block or aberrancy. The AV conduction ratio (ratio of flutter waves to QRS complexes) is usually a fixed, even number (e.g., 2:1, 4:1), but AV conduction can be variable (e.g., 2:1 and 4:1 in the same tracing). Odd-numbered conduction ratios (1:1, 3:1) are uncommon. Atrial flutter with 1:1 AV conduction often conducts aberrantly, resulting in a wide QRS tachycardia that may be confused for VT. In untreated patients, conduction ratios 1:4 or greater suggest the presence of AV conduction system disease. Carotid sinus massage can unmask flutter waves and help confirm the diagnosis of atrial flutter with 2:1 AV block but does not convert the arrhythmia; discontinuation of carotid sinus massage usually results in return to the original ventricular rate. Flutter rate may be slower (200–240 per minute) in the presence of Type IA, 1C, III antiarrhythmic drugs, or massively dilated atria, and atypical atrial flutter can exhibit upright F-waves in the inferior leads.

C. Treatment. Cardioversion is required if there is associated hemodynamic compromise (initial synchronized monophasic shock of 50 J or an appropriate biphasic energy dose [e.g., device specific], preceded by brief anesthesia or conscious sedation). Ibutilide should be avoided in ACS due to the increased risk of torsade de pointes. IV and oral amiodarone can be used to maintain sinus rhythm if atrial flutter recurs after cardioversion. Beta-blockers are recommended for rate control in persistent atrial flutter. Anticoagulation should be considered for 3 weeks prior to attempted cardioversion for atrial flutter >48 hours in duration unless the patient is already receiving IV anticoagulation.

ATRIAL FIBRILLATION

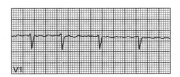

A. **Overview.** Atrial fibrillation (AF) occurs in 6% to 15% of patients with acute MI. Risk factors include age >70 years, acidosis, hypoxemia, hypokalemia, hypomagnesemia, large anterior MI, or MI complicated by heart failure, pericarditis, atrial infarction, or acute mitral regurgitation with left atrial distension. AF often occurs within the first 24 hours of symptom onset, and episodes are frequently transient but may recur. The incidence of systemic embolization is 2% in paroxysmal AF and <1% in sustained AF. Most embolic events occur by day 4% and 50% occur within the first 24 hours. AF portends a worse prognosis in acute MI and in long-term follow-up.

B. **ECG Characteristics.** P-waves are absent, and atrial activity (best seen in leads V_1, V_2, II, III, and aVF) is totally irregular and represented by fibrillatory (f) waves of varying amplitude, duration, and morphology, which cause random oscillation of the baseline. The ventricular rhythm is irregular in most cases but can be regular in the presence of complete heart block (e.g., digitalis toxicity). Ventricular rates are 100–180 per minute in the absence of AV nodal blocking agents. Ventricular rates <100 per minute suggest coexistent AV conduction system disease; rates >200–220 per minute suggest the presence of an accessory pathway.

C. **Treatment.** No treatment is required for brief, well-tolerated episodes. Immediate synchronized cardioversion with an initial monophasic shock of 200 J or an appropriate biphasic dose (preceded by brief general anesthesia or conscious sedation) is required for AF resulting in ischemia, hypotension, or heart failure. Hemodynamically significant persistent AF or AF that recurs after brief sinus rhythm should be treated with amiodarone and/or digoxin. Patients with sustained AF with ongoing ischemia but without hemodynamic compromise should be treated with beta-blockers (preferred), verapamil or diltiazem, and/or synchronized cardioversion (200 J). For sustained AF in patients without ischemia or hemodynamic compromise, rate control and anticoagulant therapy are indicated. Cardioversion to sinus rhythm can be considered for patients with a history of AF or atrial flutter prior to MI. Sustained AF requires anticoagulation with IV heparin to maintain the PTT at 50–70 seconds. Recent data from the AFFIRM study showed that among 4060 patients with atrial fibrillation and a high risk of stroke or death, rate control plus anticoagulation resulted in a trend toward lower mortality at 5 years (21.3% versus 23.8%, p = 0.08) and significantly less rehospitalization and fewer adverse drug reactions than did rhythm control with antiarrhythmic drugs. For AF >48 hours in duration when sinus rhythm is preferred, warfarin is recommended for 3 weeks prior to attempted cardioversion, unless transesophageal echocardiography (TEE) confirms the absence of LV or atrial clot. With or without TEE, anticoagulation is required during and for a minimum of 4 weeks after cardioversion. Correction of acidosis, hypoxemia, and electrolyte disturbances is mandatory for all patients.

ACCELERATED IDIOVENTRICULAR RHYTHM

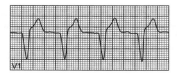

A. **Overview.** Accelerated idioventricular rhythm (AIVR) is common in the early period after ACS. It is likely due to automaticity and usually self-terminates. It is not associated with an increased risk of late mortality. In the setting of ACS, common causes include myocardial ischemia and coronary reperfusion. AIVR can also be caused by digitalis toxicity.

B. **ECG Characteristics.** AIVR is a regular wide-complex rhythm with a ventricular rate greater than the atrial rate but less than 100 beats per minute. A wide-complex rhythm ≥100 bpm with atrioventricular dissociation should be treated as ventricular tachycardia. AIVR is an imprecise and limited predictor of reperfusion. AV dissociation, ventricular capture complexes, and fusion beats are common because of the competition between normal sinus and ectopic ventricular rhythms.

C. **Treatment.** No treatment is usually necessary, and prophylaxis against VF is not recommended.

VENTRICULAR TACHYCARDIA

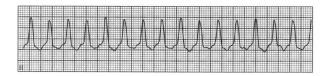

A. **Overview.** Most episodes of VT associated with acute MI occur within the first 48 hours of symptom onset. In contrast to early VT, which has no impact on prognosis after hospital discharge, VT after 48 hours increases the risk of late mortality and is an indication for cardiac catheterization. Nonsustained VT occurs in two-thirds of patients within the first 12 hours of MI and is not associated with increased mortality. VT can also be induced by electrolyte disturbances (hypokalemia, hyperkalemia, hypomagnesemia), hypoxemia, acidosis, drug toxicity (e.g., digitalis), and LV aneurysm or scar.

B. **ECG Characteristics.** Rapid succession of three or more ventricular premature complexes at a rate >100 per minute. Nonsustained VT lasts <30 seconds; sustained VT lasts ≥30 seconds or requires intervention due to hemodynamic instability. The RR interval is usually regular but can be irregular, especially in the first several beats. AV dissociation can be difficult to discern on the electrocardiogram and is present in approximately one-third of wide-complex tachycardias due to VT. Retrograde atrial activation, fusion complexes, and ventricular capture complexes are occasionally seen. Rarely, VT can present as a narrow QRS tachycardia.

C. **Treatment.** For well-tolerated monomorphic VT (e.g., no hypotension or ischemic symptoms) at a rate <150 per minute, drug therapy can be attempted prior to cardioversion (synchronized electrical shocks starting at 50 J; brief anesthesia is required). Amiodarone, procainamide, sotalol, or lidocaine is recommended for patients with normal LV function, and amiodarone or lidocaine is recommended for patients with poor LV function (Amiodarone dose: 150 mg infused over 10 minutes [or 5 mg/kg], with 150-mg doses repeated every 5–10 minutes as needed. Alternative infusion: 360 mg over 6 hours [1 mg/min], then 540 mg over next 16 hours [0.5 mg/min]. The cumulative dose should not exceed 2.2 gm over 24 hours.) Poorly tolerated monomorphic VT requires immediate synchronized cardioversion with an initial monophasic shock of 100 J, followed if necessary by increasing energies; brief anesthesia in hemodynamically stable patients is recommended. Rapid, polymorphic VT should be treated the same as ventricular fibrillation (see the following). Correction of acidosis, hypoxemia, electrolyte disturbances (maintain K$^+$ >4.0 mEq/L and Mg^{++} >2.0 mEq/L), and ongoing ischemia is mandatory for all patients. See p. 118 for indications for ICD implantation.

VENTRICULAR FIBRILLATION

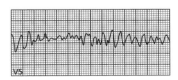

A. Overview. Primary ventricular fibrillation (VF) occurs within the first 4 hours of MI in 4% of patients and is a major cause of early mortality, but early VF is not associated with an increased risk of death after hospital discharge. Prophylaxis with lidocaine or beta-blockers reduces the incidence of primary VF, but routine lidocaine prophylaxis is not recommended due to the risk of increased overall mortality from asystole and other serious bradyarrhythmias. VF can usually be converted into a more stable rhythm when defibrillation occurs within the first minute (the electrical phase). Unfortunately, defibrillation is successful in less than 25% of cases when initiated after 4 minutes (the circulatory phase—when chest compressions and high-quality cardiopulmonary resuscitation may take priority).

B. ECG Characteristics. VF is an extremely rapid and irregular ventricular rhythm with chaotic, irregular deflections of varying amplitude and contour and the lack of distinct QRS complexes.

C. Treatment. VF requires ACLS and immediate defibrillation (if witnessed), starting with an unsynchronized electrical shock with 200 J monophasic or an appropriate biphasic shock energy (device specific). Current ACLS guidelines recommend immediate resumption of cardiopulmonary resuscitation (CPR) for 2 minutes or five cycles (100 compressions per minute). Epinephrine 1 mg IV push every 3–5 minutes or vasopressin 40 U IV push one time only should be administered for persistent VF. Every attempt should be made to minimize the interruption of chest compressions. After five cycles of CPR, if VF persists, another shock should be delivered. Amiodarone (300 mg or 5 mg/kg, IV bolus) is reasonable for VF not responding to initial electrical shocks and vasopressor therapy. Magnesium (1–2 gm IV bolus over 5 minutes) may be useful for torsades de pointes or hypomagnesemia. Procainamide is an option for intermittent or recurrent VF but is not recommended acutely due to its long administration time. Serum K^+ and Mg^{++} levels should be maintained above 4.0 mEq/L and 2.0 mEq/L, respectively, and acidosis, hypoxemia, ongoing ischemia, and heart failure must be treated aggressively. Routine prophylactic lidocaine has been associated with a trend toward increased mortality and is not recommended. See p. 118 for indication for ICD implantation. (For asystole, which may be difficult to distinguish from fine VF, vasopressin 40 IU was superior to epinephrine 1 mg in a randomized trial of out-of-hospital cardiac resuscitation.)

Note: Once a victim of ventricular fibrillation arrest has been successfully resuscitated consideration should be given to therapeutic hypothermia if the patient remains comatose. Randomized controlled trials of cooling to 32°–34° (90°–93°F) C for 12–24 hours in comatose survivors of out-of-hospital cardiac arrest have demonstrated improved neurologic recovery (number needed to treat = 4). Although randomized trials have not been conducted for survivors of in-hospital arrest, the risk-benefit profile appears favorable.

AV BLOCK, 1°

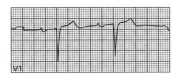

A. **Overview.** AV block, 1° is more common with inferior MI, due to associated high vagal tone. It can also be drug induced (e.g., digitalis, quinidine, procainamide, flecainide, propafenone, amiodarone, sotalol, beta-blockers, diltiazem, verapamil) and can occur in normal individuals.

B. **ECG Characteristics.** PR interval >0.20 seconds and each P-wave is followed by a QRS complex. The PR interval is usually 0.21–0.40 seconds but can be up to 0.80 seconds in duration. A prolonged PR interval with a narrow QRS complex identifies the site of block in the AV node. If the QRS is wide, conduction delay or block is usually in the His-Purkinje system, although block in the AV node with underlying bundle branch block or aberrancy can present in a similar fashion.

C. **Treatment.** No treatment is usually required. Patients with rare, very long (>0.40 sec) PR intervals and symptoms of low cardiac output may benefit from AV sequential pacing.

AV BLOCK, 2°—MOBITZ TYPE I (WENCKEBACH)

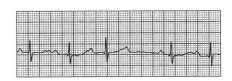

A. **Overview.** In the setting of ACS, common causes include myocardial infarction (especially inferior MI) and drugs (digitalis, beta-blockers, nondihydropyridine calcium antagonists, flecainide, sotalol, amiodarone, propafenone). Type I block is generally benign and usually occurs at the level of the AV node, resulting in a narrow QRS complex. (In contrast, Mobitz Type II block usually occurs within or below the bundle of His, resulting in a wide QRS complex in 80% and requires pacing.) A Type I block can also occur in normal individuals.

B. ECG Characteristics. Progressive lengthening of the PR interval and progressive shortening of the RR interval until a P-wave is blocked. Additionally, the RR interval containing the nonconducted P-wave is less than two PP intervals. Classical Wenckebach periodicity is not always evident, especially when sinus arrhythmia is present or an abrupt change in autonomic tone occurs (e.g., vagal reaction). In a Type I block with high conduction ratios (e.g., infrequent pauses), the PR interval of the beats immediately preceding the blocked P-wave may be equal to each other, suggesting a Type II block. In these situations, it is best to compare the PR interval immediately before and after the blocked P-wave; a difference in the PR interval suggests a Type I block, whereas a constant PR interval suggests a Type II block. Mobitz Type I AV block, 2° results in "group" or "pattern beating" due to the presence of nonconducted P-waves. Other causes of group beating include blocked APCs, Type II second-degree AV block, and concealed His-bundle depolarizations.

C. Treatment. No treatment is recommended in asymptomatic patients, although application of transcutaneous pacing patches is reasonable (Table 11.1, p. 117). Atropine (0.6–2.0 mg) followed by pacing can be used to treat symptomatic patients with frequent nonconducted beats and associated hypotension, heart failure, or other low-output symptoms.

AV BLOCK, 2°—MOBITZ TYPE II

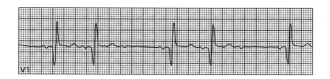

A. Overview. A Mobitz Type II block is almost always due to a serious conduction system disease and is associated with an increased risk of progression to complete heart block.

B. ECG Characteristics. Regular sinus or atrial rhythm with intermittent nonconducted P-waves and no evidence for atrial prematurity. The PR interval in the conducted beats is constant, and the RR interval containing the nonconducted P-wave is equal to two PP intervals. A Type II block may be confused for a Type I block with high conduction rates (e.g., 10:9 conduction). In these situations, it is best to compare the PR interval immediately before and after the blocked P-wave; a difference in the PR interval suggests a Type I block, whereas a constant PR interval suggests a Type II block.

C. Treatment. Temporary followed by permanent pacing is indicated for a Mobitz Type II block, regardless of the presence or absence of symptoms. In the case of infranodal block, atropine may increase the sinus rate without affecting infranodal conduction. This may lead to more nonconducted sinus beats and effectively, a slower ventricular rate.

AV BLOCK, 3° (COMPLETE HEART BLOCK)

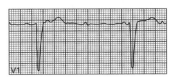

A. **Overview.** Complete heart block occurs in 5% to 15% of patients with acute MI. In inferior MI, complete heart block is usually preceded by first-degree AV block and typically occurs at the level of the AV node. In these cases, heart block is often associated with a stable junctional escape rhythm (narrow QRS complex at a rate >40 per minute) and usually lasts <1 week. In anterior MI, complete heart block occurs as a result of extensive damage to the left ventricle and is often preceded by a Type II second-degree AV block or bifascicular block. Mortality rates are very high (up to 70%) due to pump failure rather than heart block, per se.

B. **ECG Characteristics.** Atrial impulses consistently fail to reach the ventricles, resulting in independent atrial and ventricular rhythms. This manifests as a varying PR interval with constant PP and RR intervals. The P-wave may precede, be buried in, or follow the QRS. Ventricular rhythm is maintained by a junctional or idioventricular escape rhythm or a ventricular pacemaker. Ventriculophasic sinus arrhythmia (e.g., PP interval containing a QRS complex is shorter than the PP interval without a QRS complex), due to hemodynamically mediated alterations in sinus node automaticity, occurs in 30% to 50%.

C. **Treatment.** The site and stability of the escape rhythm determines the need and urgency for intervention. No treatment is usually necessary for stable patients with narrow escape complexes. For symptomatic patients and those with wide-complex escape rhythms, temporary pacing is indicated. Permanent pacing is usually required for persistent heart block >5 days and for complete heart block preceded by a Mobitz Type II second-degree AV block or accompanied by bundle branch block. It is important to exclude reversible causes of complete heart block, including digitalis toxicity and hyperkalemia.

LEFT ANTERIOR OR LEFT POSTERIOR FASCICULAR BLOCK

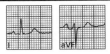

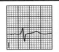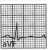

LAFB   *LPFB*

A. Overview. Compared to the left anterior fascicle, the left posterior fascicle is shorter and thicker and receives dual blood supply from both the left and right coronary arteries. In acute MI, the incidence of isolated left anterior fascicular block (LAFB) and isolated left posterior fascicular block (LPFB) is 4% and 0.4%, respectively. LAFB usually occurs in the setting of anteroseptal or anterolateral infarction, and the LAD is typically the infarct vessel. When LPFB develops during acute MI, multivessel disease with extensive infarction is usually present and the prognosis is poor.

B. ECG Characteristics. *LAFB:* Left axis deviation with mean QRS axis between −45 and −90 degrees; qR complex (or an R-wave) in leads I and aVL; rS complex in lead III; normal or slightly prolonged QRS duration (0.08–0.10 seconds); and no other factors responsible for left axis deviation (e.g., LVH, inferior MI, chronic lung disease, left bundle branch block, ostium premium atrial septal defect, severe hyperkalemia). *LPFB:* Right axis deviation with mean QRS axis between 100 and 180 degrees; normal or slightly prolonged QRS duration (0.08–0.10 seconds); rS complex in leads I and VL; qR complex in lead III; and no other factors responsible for right axis deviation (e.g., RVH, vertical heart, chronic lung disease, pulmonary embolism, lateral MI, dextrocardia, lead reversal, Wolff-Parkinson-White syndrome).

C. Treatment. No treatment is required for isolated hemiblock. Application of transcutaneous pacing patches is reasonable when LAFB or LPFB is accompanied by AV conduction disturbances (Table 11.1, p. 117) or right bundle branch block (see bifascicular block, p. 139).

RIGHT BUNDLE BRANCH BLOCK (RBBB)

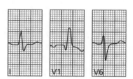

A. Overview. Complete RBBB occurs in 5% of patients with acute (usually anterior) MI, often in conjunction with left anterior fascicular block. RBBB is associated with an increased risk of death post-MI. Normal adults with RBBB (incidence 0.2%) have essentially the same prognosis as the general population.

B. ECG Characteristics. Prolonged QRS duration (≥0.12 seconds); secondary R-wave (R') in leads V_1 and V_2 (rsR' or rSR'; R' usually taller than the initial R-wave); delayed onset of intrinsicoid deflection (beginning of QRS complex to peak of R-wave >0.05 seconds) and secondary ST-T changes (T-wave inversion ≥ downsloping ST segments) in leads V_1 and V_2; and wide terminal S-waves in leads I and V_6. In RBBB, the mean QRS axis is determined by the initial unblocked 0.06–0.08 seconds of the QRS and should be normal unless a left anterior fascicular block or left posterior fascicular block is present. RBBB does not interfere with the ability to detect ventricular hypertrophy or Q-waves on ECG.

C. **Treatment.** Application of transcutaneous patches/pacing or transvenous pacing may be indicated depending on the age of RBBB and whether AV conduction abnormalities coexist (Table 11.1, p. 117).

LEFT BUNDLE BRANCH BLOCK (LBBB)

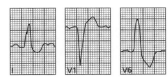

A. **Overview.** LBBB occurs in 1% to 2% of patients with acute (usually anterior) MI and is associated with an increased risk of complete heart block and death. In-hospital mortality rates up to 25% have been reported.

B. **ECG Characteristics.** Prolonged QRS duration ($\leq$0.12 seconds); delayed onset of intrinsicoid deflection (beginning of QRS to peak of R-wave >0.05 seconds) in leads V_5 and V_6; broad monophasic R-waves in leads I, V_5, and V_6, which are usually notched or slurred; secondary ST-T changes opposite in direction to the major QRS deflection (e.g., ST depression and T-wave inversion in leads I, V_5, and V_6; ST elevation and upright T-waves in leads V_1 and V_2); and rS or QS complexes in the right precordial leads. Left axis deviation may be present. LBBB interferes with the ability to detect QRS axis, ventricular hypertrophy, and acute MI on ECG.

C. **Treatment.** Application of transcutaneous patches/pacing or transvenous pacing may be indicated depending on the age of LBBB and whether AV conduction abnormalities coexist (Table 11.1, p. 117).

BIFASCICULAR BLOCK OR ALTERNATING BUNDLE BRANCH BLOCK

A. **Overview and ECG Characteristics.** RBBB with LAFB occurs in 5% of patients with acute (usually anterior) MI, and the usual infarct vessel is the LAD. RBBB with LPFB is uncommon in acute MI (incidence <1%) and indicates the presence of multivessel disease. Alternating bundle branch block is associated with an increased risk of progression to complete heart block and can present as RBBB alternating with LBBB or as RBBB with alternating LAFB and LPFB.

B. Treatment. Temporary transvenous pacing is recommended for alternating bundle branch block of any age and for new or indeterminate age bifascicular block with first-degree AV block. Permanent pacing is indicated for bifascicular or alternating bundle branch block associated with complete heart block or second-degree AV block in the His-Purkinje system, regardless of symptoms.

Chapter 14
Ischemic and Mechanical Complications

FAILED FIBRINOLYSIS

A. **Overview.** Only 50% to 60% of infarct vessels achieve TIMI-3 flow after fibrinolytic therapy, and there are no clinical markers to accurately predict reperfusion success with fibrinolysis. In small randomized trials, rescue PCI improved regional wall motion and LV function after failed fibrinolysis and reduced the risk of recurrent ischemia, heart failure, shock, and death in high-risk patients. However, early mortality was high (>30%) if rescue PTCA failed. In GUSTO-III, the use of abciximab during rescue PCI reduced mortality rates at 30 days.

B. **Treatment.** Emergency angiography should be considered for ongoing chest pain, hemodynamic instability, or persistent ST-elevation (<50% ST recovery) 90 minutes after lytic therapy especially for large anterior MI. Stents plus GP IIb/IIIa inhibitors are recommended for high-grade lesions with impaired coronary flow.

LEFT VENTRICULAR ANEURYSM

A. **Overview.** LV aneurysm develops in up to 10% of acute (usually anterior) infarctions, typically within the first 3 months. Important risk factors include LAD occlusion, a persistently occluded infarct artery, poor collateral blood flow, and female gender. Early reperfusion therapy and ACE inhibition reduce infarct expansion and LV aneurysm formation.

B. **Diagnosis.** A thinned, smooth, dyskinetic ventricular wall is evident on the echocardiogram or ventriculogram. Persistent ST-elevation in the region of the aneurysm is often present on ECG.

C. **Complications.** LV aneurysms predispose to heart failure, mitral regurgitation, late ventricular arrhythmias, and sudden death. Mural thrombus is common on autopsy, and systemic thromboembolism occurs in 2% to 5%. The risk of cardiac rupture is much greater with pseudoaneurysm (see the following) than with true aneurysm.

D. **Treatment.** Surgical resection is indicated for aneurysms causing heart failure, systemic thromboembolism, or recurrent VT/VF unresponsive to conventional therapy (Grade IIa, Level of Evidence B). Aneurysmectomy often improves ejection fraction and functional status, and resection is usually combined with CABG. Associated papillary muscle dysfunction may require mitral valve repair or replacement, and inducibility of VT may require ICD implantation. Operative mortality is approximately 10% overall, though it is 19% in those patients with an LVEF <20%. The recently completed STITCH trial, which randomized patients with ischemic cardiomyopathy with an LVEF ≤35% to CABG alone or CABG with surgical ventricular restoration, demonstrated that surgical ventricular restoration decreased ventricular volumes but did not improve symptoms, exercise tolerance, or death/hospitalization for cardiovascular causes.

LEFT VENTRICULAR PSEUDOANEURYSM

A. **Overview.** Pseudoaneurysms are contained free-wall ruptures protected from exsanguinating hemorrhage by clot in the pericardial space. In contrast to the walls of true aneurysms, which are composed of endocardial tissue and fibrosed myocardium, pseudoaneurysmal walls are composed only of pericardium and thrombus, increasing the risk of cardiac rupture. Pseudoaneurysms usually involve the anterior-apical or inferoposterior walls of the left ventricle.

B. **Diagnosis.** Narrow neck opening into the body of the pseudoaneurysm is evident on echocardiogram or ventriculogram.

C. **Treatment.** Prompt surgical resection is usually recommended, even in clinically stable patients, due to the increased risk of cardiac rupture and death.

LEFT VENTRICULAR DYSFUNCTION (ACUTE HEART FAILURE)

A. **Overview.** In the setting of acute MI, acute heart failure is often a result of both systolic and diastolic LV dysfunction (e.g., decreased contractility and impaired compliance). Other causes of low-output failure include RV infarction, mechanical defects (e.g., acute MR, VSD), bradyarrhythmias (e.g., sinus arrest, AV junctional rhythm), tachyarrhythmias (e.g., atrial fibrillation, SVT, VT), and conduction disturbances (e.g., high-degree AV block). Recovery of diastolic and systolic function can be delayed for days or weeks after successful coronary reperfusion due to stunned myocardium.

B. **Presentation.** Depending on the extent of LV dysfunction, symptoms can vary from mild pulmonary congestion to acute pulmonary edema to severe low cardiac output with cardiogenic shock.

C. **Treatment** (Figure 14.1). The immediate goals of therapy are to treat reversible factors, control symptoms, and maintain vital organ perfusion. Supplemental oxygen is recommended to maintain arterial saturation >90%.
   1. **Parenteral therapy.** Patients with normal blood pressure should be treated acutely with furosemide, sublingual nitroglycerin, and morphine. Dobutamine (and/or milrinone) and IV nitroglycerin are added if there is evidence of persistent signs and symptoms of a low-output state. Nitroprusside should be considered for afterload reduction in cases of severe hypertension or acute mitral regurgitation. Patients with

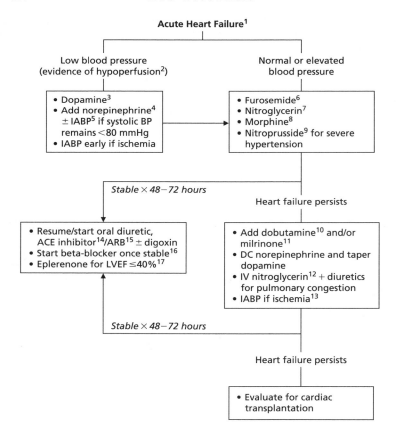

Figure 14.1. Management of Acute Heart Failure Secondary to ACS

ACE = angiotensin-converting enzyme, ARB = angiotensin receptor blocker, BP = blood pressure, DC = discontinue, IABP = intra-aortic balloon pump, PA = pulmonary artery.

1. Assess airway, breathing circulation; administer oxygen; start IV; intubate early for severe respiratory distress, acidosis, hypotension; pulse oximetry, blood pressure cuff, ECG monitor; obtain 12-lead ECG and treat arrhythmias and heart block; obtain CBC, electrolytes, portable chest X-ray, and echocardiogram; utilize arterial line for hypotension and pulmonary artery catheter when feasible; treat reversible causes and precipitating factors (e.g., ongoing ischemia, ventricular septal defect,

Figure 14.1. Management of Acute Heart Failure Secondary to ACS (cont'd)

papillary muscle rupture). PCI is preferred over fibrinolytic therapy as the primary reperfusion strategy for acute MI complicated by heart failure.

2. Cool clammy skin, impaired cognition, oliguria, azotemia.

3. Dopamine 5–15 mcg/kg/min IV infusion.

4. Norepinephrine 0.5–30 mcg/min IV infusion.

5. Intra-aortic balloon counterpulsation is contraindicated in the presence of moderate-to-severe aortic regurgitation.

6. Furosemide 0.5–1.0 mg/kg IV. Up to 100–200 mg IV may be needed for patients receiving long-term diuretic therapy. Torsemide or bumetanide can also be used. Caution: Diuretics should be given only to patients with suspected hypervolemia, because acute diuresis in the setting of relative intravascular volume depletion can precipitate cardiogenic shock.

7. Nitroglycerin 0.4 mg SL or spray every 5 minutes. Follow with IV nitroglycerin if systolic BP >100 mmHg: 10–20 mcg bolus, then infusion of 10 mcg/min, increased by 5–10 mcg every 5–10 minutes until dyspnea is relieved, mean arterial pressure is lowered by 10% in normotensive patients (30% in hypertensive patients), or heart rate increases by 10%.

8. Morphine 1–5 mg IV over 1–5 minutes; may repeat dose every 5–30 minutes × 3.

9. Nitroprusside 0.1–5.0 mcg/kg/min IV infusion.

10. Dobutamine 2–20 mcg/kg/min IV infusion.

11. Milrinone 50 mcg/kg IV bolus over 10 minutes plus 0.375–0.75 mcg/kg/min IV infusion.

12. IV nitroglycerin 10–100 mcg/min IV infusion. Tachyphylaxis can occur as early as 24 hours after continuous IV therapy.

13. IABP or ventricular assist device may be needed as a bridge to cardiac transplantation.

14. If blood pressure precludes use of ACE inhibitor, reduce/discontinue other vasodilators.

15. ARBs can be used in place of ACE inhibitors, if needed (e.g., intolerance to ACE inhibitors). The combination of an ACE inhibitor and an ARB (valsartan 20 mg/d initially, titrated to 160 mg bid; or candesartan 4–8 mg/d initially, titrated to 32 mg/d) may be considered for the long-term management of MI with symptomatic heart failure and LVEF <40% (if creatinine in ≤2.5 mg/dL in men or <2.0 mg/dL in women and serum K⁺ ≤5.0 mEq/L). Alternatively, an ACE inhibitor plus an aldosterone antagonist may be used.

16. Carvedilol, starting at 6.25 mg PO bid and advancing over 4–6 weeks to a maximum dose of 25 mg PO bid, is a reasonable choice, based on CAPRICORN and IMPACT-HF.

17. Aldosterone blockade (eplerenone 25 mg/d titrated to maximum 50 mg/d or spironolactone 25–50 mg/d) for long-term management of patients post-MI who are already receiving therapeutic doses of an ACE inhibitor and have LVEF ≤40%, plus either symptomatic heart failure or diabetes. Not recommended if creatinine >2.5 mg/dL in men or >2.0 mg/dL in women or serum K⁺ >5.0 mEq/L.

hypotension should be treated with dopamine, followed by IABP counterpulsation for persistent hypotension. Endotracheal intubation with mechanical ventilation may be required to maintain oxygenation, prevent CO_2 retention, redistribute blood flow out of the pulmonary circuit, and decrease the work of breathing. Proper management also requires treatment of ongoing ischemia, mechanical defects, arrhythmias, and conduction disturbances.

2. **Oral therapy.** Once patients have been stabilized on IV medications × for 48–72 hours, they can usually be switched to oral therapy. ACE inhibitors, beta-blockers, angiotensin II receptor blockers (ARBs), and selective aldosterone blockers (e.g., eplerenone) improve long-term outcomes.

3. **Recent trials.**

   a. **Beta-blockers.** In CAPRICORN, 1959 patients with acute MI and LV ejection fraction ≤40% were randomized within 21 days to carvedilol (beta-blocker with alpha-1-blocking properties) or a placebo. Carvedilol reduced all-cause mortality by 23% (12% versus 15%, p = 0.03) at 1.3 years and reduced cardiovascular mortality and nonfatal MI. Carvedilol is the only beta-blocker with an approved indication to reduce the risk of death in patients with acute MI complicated by LV systolic dysfunction. (It is also the only beta-blocker with approved indications for mild, moderate, and severe heart failure.) The starting dose of carvedilol is 6.25 mg twice daily, titrated over 4–6 weeks to a maximum dose of 25 mg twice daily, as tolerated.

   b. **Angiotensin Receptor Blockers.** In the VALIANT trial, 14,703 patients with acute MI complicated by LV systolic dysfunction and/or heart failure were randomized at 0.5–10 days post-MI to valsartan (ARB), captopril (ACE inhibitor), or both, in addition to standard medical therapy. At 24.7 months, there was no difference in the all-cause mortality (primary endpoint) between groups, although adverse drug effects were more common following combination therapy.

   c. **Aldosterone Antagonists.** In the EPHESUS trial, 6632 patients with acute MI, LV ejection fraction ≤40%, and heart failure (not required in diabetics) were randomized at 3–10 days to the selective aldosterone blocker eplerenone (25 mg/d titrated to a maximum of 50 mg/d) or a placebo, in addition to standard medical therapy. At 16 months, eplerenone reduced the risk of total mortality by 15% (p = 0.008), cardiovascular mortality by 17% (p = 0.005), sudden cardiac death by 21% (p = 0.03), and cardiovascular mortality/hospitalization by 13% (p = 0.002). There was also a 23% reduction in episodes of hospitalization for heart failure (p = 0.002). The absolute rate of serious hyperkalemia was increased by 1.6% in the eplerenone group (p = 0.002), and the absolute rate of hypokalemia was decreased by 4.7% (p <0.001). It was estimated that the number needed to treat (NNT) to save one life in 1 year with eplerenone was 50, and the NNT to prevent one cardiovascular event or hospitalization for a cardiovascular event in 1 year was 33, indicating an important role for eplerenone in the management of patients with LV systolic dysfunction/heart failure following acute MI.

D. **Prognosis.** In the GRACE registry, heart failure on admission for ACS patients was associated with a fourfold increase in hospital mortality (12.0% versus 2.9% without heart failure, p <0.0001) and a threefold increase in mortality at 6 months (8.5% versus 2.8%, p <0.0001). Patients with heart failure also had longer hospitalizations, more readmissions, and lower rates of cardiac catheterization (46.5% versus 54.2%, p <0.0001) and PCI (26.0% versus 31.8%, p <0.0001). They also received beta-blockers and statins less often than patients without heart failure (beta-blockers: 65.1% versus 73.4%, p <0.0001; statins: 45.7% versus 52.1%, p <0.0001). Only 63.7% of patients with heart failure received ACE inhibitors. In-hospital mortality rates were higher in patients who developed heart failure during hospitalization compared to patients who presented in heart failure (17.8% versus 12.0%, p <0.0001). In-hospital revascularization was associated with improved prognosis at 6 months. Similar results were observed in the VALIANT trial.

LEFT VENTRICULAR THROMBUS

A. **Overview.** LV thrombus develops in up to 20% of patients with acute (usually anterior) MI, typically within the first 5 days. Most embolic events occur in the first 3 months, and the risk of embolism is increased for mobile or protruding thrombi.

B. **Treatment.** Consider IV heparin during hospitalization followed by warfarin (INR 2.0–3.0) for at least 3 months (and possibly long term in the absence of increased bleeding risk), especially for mobile or protruding LV thrombi associated with anterior MI, to reduce the risk of embolization. Randomized trials are underway to examine the preferred mode of antithrombotic therapy in these patients.

MITRAL REGURGITATION: RUPTURED PAPILLARY MUSCLE/CHORDAE

A. **Overview.** Papillary muscle rupture complicates 1% of acute (usually inferior) infarctions caused by right coronary artery (most common) or left circumflex coronary artery occlusion. The posteromedial papillary muscle has a single blood supply from the posterior descending branch of the dominant coronary artery and is more likely to rupture than the anterolateral papillary muscle, which receives a dual-blood supply from the left anterior descending and left circumflex coronary arteries.

B. **Presentation.** Papillary muscle rupture or ruptured chordae should be suspected in patients who develop acute pulmonary edema 2–9 days post-MI. (Rupture is less common within the first 24 hours.) A new apical systolic mitral regurgitation murmur may be present, and the infarct can be large or small.

C. **Diagnosis.** Transthoracic or transesophageal echocardiography with Doppler imaging is used to confirm the diagnosis of ruptured papillary muscle and exclude other mechanical defects (e.g., VSD, LV aneurysm or pseudoaneurysm, free-wall rupture). Echocardiography demonstrates a flail or prolapsing mitral valve leaflet with regurgitant flow into the left atrium, although the severity of acute MR is often underestimated by echo. A prominent V-wave is frequently seen in the pulmonary capillary wedge pressure tracing.

D. **Treatment.** Emergency surgical repair is recommended, even in hemodynamically stable patients, due to the risk of acute decompensation. Stabilizing measures prior to surgery include IABP counterpulsation, sodium nitroprusside, and possibly inotropes.

E. **Prognosis.** Mortality rates are high with medical treatment (70% to 90%) or surgery (20% to 50%).

MITRAL REGURGITATION: ISCHEMIC PAPILLARY MUSCLE

A. **Overview.** Ischemic papillary muscle dysfunction is more common after inferior MI, usually involves the posteromedial papillary muscle, and can occur in large or small infarcts.

B. **Presentation.** Transient papillary muscle dysfunction can cause acute (flash) pulmonary edema in otherwise stable patients. An apical systolic murmur can be persistent, intermittent, or absent.

C. **Diagnosis.** Echocardiogram demonstrates mitral regurgitation, which can be persistent or transient (due to intermittent ischemia). A prolapsing mitral valve may be present. A prominent V-wave is sometimes seen in the pulmonary capillary wedge pressure tracing during episodes of flash pulmonary edema.

D. **Treatment.** Vasodilators should be used to stabilize the patient; if unsuccessful, IABP counterpulsation is often effective. Revascularization with PCI or CABG should be considered.

ACUTE PERICARDITIS

A. **Overview.** Acute pericarditis complicates 10% to 15% of acute MI events, and usually occurs 2–4 days following STEMI. Persistent or recurrent chest pain within the first 24 hours of acute MI is unlikely to be caused by pericarditis.

B. **Presentation.** The most common symptom is pleuritic-type chest pain, which radiates to the left trapezial ridge and is relieved by sitting forward. ECG findings include J-point elevation, PR-segment depression (and PR elevation in lead aVR), and concave upward ST-segment elevation, which can be diffuse but is more often localized to the area of transmural necrosis. A three-component pericardial friction rub may be present, but the absence of a friction rub does not exclude acute pericarditis. Pericardial effusion occurs in 40%, but cardiac tamponade is infrequent, and a small pericardial effusion can accompany acute MI in absence of pericarditis. Pericarditis does not cause an elevation in cardiac markers.

C. **Treatment.** Aspirin 160–325 mg PO q24h is recommended, and doses up to 650 mg PO q4–6h may be required. For persistent pain, it is reasonable to administer colchicine 0.6 mg PO q 12h and/or acetaminophen 500 mg PO q6h. Refractory cases often benefit from indomethacin $\geq$ corticosteroids (e.g., prednisone 60–80 mg/d $\times$ 5–7 days, then discontinued gradually), but these agents should be used sparingly because they can increase coronary vascular resistance, impair infarct healing, and possibly increase the risk of myocardial rupture. Pericarditis is a relative contraindication for anticoagulation, and anticoagulation should be immediately discontinued if pericardial effusion develops or increases. Pericarditis is a strong contraindication for fibrinolytic therapy. All patients with pericarditis require close monitoring for enlarging pericardial effusion and impending cardiac tamponade.

PERICARDITIS, DRESSLER'S SYNDROME

A. **Overview.** Dressler's syndrome is an immunologic reaction that presents as a pleuropericarditis 1–12 weeks after acute MI in 1% to 3% of patients. It is generally benign and self-limited, but recurrences are common and constrictive pericarditis can occur.

B. **Presentation.** Symptoms include fever, chest pain, and pericardial and pleural effusions. ECG findings are typical of pericarditis, with diffuse, concave upward ST-segment elevation.

C. **Treatment.** Treated the same as acute pericarditis post-MI (p. 148).

RECURRENT ISCHEMIA/INFARCTION

A. **Overview.** Postinfarct angina is more common after fibrinolysis (30%) than after primary PCI (10%) and is associated with an increased risk of reinfarction and death. In the DANAMI trial of revascularization versus medical therapy for spontaneous or inducible ischemia after fibrinolysis, revascularization reduced reinfarction, unstable angina, and the need for antianginal medications at 12–24 months.

B. **Treatment.** Recommendations include resumption of IV heparin or SQ enoxaparin (for rest angina), continuation/escalation of beta-blockers (IV, then PO) and nitrates (SL, then IV), and triage to cardiac catheterization and revascularization (PCI/CABG).

REINFARCTION

A. **Overview.** Reinfarction is more common after fibrinolytic therapy (4%) than after medical therapy or PCI for STEMI (<1% to 2%). It also is more common after NSTEMI than after STEMI. Reinfarction is associated with further reductions in ejection fraction and an increased risk of cardiogenic shock and death. Aspirin and beta-blockers reduce the risk of reinfarction.

B. Treatment. IV heparin or low molecular-weight heparin, nitroglycerin, morphine sulfate, and triage to catheterization and revascularization (PCI or CABG) are recommended. For patients with recurrent chest pain not considered candidates for revascularization or when angiography/PCI is not readily available, (re)administration of fibrinolytic therapy is reasonable. Streptokinase should not be readministrated if a nonfibrin-specific agent was given more than 5 days previously.

RIGHT VENTRICULAR INFARCTION

A. Overview. RV infarction occurs in 30% of inferior infarcts and 10% of anterior infarcts. Large RV infarcts are complicated by heart block or atrial fibrillation in 20% to 50%.

B. Presentation. Varies from mild, asymptomatic RV dysfunction to cardiogenic shock. Cardiogenic shock can occur with relatively well-preserved LV function.

C. Diagnosis. RV infarction is suggested by distended neck veins or Kussmaul's sign (jugular venous distension on inspiration) with or without clear lungs and low blood pressure in the setting of inferior MI. RV infarction should also be suspected when severe hypotension develops after sublingual nitroglycerin. ST-elevation is often present in lead V_1 and right-sided lead V_{4R}, but these findings are transient and resolve within hours in >50%. Echocardiography demonstrates a hypokinetic, dilated right ventricle with abnormal interventricular and interatrial septal motion. On pulmonary artery catheterization, right atrial pressure exceeds 10 mmHg and the ratio of right atrial pressure to wedge pressure is ≤0.8. Right-to-left shunting across a patent foramen ovale should be suspected when arterial oxygen saturation fails to respond to supplemental oxygen.

D. Treatment. The most important form of therapy is early reperfusion with PCI or fibrinolysis, which improves RV ejection fraction and reduces the risk of heart block. Other useful measures include maintenance of RV preload with aggressive volume expansion (1–2 L initially), dobutamine (preferred) or dopamine for persistent low cardiac output, AV sequential pacing for high-grade heart block or bradycardia not responding to atropine, cardioversion for hemodynamically significant SVT or atrial fibrillation, and use of an RV assist device for severe refractory shock. For concommitant LV dysfunction, therapeutic considerations include IABP counterpulsation and careful afterload reduction with ACE inhibitors. Nitrates and diuretics can worsen hemodynamics by causing further reductions in preload and should be avoided.

E. Prognosis. RV infarction increases morbidity and mortality associated with inferior MI, even though RV function recovers in most patients within days to weeks. Prognosis is closely related to LV function and residual coronary artery disease. Compared to patients with LV shock (n = 884) in the SHOCK trial registry, patients with predominantly RV shock (n = 49) were younger, had less anterior MI and more single-vessel disease, and derived similar benefit from revascularization. In-hospital mortality was 53.1%, similar to that for LV shock, emphasizing the need for aggressive management of patients with RV shock.

CARDIAC RUPTURE

A. **Overview.** Cardiac free-wall rupture (cardiorrhexis) complicates <1% of acute infarctions, however it is the second leading cause of hospital death post-MI. More than 90% of ruptures occur in the first week and up to 40% occur in the first 24 hours. Risk factors include first MI, female gender, advanced age, hypertension, anterior MI, Q-wave MI, persistent chest pain, lack of collateral circulation, no prior angina, use of NSAIDs or corticosteroids, and late (>12 hours) administration of fibrinolytic therapy. The risk of rupture is reduced by early (<12 hours) reperfusion and beta-blockers.

B. **Presentation.** Cardiac rupture presents with recurrent chest pain and acute hemodynamic collapse. Shock, electromechanical dissociation, and cardiac tamponade occur suddenly.

C. **Treatment.** Immediate surgical repair after rapid confirmation by echocardiography can be lifesaving. Pericardiocentesis should be performed for hypotension or shock en route to emergency surgery.

D. **Prognosis.** Death is often immediate.

CARDIOGENIC SHOCK

A. **Overview.** Cardiogenic shock complicates 5% to 7% of acute infarctions, usually within the first few hours, and is the leading cause of death post-MI. Cardiogenic shock develops when myocardial necrosis exceeds 40% of LV mass, but it may also result from a relatively smaller infarct complicated by hypovolemia, RV infarction, papillary muscle rupture, ventricular septal defect, or cardiac tamponade. Risk factors include large MI, previous MI, admission ejection fraction <35%, diabetes mellitus, and advanced age. The risk of cardiogenic shock is reduced by early reperfusion.

B. **Presentation.** Persistent hypotension (BP <90 mmHg) accompanied by hypoperfusion of vital organs, including impaired sensorium, oliguria, and clammy skin. When cardiogenic shock is caused by extensive myocardial necrosis, low cardiac output, elevated systemic vascular resistance and pulmonary capillary wedge pressure, and pulmonary rales are present.

C. **Treatment.** Cardiogenic shock requires aggressive therapy, given the high (70% to 90%) mortality rates associated with fibrinolytic/medical therapy alone. Immediate angiography, IABP counterpulsation, and revascularization are recommended for patients <75 years (Class I; Level of Evidence A) and select patients >75 years (Class IIa; Level of Evidence B). Revascularization is especially beneficial for those who develop shock within 36 hours of MI and when revascularization is performed within 18 hours of shock. Fibrinolytic therapy should be administered to patients who cannot undergo mechanical revascularization; it can also be considered for patients who present to a noninvasive center within 3 hours of STEMI if expected time to PCI exceeds 90 minutes, followed by prompt transfer to an invasive center. Other measures include IV fluids to optimize filling pressures, dobutamine to enhance cardiac output, dopamine to maintain vital organ perfusion, and treatment of associated mechanical defects, arrhythmias, and conduction disturbances. A left ventricular assist device (LVAD) is sometimes required as a stabilizing bridge to revascularization. Echocardiography or other invasive measures should be used to exclude mechanical complications.

D. Prognosis. In GUSTO-I, an aggressive revascularization strategy (PTCA or CABG) was independently associated with improved 30-day survival. In the randomized SHOCK trial comparing emergency revascularization (PTCA or CABG) to initial medical stabilization and later revascularization, 30-day mortality was significantly reduced using the early invasive approach in the following groups: age <75 years (41% versus 57%, p <0.05); randomization within 6 hours of symptom onset (37% versus 63%, p <0.01); and prior MI (40% versus 68%, p <0.01). Survival benefit persisted at 1 year for patients in the emergency revascularization group (47.6% versus 33.6%, p <0.03), and 83% of 1-year survivors were in NYHA heart failure class I or II. Failure to restore TIMI-3 flow during PCI was associated with higher mortality rates at 30 days (65% versus 35% if TIMI-3 flow was restored, p <0.001). Correlates of survival at 1 year included LV function, initial TIMI flow, and culprit vessel location. Data from the SHOCK trial registry indicated a survival benefit for early revascularization in select patients ≥75 years. Patients with RV and LV shock experienced similar benefit from revascularization.

VENTRICULAR SEPTAL DEFECT (VSD)

A. Overview. Acute VSD complicates 0.5% to 2% of acute infarctions, usually between days 2–5, and is more common after anterior MI than after inferior-posterior MI.

B. Presentation. VSD usually presents as a new systolic murmur. Features favoring the diagnosis of VSD over acute mitral regurgitation include a palpable thrill, absence of acute pulmonary edema, lack of a prominent V-wave in the pulmonary capillary wedge pressure tracing, and an oxygen step-up in the high right ventricle. Cardiogenic shock may ensue.

C. Diagnosis. VSDs are confirmed by echocardiography with Doppler imaging, which allows visualization of the defect and detection of the shunt. Pulmonary artery catheterization with oximetry demonstrates >5% to 7% step-up in O_2 saturation of blood between the right atrium and right ventricle.

D. Treatment. Early catheterization and surgical intervention are recommended, even in clinically stable patients, despite biased, early surgical series recommending medical stabilization prior to surgical repair. IABP counterpulsation, vasodilators, and inotropes can be used as stabilizing measures during preparation for surgery.

E. **Prognosis.** Mortality rates are high with medical therapy (90%) or surgery (40% to 60%). Survival is worse for VSDs associated with inferior-posterior MI or RV infarction and for complex septal defects.

MAJOR DEPRESSION

A. **Overview.** Major depression occurs in over 15% of patients after acute MI and is an independent risk factor for adverse long-term prognosis. Small studies have demonstrated increased risk of ventricular arrhythmias and death within the first 6 months post-MI, possibly related to altered autonomic tone.

B. **Treatment.** Selective serotonin reuptake inhibitors (SSRI) improve psychosocial functioning and exhibit mild antiplatelet effects post-ACS, but their impact on survival is unknown. Major depression should be distinguished from minor depressive symptoms, which are common after MI and represent a normal adjustment reaction that is often short-lived. Recent data indicate that SSRI treatment after ACS in depressed patients improves depression and may improve clinical outcome. In ENRICHD, cognitive behavior therapy improved psychosocial outcomes but had no effect on death or recurrent MI at 6 months (primary endpoint). Antidepressant drug use, most commonly SSRI, was associated with a 37% reduction in death or MI. Cognitive behavior therapy improves depression but does not reduce cardiac events.

SECTION 6
ACS PITFALLS

Chapter 15
ACS Pitfalls

PITFALL: DELAY IN DIAGNOSIS OF ACS

Prompt triage and early therapy improve outcomes in ACS. An abbreviated evaluation including a brief history, physical examination, and ECG should be performed immediately upon arrival, ideally within 10 minutes. The use of emergency department algorithms substantially improves time to diagnosis.

PITFALL: FAILURE TO CONSIDER NONISCHEMIC CAUSES OF CHEST PAIN AT PATIENT PRESENTATION

Pulmonary embolism, aortic dissection, and pericarditis can present similarly to ACS and possess ECG and cardiac marker abnormalities. These conditions can progress to life-threatening situations and require expedient diagnosis and treatment.

PITFALL: FAILURE TO RECOGNIZE ACUTE MI IN THE ABSENCE OF CHEST PAIN

In the National Registry of Myocardial Infarction 2, one-third of more than 400,000 patients with confirmed MI did not have chest pain on hospital presentation. Women, diabetics, the elderly, and patients with prior heart failure were disproportionately affected. MI patients without chest pain were less likely to be diagnosed on hospital admission (22% versus 50%); were less likely to receive reperfusion therapy (25% versus 74%), beta-blockers (28% versus 48%), or heparin (53% versus 83%); and were more likely to die in-hospital (23% versus 9%). Patients with STEMI presenting with 12 hours of symptom onset should be considered for reperfusion therapy regardless of pain status.

PITFALL: FAILURE TO CHECK SERIAL ECGS IN PATIENTS WITH ONGOING CHEST PAIN BUT WITHOUT ST-ELEVATION ON INITIAL ECG

Patients presenting with ACS but without ST-elevation on initial ECG occasionally develop complete coronary occlusion and ST-elevation early during their hospital stay. In patients with ongoing or changing ischemic symptoms, serial ECGs should be used to monitor ST-segment shifts. Patients who develop ST-elevation should be considered for reperfusion therapy.

PITFALL: FAILURE TO CHECK A RIGHT-SIDED ECG IN AN INFERIOR MI
TO IDENTIFY A RIGHT VENTRICULAR INFARCTION

RV infarction is often associated with inferior MI and can be diagnosed early by documenting ≤ 1 mm ST-elevation in lead V_{4R}. ST segment elevation in lead III $>$aVF $>$II is suggestive of RV involvement. RV injury may also present with ST-elevation in lead V_1. Early recognition of RV infarction can minimize or prevent adverse hemodynamic consequences by alerting clinicians of the need for aggressive intravenous fluid administration and avoidance of nitrates and other vasodilators. The most important form of therapy for RV infarction is early reperfusion therapy, which improves RV ejection fraction and reduces the risk of heart block. Other useful measures include maintenance of RV preload with 1–2 liters of normal saline, dobutamine (preferred) or dopamine for persistent low cardiac output, AV sequential pacing for high-grade heart block or bradycardia unresponsive to atropine, cardioversion for hemodynamically significant SVT or atrial fibrillation, and use of an RV-assist device for refractory shock. Nitrates and diuretics can worsen hemodynamics by further reducing the RV preload.

PITFALL: DELAY IN INITIATING REPERFUSION THERAPY

A number of analyses from randomized clinical trials have demonstrated improved clinical outcomes associated with prompt reperfusion therapy, including smaller infarct size, less ventricular dysfunction, and better survival. For every hour saved in time from symptom onset to treatment, there is an approximate 1% reduction in 30-day mortality. Early symptom recognition and triage are critical components of the overall treatment strategy for ACS. AHA/ACC guidelines have targeted a door-to-needle time within 30 minutes and a door-to-balloon inflation time within 90 minutes as the preferred quality benchmarks for STEMI patients treated with reperfusion therapy.

PITFALL: UNDERUSE OF REPERFUSION THERAPY IN STEMI

Reports from the GRACE and NRMI registries indicate that one-third of patients with STEMI do not receive reperfusion therapy. Common reasons for withholding therapy included advanced age, absence of chest pain, or a history of heart failure, MI, or CABG, none of which is a contraindication to reperfusion therapy. For every 1000 patients treated with fibrinolytic therapy, approximately 20 lives are saved. Furthermore, these benefits are long lasting: In the 10-year follow-up of the GISSI-I trial, 18 lives were saved for every 1000 patients treated with streptokinase. Similar or greater benefits exist for primary percutaneous coronary intervention. Reperfusion therapy is indicated for all patients with STEMI $<$12 hours.

PITFALL: UNDERUSE OF REPERFUSION THERAPY IN ACUTE MI PATIENTS WITH LEFT BUNDLE BRANCH BLOCK (LBBB)

LBBB interferes with the ability to identify STEMI on ECG. Patients with prolonged ischemic chest pain and new LBBB have high (20% to 25%) in-hospital mortality rates and derive substantial benefit from fibrinolytic therapy (49 lives saved for every 1000 patients treated). However, patients with LBBB are 78% less likely to receive reperfusion therapy than patients with ST-elevation. Because of their increased risk, patients with new LBBB and symptoms consistent with ACS should receive direct PCI (preferred) or fibrinolytic therapy.

PITFALL: UNDERUSE OF REPERFUSION THERAPY IN ELDERLY PATIENTS

Patients over age 75 are six times less likely to receive fibrinolytic therapy despite a high risk of death and reinfarction. Although these patients are at increased risk of intracranial hemorrhage when treated with fibrinolytic therapy compared with younger patients, they are also at higher risk of death after MI. Unless specific contraindications exist, patients over age 75 with ST-elevation or new LBBB should undergo primary PCI; if not readily available, the risks and benefits of fibrinolytic therapy should be carefully weighed in this high-risk population.

PITFALL: INAPPROPRIATE DOSING OF HEPARIN, ESPECIALLY IN THE SETTING OF FIBRINOLYTIC THERAPY

Most current fibrinolytic regimens call for concomitant antithrombin therapy with unfractionated heparin, and judicious dosing of heparin is especially important in this setting. Intravenous heparin dosing and the degree of anticoagulation are directly related to clinical outcomes: The probability of 30-day mortality and reinfarction rises for aPTT values below 50 seconds and above 70 seconds in a classic "J-shaped" therapeutic curve. Higher aPTT values are strongly related to lower patient weight, older age, female gender, and lack of cigarette smoking. These observations have prompted a revision of the AHA/ACC guidelines for heparin dosing in the setting of acute MI. For patients receiving fibrinolytic therapy, intravenous unfractionated heparin is recommended as a 60 U/kg IV bolus followed by an IV maintenance infusion of 12 U/kg/hr (not to exceed 4000 U bolus and 1000 U/hr infusion), adjusted to aPTT of 1.5–2.0 times control (50–70 seconds).

PITFALL: MISUSE OF CARDIAC TROPONINS FOR RISK STRATIFICATION

Cardiac troponins are more sensitive markers of myocardial injury than CK-MB, but troponins are not generally detectable above the upper limit of normal for 6–8 hours. A single initial negative value does not imply low risk and may, in fact, mask a troponin-positive, high-risk patient. The tendency to minimize the importance of a positive troponin in renal insufficiency is another important and possibly more widespread problem. Troponin values independently predict early outcome and identify patients most likely to benefit from GP IIb/IIIa receptor antagonists and the early invasive approach to management.

PITFALL: NOT RECOGNIZING THE HIGH RISK ASSOCIATED WITH NSTEMI

Compared with STEMI, NSTEMI is associated with less myocardial necrosis (smaller infarct), better preservation of LV function, and lower in-hospital mortality. However, because non-ST-elevation infarcts are usually associated with residual viable myocardium supplied by a coronary artery with a high-grade but nonocclusive stenosis, reinfarction rates are higher than after STEMI. In the GUSTO-IIb study, 1-year mortality rates did not significantly differ between STEMI and NSTEMI. The substantial increase in late mortality and reinfarction associated with NSTEMI underscores the need for close follow-up and secondary prevention measures.

PITFALL: UNDERUSE OF GP IIB/IIIA INHIBITORS IN HIGH-RISK PATIENTS WITH NSTE-ACS

Randomized clinical trials have consistently demonstrated significant reductions in death or MI with a favorable safety profile when intravenous GP IIb/IIIa inhibitors are added to conventional therapy for patients with NSTE-ACS and positive cardiac troponins (Tables 9.2 and 9.3, pp. 92, 93).

PITFALL: UNDERUSE OF ACE INHIBITORS IN ACUTE MI

Randomized trials support early administration of ACE inhibitors to all patients with acute MI regardless of LV function or heart failure symptoms. Oral ACE inhibitors should be initiated once reperfusion has occurred and blood pressure has stabilized, usually no sooner than

6 hours after presentation, and then titrated upward over 12–24 hours. ACE inhibitors should be continued long term in patients with heart failure, left ventricular dysfunction (EF <0.40), hypertension, or diabetes, and possibly for all patients based on a 22% reduction in stroke, MI, or death at 5 years in the HOPE trial.

PITFALL: UNDERUSE OF BETA-BLOCKERS FOLLOWING ACUTE MI

Beta-blocker therapy is associated with a significant reduction in mortality following acute MI. The benefit is seen across many subgroups, including patients with conditions previously considered contraindications to beta-blockers (e.g., heart failure, pulmonary disease, diabetes, advanced age). Diabetics demonstrate twice the mortality benefit of beta-blocker therapy post-MI compared with nondiabetics. Despite marked benefits, only one-third of patients with acute MI receive beta-blockers. Unless there is an absolute contraindication, all patients should be treated with a beta-blocker early after MI. Patients with relative contraindications (e.g., mild obstructive airway disease) can be started on a low dose of a short-acting beta-blocker, with cautious upward titration. With respect to the use of acute intravenous beta-blockers, some caution should be exercised. The COMMIT trial, which randomized 45,852 patients with suspect myocardial infarction to a strategy of early, aggressive beta-blockade (metoprolol 15 mg IV over 15 min, then 200 mg PO daily) versus a placebo demonstrated that acute beta-blocker therapy was associated with a decrease in the incidence of ventricular fibrillation or reinfarction. However, patients treated with acute IV beta-blockade also experienced an increased risk of cardiogenic shock. In total, for every 1000 patients treated with acute beta-blockade, the authors estimated five cases of ventricular fibrillation and five cases of rein-farction would be avoided, but at the expense of 11 additional cases of cardiogenic shock. Accordingly, the 2007 ACC/AHA NSTE and STEMI guidelines have been amended to recommend the initiation of oral beta-blockers within 24 hours of MI for patients who do not have any of the following: (1) signs of heart failure, (2) evidence of a low output state, (3) increased risk for cardiogenic shock, or (4) other relative contraindications to beta-blockade (e.g., PR >240 msec, asthma, etc).

PITFALL: ROUTINE USE OF IV NITROGLYCERIN IN ACUTE MI TO THE EXCLUSION OF OTHER MORE EFFECTIVE DRUGS

Existing data support the use of IV nitroglycerin for 24–48 hours in patients with anterior MI, heart failure, persistent ischemia, or hypertension. The usefulness of this medication has not been demonstrated for patients without these clinical features. A drawback to the routine use of IV nitroglycerin is that it may preclude the use of more effective therapies, such as beta-blockers and ACE inhibitors, due to its blood pressure–lowering effects. IV nitroglycerin is contraindicated in preload-dependent conditions (e.g., right ventricular infarction) and within 24 hours of sildenafil (Viagra), due to the risk of profound hypotension. There is no evidence to support the use of IV nitroglycerin beyond 48 hours in the absence of recurrent ischemia or persistent pulmonary edema.

PITFALL: FAILURE TO TREAT ACS PATIENTS INDEFINITELY WITH ASPIRIN

Despite a 40% reduction in the risk of in-hospital death, many patients with ACS either do not receive or experience substantial delays in receiving aspirin. In ISIS-2, the mortality benefit of aspirin for acute MI was comparable to fibrinolytic therapy. In addition, long-term therapy with aspirin reduces vascular mortality by 17%, stroke by 30%, and recurrent infarction by 30% in patients with prior MI. Despite these convincing data, in one study nearly half of the patients presenting to an emergency room with acute MI did not receive aspirin therapy. All MI patients without a serious aspirin allergy should receive aspirin 81–325 mg (PO) q24h indefinitely.

PITFALL: PREMATURE DISCONTINUATION OF DUAL-ANTIPLATELET THERAPY WITH ASPIRIN PLUS CLOPIDOGREL IN PATIENTS WITH AND WITHOUT PCI

Several recent studies have established an important role for dual-antiplatelet therapy in ACS. In CURE, 12,562 patients with unstable angina or NSTEMI were treated with aspirin (75–325 mg PO q24h) and randomized to clopidogrel (300 mg loading dose followed by 75 mg/day) or a placebo for 3–12 months (average 9 months). Dual-antiplatelet therapy resulted in a highly significant 20% reduction in the primary composite endpoint of cardiovascular death, MI, or stroke (9.3% versus 11.5%, $p < 0.001$). In PCI-CURE and CREDO, long-term (CURE: 8 months; CREDO: 1 year) therapy with aspirin plus clopidogrel improved event-free survival compared to short-term (4-week) therapy with aspirin plus clopidogrel followed by aspirin alone. Preliminary cost analysis indicates that chronic use of clopidogrel after ACS falls in the range of societal standards with regards to cost effectiveness. These data indicate that clopidogrel should be added to aspirin for at least 9 months in NSTE-ACS patients in whom a noninterventional or interventional approach is planned. In patients who have received a drug-eluting stent, the continuation of dual-antiplatelet therapy is even more important. Observational data from multiple registries has demonstrated an increased risk of stent-thrombosis and mortality following premature discontinuation of clopidogrel after placement of a drug-eluting stent. While the optimal duration of dual-antiplatelet therapy is unknown, given the significant risks associated with stent thrombosis, a conservative approach calls for indefinite dual-antiplatelet therapy in patients with drug-eluting stents who have demonstrated an ability to tolerate therapy without significant bleeding.

PITFALL: FAILURE TO INITIATE INTENSIVE STATIN THERAPY DURING HOSPITALIZATION FOR ACS

Recent results from PROVE IT indicate that compared to standard statin therapy (LDL 95 mg/dL), more intensive statin therapy (LDL 62 mg/dL) provides greater protection against death or major cardiovascular events at 18–36 months following ACS. In PROVE IT, 4162 patients hospitalized for ACS within 10 days were randomized to atorvastatin 80 mg/d (intensive therapy) or pravastatin 40 mg/d (standard therapy). At a mean follow-up of 24 months, atorvastatin reduced the primary endpoint (death, MI, unstable angina requiring hospitalization, revascularization ≥30 days after randomization, stroke) by 16% compared to pravastatin (22.4% versus 26.3%, p = 0.005) (Table 9.8, p. 105). Benefits were evident as early as 30 days and continued throughout the study. Statins were also well-tolerated and very safe. Based on these compelling results, intensive statin therapy is recommended for all ACS patients, starting in-hospital (once stable) and continued long term, to reduce the early and late risk of death or recurrent ischemia. See the discussion on pp. 104–105.

PITFALL: UNDERUTILIZATION OF ICD PROPHYLAXIS FOR PATIENTS WITH MI AND LV SYSTOLIC DYSFUNCTION

Two randomized controlled trials have demonstrated markedly improved survival for patients with severe LV dysfunction receiving ICD prophylaxis. In MADIT-2, 1232 patients with prior MI and LV ejection fraction ≤0.30 were randomized without EP testing to ICD or medical therapy. At 20 months, the risk of death was reduced by 31% with prophylactic ICD (14.2% versus 19.8%, p = 0.016). In SCD-HeFT, 2521 patients with LV ejection fraction ≤35% (ischemic or nonischemic cardiomyopathy) and class 2–3 heart failure were randomized to ICD, amiodarone, or placebo. At 5 years, ICDs reduced the risk of death by 23% (28.9% versus 35.8%, p = 0.007). These data indicate significant survival benefit for ICD prophylaxis in patients with prior MI and LV dysfunction. Based on MADIT-2, there are 3–4 million potential ICD candidates now and 400,000 new candidates each year. Indications for ICD implantation following acute MI are shown in Figure 12.1 (p. 122). Of note, patients with ACS should be screened for eligibility for primary prevention ICD therapy typically 3 months after the ACS event, since trials of primary prevention ICD therapy immediately following MI and revascularization have not demonstrated a benefit.

PITFALL: FAILURE TO APPROPRIATELY DOSE ANTITHROMBOTIC MEDICATIONS BASED ON RENAL FUNCTION

Chronic kidney disease and impaired creatinine clearance are common in patients with ACS. Many antithrombotic and other medications used in the treatment of ACS undergo renal elimination, therefore, estimation of creatinine clearance is an essential part of safe and effective ACS management. Two commonly used formulas for the estimation of glomerular filtration rate (GFR) are the Cockcroft-Gault formula and the Modified Diet in Renal Disease (MDRD) formula. An analysis of 46,942 ACS patients demonstrated that GFR calculations disagree in as many as one in five patients. These discrepancies in estimated GFR often lead to significant changes in anticoagulant dosing. Since the majority of dosing studies for anti-thrombotic agents have used the Cockcroft-Gault formula, dosing based on the Cockcroft-Gault formula is preferred, particularly in smaller, female, or elderly patients.

PITFALL: FAILURE TO DISCUSS SMOKING CESSATION REGULARLY AND SYSTEMATICALLY WITH PATIENTS

Continued cigarette smoking is a major risk factor for recurrent events in patients with coronary artery disease, and less than one-third of smokers quit smoking following an acute coronary event. Regular and systematic discussion of the importance of smoking cessation can increase the discontinuation rate to almost 60% and is a critical component of the care of smokers. Even a single physician recommendation to quit smoking has a significant impact on the likelihood of successful abstinence. Patients who experience difficulty quitting should be offered counseling and nicotine preparations or bupropion hydrochloride (Zyban).

PITFALL: FAILURE TO RECOGNIZE AND TREAT DEPRESSION FOLLOWING MI

Major depression occurs in up to 25% of patients after MI and has been associated with an increased risk for malignant ventricular arrhythmias and death, possibly due to altered autonomic tone. Major depression should be distinguished from minor depressive symptoms, which are common after MI and are typically short-lived. Major depression is defined by a depressed mood or loss of interest in nearly all activities for a minimum of 2 weeks, plus at least three of the following symptoms: insomnia or hypersomnia; feelings of worthlessness or excessive guilt; fatigue or loss of energy; impaired ability to think or concentrate; significant change in appetite; psychomotor agitation or retardation; recurrent thoughts of death or suicide. For patients with moderate or severe symptoms who are unlikely to recover in 2–4 weeks with support and encouragement, a trial of selective serotonin reuptake inhibitors may improve psychosocial functioning, although their impact on survival is unknown. Tricyclic anti-depressants should generally be avoided due to the increased risk of postural hypotension, arrhythmias, and conduction abnormalities. To help identify depression in a likely patient, the following two questions should be asked: Do you have little interest or pleasure in doing things you usually enjoy? Are you feeling down, depressed, or helpless?

**PITFALL: FAILURE TO REFER ACS PATIENTS FOR CARDIOPULMONARY
REHABILITATION AT DISCHARGE**

Cardiopulmonary rehabilitation has been shown to improve exercise tolerance, lipid profiles, psychological well-being, and reduces morbidity and mortality. Accordingly, cardiopulmonary rehabilitation is a Class I recommended treatment after ACS (both STEMI and UA/NSTEMI). Unfortunately, epidemiologic studies suggest that less than 40% of patients participate in cardiac rehab programs after myocardial infarction. In order to maximize cardiac rehabilitation utilization and postdischarge outcomes, patients should be referred to cardiac rehab before discharge.

SECTION 7
DRUG SUMMARIES

This section contains prescribing information for drugs used in the management of acute coronary syndromes. The recommendations are offered as general guidelines, not specific instructions for individual patients. Clinical judgment should always guide the physician in the selection, dosing, and duration of drug therapy for individual patients. Unless otherwise stated, the dosing recommendations apply to patients with normal renal and hepatic function, not to patients with renal dysfunction, hepatic insufficiency, or other circumstances that may require dosing adjustment. Not all medications have been accepted by the U.S. Food and Drug Administration for indications cited in this section, and drug recommendations are not necessarily limited to indications in the package insert. The use of any drug should be preceded by a careful review of the package insert, which provides indications and dosing approved by the U.S. Food and Drug Administration. The information provided is not exhaustive, and the reader is referred to other drug information references and the manufacturer's product literature for further information. Clinical use of the information provided and any consequences that may arise from its use are the responsibilities of the prescribing physician. The authors, editors, and publisher do not warrant or guarantee the information contained in this section, and do not assume and expressly disclaim any liability for errors or omissions or any consequences that may occur from such.

Chapter 16

Drug Summaries

This chapter details acute and chronic medical therapy for ACS.

Table 16.1. Medical Therapy for ACS

	Beneficial Effect	**Possible Detrimental Effect**

Acute therapy All patients	• Aspirin
	• Anticoagulants
	  • Heparin
	  • Enoxaparin
	  • Fondaparinux
	• Beta-blockers (PO)^
	• ACE inhibitors
	• Clopidogrel
	• IV nitrates for large MI*
		• Immediate-release nifedipine
		• Prophylactic lidocaine
		• Nitrates for RV infarction or within 24 hours of sildenafil (Viagra) or vardenafil (Levitra), or within 48 hours of tadalafil (Cialis)

STEMI	• Fibrinolytic therapy • GP IIb/IIIa inhibitors as adjuncts to PCI*	• See "all patients"
NSTE-ACS	• Clopidogrel • Fondaparinux • GP IIb/IIIa inhibitors • Enoxaparin	• Fibrinolytic therapy • See "all patients"
Chronic therapy (>48–72 hours)	• Aspirin • Clopidogrel • Beta-blockers • ACE inhibitors/ARBs† • Statins • Warfarin for mobile LV thrombus* or AF • Aldosterone antagonists‡ • Diltiazem or verapamil§	• Hormone replacement therapy during first year

^   Acute beta-blocker therapy should be used with caution in those patients with signs and symptoms of heart failure. Acute IV beta-blockade is contraindicated in patients with Killip III/IV myocardial infarction.

*   Possible benefit, AF = atrial fibrillation, RV = right ventricular.

†   ARBs for intolerance to ACE inhibitors or as alternative to ACE inhibitors in MI patients with heart failure (radiographic or clinical) or LVEF <40%.

‡   Aldosterone antagonists (eplerenone, spironolactone) for MI patients on therapeutic doses of an ACE inhibitor who have LVEF <40% plus either heart failure or diabetes.

§   Diltiazem or verapamil for non-Q-wave MI without pulmonary congestion.

ACE INHIBITORS

Indications and Dose: Acute MI within the first 24 hours; hypertension; heart failure; LV dysfunction: Start PO at low dose as soon as the patient is stabilized from MI (after lytics/PCI and blood pressure has stabilized, no sooner than 6 hours post-MI but usually within 24 hours); titrate upward over 1–4 days, as tolerated. Doses (PO): Captopril 6.25 mg q8h, titrated to 50 mg q8h; lisinopril 2.5 mg q24h, titrated to 10–20 mg q24h; ramipril 2.5 mg q12h, titrated to 5 mg q12h; enalapril 2.5 mg q12h, titrated to 10–20 mg q12h. For patients unable to take PO medications, IV enalapril can be given at 1.25 mg over 5 minutes, then 1.25–5 mg q6h (avoid in first 24 hours). Other ACE inhibitors are probably as effective. Continue long-term therapy for secondary prevention.

Contraindications: Do not administer if systolic BP <90–100 mmHg or there are contraindications to ACE inhibitors (e.g., renal failure, bilateral renal artery stenosis, known allergy).

Clinical Trials: Following acute MI, ACE inhibitors reduce the risk of recurrent MI, progression to heart failure, the need for rehospitalization, and death (4.6 fewer deaths for every 1000 patients treated). Survival benefit is evident on the first day and is greatest for patients with anterior MI, prior MI, heart failure, or LV dysfunction (EF <0.40). In a meta-analysis of ACE inhibitors for LV dysfunction after acute MI, there were 23 fewer deaths for every 1000 patients treated. In HOPE, ramipril (10 mg/d) reduced the risk of MI, stroke, or death by 22% at 5 years in patients with atherosclerotic vascular disease, including those with prior MI. (In lower-risk patients with stable CHD, perindopril reduced the risk of MI, cardiovascular death, and resuscitated cardiac arrest by 20% at 4.2 years in EUROPA; in PEACE, no benefit was demonstrated with trandolapril.) For acute MI complicated by LV dysfunction/heart failure, captopril and valsartan (angiotensin II receptor blocker) resulted in similar cardiovascular outcomes at 2 years in VALIANT.

Comments: Ensure adequate hydration before starting ACE inhibitors. Avoid IV enalaprilat acutely (first 24 hours) due to a lack of benefit and possible harm in CONSENSUS II. For patients with acute MI who are intolerant of ACE inhibitors and have heart failure (radiographic or clinical) or LVEF <40%, an ARB (valsartan, candesartan) should be administered.

ADENOSINE

Indications and Dose: Termination of sinus node reentrant tachycardia, AV nodal reentrant tachycardia, or reentrant tachycardias utilizing an accessory pathway: 6-mg IV bolus over 1–2 seconds. If needed, a 12-mg IV bolus can be given 1–2 minutes later, followed by another

12-mg IV bolus 1–2 minutes after the second dose. Each IV dose should be followed with a rapid saline flush (20 cc) and elevation of the extremity.

Contraindications: Avoid in drug-induced tachycardias, wide QRS tachycardias of unknown origin, and patients taking dipyridamole.

Comments: Generally does not convert atrial fibrillation, atrial flutter, or VT. Transient side effects include flushing, chest pain, dyspnea, brief asystole, bradycardia, VPCs. Transient sinus bradycardia and VPCs are common after conversion to sinus rhythm.

ALDOSTERONE ANTAGONISTS

Indications and Dose: Post-MI patients who are receiving therapeutic doses of an ACE inhibitor and have LVEF ≤40% plus either symptomatic heart failure or diabetes: Eplerenone 25 mg/d titrated to maximum 50 mg/d or spironolactone 25–50 mg/d; start 3–10 days post-MI and continue long term.

Contraindications: Do not administer if creatinine >2.5 mg/dL in men or 2.0 mg/dL in women or K^+ >5.0 mEq/L. Close monitoring of K^+ levels is indicated in patients with renal dysfunction.

Clinical Trials: In EPHESUS, eplerenone (starting 3–10 days post-MI; target dose 50 mg/d) reduced total mortality, cardiovascular mortality, and cardiac hospitalization by 15% to 20% at 16 months in post-MI patients with LVEF <40% plus either heart failure or diabetes managed with optimal therapy, including ACE inhibitors. In RALES, spironolactone (25–50 mg/d) reduced all-cause mortality by 24% at 2 years in patients with class III–IV heart failure, 55% of whom had ischemic heart disease as the cause of heart failure and 95% of whom were being treated with ACE inhibitors.

AMIODARONE

Indications and Dose: Cardiac arrest (VF or pulseless VT): Initial IV bolus of 300 mg. Can repeat 150-mg bolus doses as needed up to a total maximum dose of 2.1 gm in 24 hours. Recurrent/refractory VF/VT, life-threatening VF, hemodynamically unstable VT, stable wide-complex tachycardia: Begin with IV infusion of 150 mg over no less than 10 minutes. This may be followed by an infusion of 1 mg/min × 6 hours, then a maintenance infusion of 0.5 mg/min × 18 hours or until the switch to oral amiodarone can be made. Additional bolus infusions of 150 mg over no less than 10 minutes can be administered for breakthrough events. Oral dosing for life-threatening recurrent VF or recurrent hemodynamically unstable

VT not responsive to other antiarrhythmics: Loading dose of 800–1600 mg/d × 1–3 weeks (occasionally longer) until the arrhythmia is controlled or prominent side effects occur. The dose should then be reduced to 600–800 mg/d × 1 month, followed by the usual maintenance dose of 400 mg/d. Amiodarone should be administered once daily (or in divided doses with meals for total daily doses ≤800 mg or GI intolerance). Use lowest effective dose.

Contraindications: Severe sinus node dysfunction causing marked sinus bradycardia; second- or third-degree AV block; symptomatic bradyarrhythmias without a functioning pacemaker. Use with caution in patients with a preexisting lung disease (including COPD) and with other drugs that prolong the QT interval. Avoid in patients with hepatic dysfunction.

Clinical Trials: Amiodarone-reduced VF or arrhythmic death in patients with acute MI and frequent PVCs or LV dysfunction (EF <0.40) but had no effect on total mortality.

Comments: Not recommended chronically unless the risk of recurrent hemodynamically unstable ventricular arrhythmias is high. The most common serious side effects include hypotension, bradycardia, AV block, torsade de pointes (<2%), ARDS (2%), and negative inotropic effects in some. Exclude amiodarone-induced hyperthyroidism with new signs of arrhythmia. Therapy should be initiated in the hospital after withdrawal of other antiarrhythmic drugs when starting amiodarone. Liver, lung (chest X-ray and pulmonary function tests with DLCO), and thyroid function should be evualuated at baseline and periodically thereafter. Plasma concentrations (normal: 1–2.5 mcg/mL) may be helpful in evaluating nonresponsiveness or unexpected severe toxicity. Patients should be monitored closely after dosage adjustments due to amiodarone's long half-life (9–44 days). Amiodarone can increase serum levels of digoxin, quinidine, procainamide, flecainide, cyclosporine, and warfarin (follow prothrombin times closely). Due to an increased risk of rhabdomyolysis, concomitant doses of simvastatin >20 mg should be avoided. Phenytoin and cholestyramine can reduce amiodarone levels. Amiodarone can also be used as an adjunct to cardioversion for SVT, for rate control of ectopic or multifocal atrial tachycardia in patients with preserved LV function, and for rate control of atrial fibrillation or flutter when other therapies are ineffective.

ANGIOTENSIN II RECEPTOR BLOCKERS (ARBS)

Indications and Dose: Post-MI patients who are intolerant of ACE inhibitors and have heart failure (clinical or radiographic) or LVEF <40%: valsartan 20 mg (PO) qd, titrated to 160 mg bid, based on VALIANT (see the following clinical trials); candesartan 4–8 mg (PO) qd, titrated to 32 mg qd, based on the CHARM trials.

Contraindications: Do not administer if systolic BP <90–100 mmHg or there are contraindications to ACE inhibitors (e.g., renal failure, bilateral renal artery stenosis, known allergy).

Clinical Trials: In VALIANT, there was no difference in mortality at 24.7 months in post-MI patients with LV dysfunction randomized to valsartan (up to 160 mg bid), captopril (target 50 mg tid), or combination therapy. In the CHARM trials, candesartan (target 32 mg/d) improved event-free survival in patients with chronic heart failure and LVEF ≤40% who were intolerant of ACE inhibitors (CHARM-Alternative) or had ARBs added to ACE inhibitors (CHARM-Added).

Comments: ARBs may be considered as an alternative to ACE inhibitors for post-MI patients with heart failure or LVEF <40%, but there is more experience using ACE inhibitors. ARBs can also be used in combination with ACE inhibitors for post-MI heart failure/LV dysfunction; candesartan is preferred in this setting based on CHARM-Added. Note that triple combination of ACE inhibitors, ARBs, and aldosterone blockade is not recommended.

ASPIRIN

Indications and Dose: All ACS patients: 162–325 mg of a nonenteric-coated preparation chewed acutely, followed by 75–325 mg (PO) q24h of an enteric- or nonenteric-coated preparation long term. Rectal suppositories (325 mg) can be used for patients unable to take oral medications. Recent evidence suggests that lower doses (162 mg for ACS, 81 mg for 1°/2° prevention) have similar efficacy and may have less bleeding.

Contraindications: Active bleeding; aspirin allergy; severe hypertension; active peptic ulcer disease. Not recommended in the third trimester of pregnancy. Can precipitate gout.

Clinical Trials: Aspirin reduces vascular death, MI, and stroke by 29% at 1 month and 24% at 2 years following acute MI and by 36% at 6 months following unstable angina. Aspirin enhances coronary reperfusion after fibrinolytic therapy, and it reduces the risk of reocclusion after fibrinolytic therapy, PCI, and CABG. It has been estimated that aspirin prevents 24 deaths, 12 reinfarctions, and two strokes for every 1000 patients treated post-MI.

Comments: Aspirin inhibits platelet function via irreversible acetylation of platelet cyclooxygenase and subsequent impaired formation of thromboxane A_2. Enzyme inhibition lasts for the lifespan of the platelet (~10 days). Aspirin does not prevent platelet adhesion or platelet aggregation in response to ADP, collagen, thrombin, or epinephrine. Aspirin blocks the formation of bradykinin, raising concern over a possible aspirin-ACE inhibitor antagonism. However, most studies indicate that this interaction is not clinically relevant, and that aspirin should not be withheld in patients receiving ACE inhibitors. Long-term administration of nonsteroidal anti-inflammatory agents (NSAIDS), including the cyclooxygenase-2 (COX-2) selective inhibitors may interfere with the cardiovascular protective effects of aspirin. Buccal absorption of chewed aspirin is the fastest route for platelet inhibition. Enteric-coated preparations should be avoided acutely due to delays in GI absorption and platelet inhibition.

Up to 10% of patients with coronary artery disease are aspirin resistant, and the antiplatelet effects of aspirin may diminish over time.

ATROPINE

Indications and Dose: Ventricular asystole; pulseless electrical activity: 1 mg IV push (may repeat). Symptomatic sinus bradycardia or intranodal (Mobitz type I) AV block; nausea and vomiting caused by morphine: 0.5–1.0 mg. This may be repeated up to a total dose of 3 mg. Tracheal dose/route: 1–2.5 mg in 10–25 cc normal saline.

Contraindications: Use with caution in ACS (increased heart rate can provoke myocardial ischemia, acute MI, and rarely VT or VF). Avoid in patients with cardiac denervation (e.g., transplant patients) and those taking dipyridamole.

Comments: Atropine can worsen infranodal (Mobitz type II) second-degree AV block. Low doses (<0.5 mg) can cause a paradoxical slowing of heart rate.

BETA-BLOCKERS, ACUTE

Indications and Dose: All ACS patients: Start PO therapy unless there is a compelling reason to give IV (e.g., ventricular arrhythmias, significant hypertension). Metoprolol: Begin with 12.5 or 25 mg (PO) q12h × 1, 50 mg q12h × 2, then 100 mg (PO) q12h, as tolerated. If IV metoprolol is indicated, 5 mg over 1–2 minutes, repeated every 5 minutes to a total dose of 15 mg before transitioning to PO therapy. Initial doses can be reduced to 1–2 mg if a conservative regimen is desired. Alternatively Esmolol may be preferred due to its brief half-life: 0.1 mg/kg/min (IV) infusion, titrated in increments of 0.05 mg/kg/min every 5–15 minutes (as tolerated by blood pressure) until the desired therapeutic response is achieved, limiting symptoms develop, or a dose of 0.25 mg/kg/min is reached. For more rapid onset of action, a loading dose of 0.5 mg/kg can be given IV over 2–5 minutes followed by the usual maintenance dose. For patients with LVEF ≤40% post-MI, carvedilol (starting dose 6.25 mg bid, titrated over 4–6 weeks to 25 mg bid as tolerated) is reasonable, based on CAPRICORN and IMPACT-HF. For patients unable to tolerate beta-blockers during hospitalization, attempts to reinitiate therapy after 1–2 weeks of clinical stability is strongly recommended.

Contraindications (relative): Systolic BP <100 mmHg; HR <50 bpm; severe, decompensated heart failure; PR interval >0.24 seconds; greater than first-degree AV block or sick sinus syndrome without a functioning pacemaker; history of clinically important bronchospasm. Concurrent use with verapamil or diltiazem can result in severe hypotension or heart failure.

Clinical Trials: Beta-blockers reduce myocardial oxygen demand and can ameliorate angina. Early work demonstrated that early administration of beta-blockers limits infarct size, reduces ventricular fibrillation and cardiac rupture, decreases reinfarction and intracranial hemorrhage after fibrinolytic therapy, and reduces mortality by 15% within the first week. For unstable angina, beta-blockers reduce MI by 13%. Beta-blockers control ischemic pain in some patients. However, recent trial evidence has again shown that early beta-blockade in acute MI reduces the risks of recurrent myocardial infarction and ventricular fibrillation, but increases the risk of cardiogenic shock, especially in the first 24–48 hours after admission. Accordingly, acute beta-blocker therapy should be withheld in patients with any evidence of congestion or hemodynamic instability. Oral beta-blockers (Class I) are preferred to intravenous administration (Class IIa).

Comments: Monitor the heart rate, blood pressure, and ECG; evaluate the lungs for rales and wheezing. For mild wheezing or COPD, consider using low doses of a beta-1-selective agent (e.g., metoprolol). Patients with a contraindication to beta-blockers in the first 24 hours should be reevaluated for candidacy later in the hospital course.

BETA-BLOCKERS, CHRONIC

Indications and Dose: All ACS patients, except those with symptomatic bradycardia, high-grade heart block, decompensated heart failure, or significant bronchospasm should be treated with Timolol 10 mg (PO) q12h, atenolol 50–200 mg (PO) q24h, metoprolol 50–200 mg (PO) q12h, or another beta-blocker. Titrate dose to a target heart rate of 50–60 bpm.

Clinical Trials: Long-term therapy reduces the risk of reinfarction and death (primarily sudden death) by 25% to 45% at 1 year and by 20% up to 6 years after MI, especially in high-risk patients with anterior MI. Benefits are also apparent in patients with conditions often considered as contraindications to beta-blocker therapy: advanced age, pulmonary disease, and heart failure.

Comments: There is no difference between nonselective and selective agents, although beta-blockers without intrinsic sympathomimetic activity (ISA) may be more effective than beta-blockers with ISA. For patients with LV dysfunction, carvedilol beta-blocker, starting at 6.25 mg bid and titrated over 4–6 weeks to maximum dose of 25 mg bid, is recommended long term, based on the results of CAPRICORN and IMPACT-HF. Based on the results of MERIT-HF, and CIBIS-II metoprolol succinate or bisoprolol are also appropriate for patients with left ventricular dysfunction and heart failure symptoms.

BIVALIRUDIN

Indications and Dose: In patients with ACS (STE and non-STE/UA) who are being managed with an early invasive approach, initiate therapy with an IV bolus of 0.1 mg/kg followed by a 0.25 mg/kg/hr infusion. Before percutaneous intervention, give an additional bolus of 0.5 mg/kg, followed by an infusion of 0.25 mg/kg/hr. Continuation of the infusion 4 hours after percutaneous intervention can be considered.

Precautions: Bivalirudin is renally eliminated. An infusion dose (not a bolus dose) adjustment is required when CrCl <30 ml/min.

Clinical Trials: In ACUITY, in which randomized patients with moderate or high-risk ACS were treated with an early invasive approach, rates of ischemia and bleeding were similar between those patients randomized to bivalirudin or heparin on a common background of glycoprotein IIb/IIIa inhibition. However, bivalirudin alone (no IIb/IIIa) was associated with similar rates of ischemia and less bleeding (all major bleeding: 11.8% versus 9.1%).

Comments: Bivalirudin is an intravenous direct thrombin inhibitor with a half-life of 25 minutes. The greatest advantage of bivalirudin monotherapy (e.g., no glycoprotein IIb/IIIa inhibitor) appears to be reduced bleeding, particularly in elderly patients. As with all direct thrombin inhibitors, the patient is also spared the potential risk of heparin-induced thrombocytopenia, which is associated with a significant risk of inpatient mortality.

CALCIUM ANTAGONISTS

Indications and Dose: Relief of ongoing or recurrent ischemia when beta-blockers are contraindicated or ineffective; ACS due to variant angina; possibly for NSTE-ACS with preserved LV function: Diltiazem 120–320 mg/d or verapamil 120–480 mg/d PO in single or divided doses depending on the preparation. If used for NSTE-ACS, calcium antagonists should be started early (2–5 days) and continued for up to 1 year. Nondihydropyridine calcium channel blockers (e.g., nifedipine, nicardipine) must be used in conjunction with a beta-blocker to prevent reflex tachycardia. To slow the ventricular response to atrial fibrillation/flutter: *Diltiazem:* Initial IV bolus of 0.25 mg/kg (~20 mg) over 2 minutes. If the response is inadequate, a second bolus of 0.35 mg/kg (~25 mg) can be given 15 minutes later. For a continued reduction of ventricular rate (up to 24 hours), an IV infusion of 5–15 mg/hr can be started immediately after the bolus and titrated to heart rate. Infusion rates >15 mg/hr are not recommended. *Verapamil:* See the following dose for paroxysmal SVT. To terminate paroxysmal SVT after adenosine in patients with good blood pressure and preserved LV function: *Diltiazem:* Initial IV bolus of 0.25 mg/kg IV over 2 minutes. If SVT persists, a second bolus of 0.35 mg/kg can be given 15 minutes later. *Verapamil:* Initial IV bolus of 2.5–5.0 mg over 1–2 minutes (3 minutes in the elderly); peak effect in 3–5 minutes. If needed, a second bolus of 5–10 mg can be given 15–30 minutes after the first dose or 5-mg bolus doses can be repeated every 15 minutes up to a total cumulative dose of 30 mg.

Contraindications: Diltiazem and verapamil should be used with extreme caution, if at all, with IV beta-blockers or in patients with heart failure, significant LV dysfunction, or sick sinus syndrome or greater than first-degree AV block without a functioning pacemaker. Neither agent should use IV to slow the ventricular response to atrial fibrillation or flutter in Wolff-Parkinson-White syndrome (increased risk one-to-one conduction and subsequent VF) or to treat VT (increased risk of fatal hypotension). Rapid-release, short-acting nondihydropyridines should never be used due to the increased risk of reinfarction and death.

Clinical Trials (Acute MI): Diltiazem reduced early reinfarction and recurrent angina in NSTE-ACS and in STEMI treated with fibrinolytic therapy but increased mortality in patients with heart failure or severe LV dysfunction.

Comments: The primary benefit of calcium antagonists in unstable angina is the prevention and relief of ischemia. Side effects include hypotension, heart failure, and bradycardia. Verapamil can increase serum digitalis levels. IV calcium chloride (8–16 mg/kg for overdose; 2–4 mg/kg for prophylaxis) can be used to restore/prevent the drop in blood pressure associated with calcium antagonists. Amlodipine or felodipine can be safely administered to patients with chronic LV dysfunction, but their role in acute MI awaits definition.

CLOPIDOGREL

Indications and Dose: NSTE-ACS: For patients <75 years 300 mg (PO) loading dose, in conjunction with aspirin, started as soon as possible on admission and continued at 75 mg (PO) q24h for at least 9 months (see "precautions"). There is not data for a loading dose in patients 75 years and older. Coronary stenting: 300 mg (PO) loading dose prior to PCI followed by 75 mg (PO) q24h × 1 year (or longer if patient has received a drug-eluting stent). Aspirin-allergic or intolerant patients: 75 mg (PO) q24h long term.

Precautions: Use with caution in conjunction with NSAIDs or warfarin (increased risk of bleeding). Clopidogrel should be discontinued 5–7 days prior to CABG, if possible, to minimize the risk of perioperative bleeding. In patients submitted for urgent angiography and revascularization, it is reasonable to withhold clopidogrel until it is known that CABG will not be required.

Clinical Trials: In the CLARITY trial, STEMI patients treated with fibrinolysis who received clopidogrel had a 36% reduction in infarct-related artery occlusion (TIMI 0/1), death, or recurrent MI. In CURE and PCI-CURE, dual-antiplatelet therapy with aspirin plus clopidogrel resulted in 20% to 30% reductions in cardiovascular death, MI, or stroke in non-ST-elevation ACS compared to aspirin alone (pp. 84–85). In CAPRIE, clopidogrel showed a small (8.7%) but significant relative reduction in ischemic stroke, MI, or vascular death at 1.9 years compared to aspirin in high-risk patients with recent ischemic stroke, recent MI, or symptomatic peripheral arterial disease (pp. 84–87).

Comments: Clopidogrel inhibits platelet activation and subsequent aggregation by irreversibly binding to the platelet $P2Y_{12}$ receptor and impairing subsequent ADP-mediated activation of the platelet GP IIb/IIIa receptor complex. Due to the irreversible binding, platelets exposed to clopidogrel are affected for the remainder of their lifespan. The safety profile of clopidogrel is similar to low-dose aspirin, with a rare incidence of thrombotic thrombocytopenia purpura (TTP) (11 cases in 3 million patients in one report). The most frequent side effects include diarrhea, rash, and pruritus. Antiplatelet effects are not diminished by concomitant use of atorvastatin, but may be affected by proton pump inhibition.

DOBUTAMINE

Indications and Dose: Acute heart failure without shock; hemodynamically significant RV infarction not responding to volume loading: 2–20 mcg/kg/min IV infusion titrated to cardiac output or clinical effect. Although doses up to 40 mcg/kg/min have been used, a dose as low as 0.5 mcg/kg/min may be effective. Use the lowest effective dose, because tachycardia is more likely to develop at higher doses. Taper gradually upon discontinuation.

Contraindications: Avoid in cardiogenic shock, severe aortic stenosis, idiopathic hypertrophic subaortic stenosis (IHSS), and sulfite allergy (possible anaphylaxis).

Comments: Dobutamine is a potent inotropic agent with mild peripheral vasodilating effects; the net hemodynamic effect is similar to dopamine plus a vasodilator. Tolerance can occur with prolonged (>24 hour) use, requiring an increase in dose. Myocardial ischemia and arrhythmias can occur if tachycardia is induced. Dobutamine is inactivated if mixed with solutions containing sodium bicarbonate. Hemodynamic monitoring with a pulmonary artery catheter is recommended during dobutamine infusions. As with all inotropes, dobutamine is associated with increased mortality in patients with heart failure; therefore, its use should be kept as brief as possible.

DOPAMINE

Indications and Dose: Severe hypotension: Initial IV infusion of 2–5 mcg/kg/min, titrated based on blood pressure; usually effective below rates of 15 mcg/kg/min. Use the lowest effective dose, because tachycardia and systemic/splanchnic vasoconstriction are more likely to develop at higher doses. Taper gradually upon discontinuation; additional IV fluids may be required during taper.

Contraindications: Avoid in patients with pheochromocytoma, VF, sulfite allergy (possible anaphylaxis).

Comments: Dopamine can constrict pulmonary veins, which can increase pulmonary capillary wedge pressure and worsen pulmonary congestion despite improving cardiac output; this effect can be offset with concomitant use of a vasodilator (e.g., nitroglycerin, nitroprusside). Tachyphylaxis can occur with prolonged use, requiring an increase in dose. Only 10% of the usual dopamine dose should be given to patients receiving MAO inhibitors (MAO inhibitors can increase the pressor response to dopamine by six- to twentyfold). Subcutaneous extravasation can cause skin sloughing and should be treated with local infiltration of phentolamine. Dopamine can also be used for symptomatic bradycardia unresponsive to atropine. Dopamine is inactivated when mixed with solutions containing sodium bicarbonate.

EPINEPHRINE

Indications and Dose: Asystole; pulseless electrical activity; VF or pulseless VT resistant to defibrillation; severe hypotension; anaphylaxis; symptomatic bradycardia after atropine. Cardiac arrest: 1 mg (10 cc of 1:10,000 solution) IV bolus or 2 mg (diluted in 10 cc normal saline) via endotracheal tube. May be repeated every 3–5 minutes. Higher doses (up to 0.2 mg/kg) are not recommended. Each IV bolus should be followed by a saline flush (20 cc). Profound bradycardia or hypotension: 2–10 mcg/min IV infusion.

Comments: Epinephrine can precipitate myocardial ischemia even at low doses. Epinephrine may be inactivated if mixed in the same solution as bicarbonate. If subcutaneous extravasation occurs, tissue necrosis can develop. Inadvertent overdose can be counteracted by phentolamine. Discontinue if paradoxical worsening of respiratory function occurs in sulfite-allergic patients (epinephrine contains sulfite).

FIBRINOLYTIC THERAPY (TPA, RPA, TNK-TPA, STREPTOKINASE)

Indications and Dose: Acute MI <12 hours with ST-elevation or LBBB (new or presumably new) on ECG and no contraindications to fibrinolytic therapy. See pp. 44–58 for dosing regimens.

Clinical Trials: Randomized trials demonstrated a 21% relative risk reduction in 35-day mortality compared to standard medical therapy (Chapter 5). Mortality benefits are greatest when lytics are given within 6 hours, intermediate at 7–12 hours, and there is little or no benefit after 12 hours unless there is persistent ischemia or recurrent ST-elevation. All patient subgroups benefit regardless of gender, race, or age but patients with hypotension, tachycardia, diabetes mellitus, or prior MI derive the greatest benefit.

Comments: Conversion of single-chain plasminogen to double-chain plasmin by fibrinolytic agents results in degradation of fibrin and dissolution of clot. See pp. 44–58 for fibrinolytic agents, dosing regimens, adjunctive pharmacotherapy, contraindications, and complications.

FONDAPARINUX

Indications and Dose: In patients with ACS (STE and non-STE/UA), give fondaparinux 2.5 mg subcutaneously daily.

Precautions: Fondaparinux is renally eliminated. Avoid its use if severe renal impairment is present (CrCl <30 ml/min). Patients treated with fondaparinux appear to be at a small but increased risk of catheter thrombosis during percutaneous intervention. If patients are taken to the cath lab for percutaneous intervention, 1000 U heparin should be given in the lab to decrease this risk.

Clinical Trials: In OASIS 5, patients with NSTE-ACS treated with fondaparinux had less bleeding and experienced a 17% reduction in all-cause mortality compared to enoxaparin. Similarly, in OASIS 6, fondaparinux significantly reduced death and reinfarction (11.2% versus 9.7%).

Comments: Fondaparinux is a synthetic, pentasaccharide, indirect Factor Xa inhibitor with a long half-life (17–21 hours). Its fixed-dose, once-daily administration, decreased risk of bleeding, and consistent anticoagulation profile all represent significant advantages, particularly in patients managed with a noninvasive strategy.

FUROSEMIDE

Indications and Dose: Acute treatment of pulmonary congestion associated with LV dysfunction: 20–40 mg IV over 1–2 minutes. If no response, doses up to 2 mg/kg may be needed.

Comments: Diuretic effect peaks at 30 minutes and lasts for 6 hours. Reductions in venous return and central venous pressure occur before the onset of diuresis. Furosemide can induce hypotension, especially in patients with hypovolemia, RV infarction, or concurrent use of morphine or vasodilators. Potassium, calcium, and magnesium levels should be monitored to minimize the risk of arrhythmias.

GP IIB/IIIA INHIBITORS (ABCIXIMAB, EPTIFIBATIDE, TIROFIBAN)

Indications: Eptifibatide or tirofiban as primary medical therapy for NSTE-ACS in patients at high risk of thrombotic complications (e.g., ongoing ischemic pain, elevated cardiac troponins, dynamic ST-segment changes). Abciximab, eptifibatide, or tirofiban as an adjunct to PCI for ACS.

Dose: See Table 9.4, p. 94.

Clinical Trials: In a meta-analysis of 14 large-scale, randomized, placebo-controlled trials, GP IIb/IIIa inhibitors resulted in a significant reduction in death or MI at 30 days when used as an adjunct to PCI (36%; p <0.001) or as primary medical therapy for NSTE-ACS (9%; p = 0.015) (see Table 9.2, p. 92). Risk reduction was greatest for troponin-positive patients. They have also been shown to reduce mortality at 3 and 6 months when used as an adjunct to PCI (see Table 9.3, p. 93). The role for GP IIb/IIIa inhibitors in conjunction with low-dose fibrinolytic therapy for STEMI has recently been evaluated in ASSENT-3 and GUSTO-V (p. 57).

Comments: See pp. 90–96 for dosing and administration guidelines, use of adjunctive aspirin and heparin, management of complications, and trial results. The recent EARLY-ACS trial demonstrated that routine, early eptifibatide administration compared with delayed, provisional eptifibatide at PCI did not significantly reduce a composite of death, myocardial infarction, recurrent ischemia, or procedural complications. Accordingly, in high-risk NSTE-ACS patients, it is reasonable to delay glycoprotein IIb/IIIa inhibition until PCI.

HEPARIN, LOW MOLECULAR-WEIGHT (LMWH)

Indications and Dose: Primary medical therapy for NSTE-ACS: Enoxaparin 1 mg/kg SQ q12h. The optimal duration of therapy is unknown, but most patients receive enoxaparin for 2–8 days. If creatinine clearance <30 ml/min, decrease to 1 mg/kg q24h or 0.65 mg/kg q12h. Adjunct to PCI: Enoxaparin 0.75 mg/kg IV if a GP IIb/IIIa inhibitor is to be used; 1 mg/kg IV if *no* GP IIb/IIIa inhibitor is planned. If the patient has been treated with SQ enoxaparin and the last SQ dose is <8 hours, no additional enoxaparin is required prior to PCI; if the last SQ dose is >8 hours, an additional 0.3 mg/kg IV should be given just before PCI.

Clinical Trials: As the primary medical therapy for NSTE-ACS, two enoxaparin versus UFH trials (ESSENCE, TIMI 11b) showed a significant (20%) reduction in death or MI at 1 and 6 weeks with enoxaparin (see Table 9.5, p. 95). In contrast, dalteparin (FRIC) and nadroparin (FRAXIS) failed to show a benefit over UFH. As an adjunct to PCI, observational studies (NICE-1, NICE-3, NICE-4) and randomized trials (ACUTE II, CRUISE, INTERACT, A-to-Z, SYNERGY) have shown enoxaparin to be a safe and effective alternative to UFH for procedural anticoagulation (with or without GP IIb/IIIa inhibitors); compared to UFH, enoxaparin was more convenient to use and resulted in similar rates of ischemic events and major bleeding complications.

In the ASSENT 3 trial of enoxaparin versus UFH as an adjunct to TNK-tPA for STEMI, enoxaparin resulted in better event-free survival at 30 days (see p. 57).

Comments: LMWHs are homogeneous glycosaminoglycans with a mean molecular weight of 4000–6000 formed by controlled enzymatic or chemical depolymerization of unfractionated heparin (UFH). Advantages over UFH include better inhibition of thrombin generation (higher anti-Xa to anti-IIa activity), lack of a need to monitor aPTT (excellent bioavailability results in reliable anticoagulation), ease of administration (subcutaneous route), and less heparin-induced thrombocytopenia. In clinical trials, LMWHs were associated with more minor bleeding than UFH but no increase in major bleeding complications. See pp. 96–103 for the use of enoxaparin in NSTE-ACS, the monitoring, and the management of complications. To minimize the risk of vascular bleeding, vascular access sheaths should remain in place for 6–8 hours after the last enoxaparin dose, and the next enoxaparin dose should be given no sooner than 6–8 hours after sheath removal. Hemoglobin, hematocrit, and platelet counts should be monitored daily, and enoxaparin should be discontinued if the platelet count falls below 100,000 mm^3.

HEPARIN, UNFRACTIONATED (UFH)

Indications and Dose: Adjunct to tPA, rPA, TNK-tPA: 60 U/kg IV bolus (max. 4000 U) followed by 12 U/kg/hr IV maintenance infusion (max. 1000 U/hr), adjusted to aPTT of 1.5–2.0 times control (50–70 sec) × 48 hours (or until angiography or longer in patients at high risk of thromboembolism). Primary medical therapy for NSTE-ACS: IV bolus plus infusion as for tPA, just listed. During PCI: 60–100 U/kg IV bolus to achieve an intraprocedural ACT of 300–350 seconds. When a GP IIb/IIIa inhibitor is used, a 60 U/kg IV bolus is given to achieve an intraprocedural ACT of 200–250 seconds. All patients not being treated with IV heparin during periods of prolonged immobilization: 5000 units (SQ) q8h (or enoxaparin 1 mg/kg SQ ql2h).

Contraindications: Active bleeding; severe, uncontrolled hypertension; recent intracranial, intraspinal, or eye surgery; heparin-induced thrombocytopenia (HIT). Use caution in patients with bacterial endocarditis or potential sources of severe bleeding.

Clinical Trials: Compared to aspirin alone, IV heparin reduces the risk of death or reinfarction by 30% to 50% in NSTE-ACS and by 17% to 22% in ST-elevation ACS. IV heparin is probably necessary for the 1% mortality benefit associated with accelerated tPA versus streptokinase, but routine heparin is probably not necessary with streptokinase due to an increased risk of bleeding without a reduction in death or reinfarction. Subcutaneous heparin has been shown to reduce the incidence of mural thrombus post-MI by 58% to 72%.

Comments: Heparin is a heterogeneous mucopolysaccharide that binds to antithrombin to potentiate the inhibition of clotting factors IIa (thrombin) and Xa. Heparin binds to plasma proteins, endothelial cells, and macrophages, resulting in variable anticoagulant effects and the need to monitor aPTT or ACT. Other disadvantages include inhibition by platelet factor IV, an inability to inactivate clot-bound thrombin, and the development of heparin-induced thrombocytopenia (HIT). The optimal duration of heparin therapy is unknown, but most ACS patients receive treatment for 2–5 days. (No additional heparin is usually given after successful PCI.) aPTT levels should be obtained 6 hours after starting or changing the heparin dose (see Table 5.4, p. 51, for dose-adjustment nomogram); when two consecutive aPTT levels are therapeutic, they should be checked once daily thereafter, along with hemoglobin, hematocrit, and platelet counts. In patients with HIT, anticoagulation may be achieved with direct thrombin inhibition: argatroban at 2 mcg/kg/min, lepirudin at 0.4 mg/kg (max. 44 mg) bolus over 15–20 seconds followed by 0.15 mg/kg/hr (max. 16.5 mg/hr), or bivalirudin (IV bolus of 0.75 mg/kg prior to balloon inflation followed immediately by an IV infusion of 2.5 mg/kg/hr continued up to 4 hours postprocedure. If ACT <225 seconds 5 minutes after bolus, additional 0.3 mg/kg boluses are given as needed until ACT = 225 seconds).

LIDOCAINE

Indications and Dose: VF or pulseless VT resistant to defibrillation and epinephrine; hemodynamically stable VT; hemodynamically unstable VPCs: (1) Normal LV function and no hepatic impairment: loading dose of 75 mg IV followed by 50 mg IV every 5 minutes × 3 (total dose 225 mg); maintenance infusion of 2 mg/min. (2) Moderate decrease in LV function: loading dose of 75 mg IV followed by 50 mg IV every 5 minutes × 1 (total dose 125 mg); maintenance infusion of 1 mg/min. (3) Severe decrease in LV function or significant hepatic impairment: loading dose of 50–75 mg IV × 1; maintenance infusion of 0.5 mg/min. A single IV bolus of 1.5 mg/kg is acceptable for cardiac arrest. Tracheal administration: 2–4 mg/kg.

Clinical Trials: Prophylactic lidocaine for acute MI is not recommended (increased risk of death primarily from asystole).

Comments: Monitor for lidocaine toxicity: confusion, drowsiness, respiratory depression, perioral numbness, and seizures; may cause bradycardia or sinus arrest. Do not give for ventricular escape beats or rhythm (increased risk of asystole).

MAGNESIUM SULFATE

Indications and Dose: Cardiac arrest due to torsades de pointes: 1–2 gm IV push over 1–2 minutes in 10 cc D_5W. Torsade de pointes (not in cardiac arrest): 1–2 gm in 50–100 cc D_5W IV over 5–60 minutes. Consider an additional 2 gm IV over the next several hours. Regimens vary.

Clinical Trials: Several randomized trials suggested a mortality benefit for IV magnesium for acute MI, especially in high-risk patients not receiving reperfusion therapy and in elderly patients following fibrinolysis. In contrast, no benefit was observed in ISIS-4, which enrolled 58,050 patients, although the low mortality rate in control group (7.2%) and late administration of IV magnesium (e.g., after fibrinolytic therapy) were important limitations of this study. Recent results from the NHLBI-sponsored MAGIC trial, which randomized 6213 patients with acute

MI to IV magnesium or placebo, failed to show a benefit for magnesium.

Comments: Magnesium is a coronary vasodilator, has antiplatelet and antiarrhythmic effects, and can prevent calcium overload of reperfused myocytes. Magnesium may be of benefit for refractory VT after lidocaine and amiodarone and for life-threatening ventricular arrhythmias due to digitalis toxicity. It is not routinely recommended for acute MI unless magnesium deficiency is documented.

MORPHINE SULFATE

Indications and Dose: Ischemic chest pain; acute pulmonary edema associated with LV dysfunction: 2–4 mg IV over 1–5 minutes; 2–8 mg repeated every 5–15 minutes as needed.

Contraindications: Use with caution in severe, chronic lung disease (increased risk of respiratory depression). Use with caution in RV infarction or volume-depleted patients (may induce hypotension).

Comments: In addition to analgesic properties, morphine dilates peripheral venous and arterial beds, reducing preload, afterload, and myocardial oxygen consumption. Adverse effects include hypoventilation, hypotension, and nausea/vomiting. Hypoventilation can be reversed with naloxone (0.4–2.0 mg IV). Hypotension usually responds to lower extremity elevation and an IV saline (250–500 cc bolus in absence of pulmonary congestion). Bradycardia, nausea, and vomiting may improve with atropine (0.5–1.0 mg IV).

NITROGLYCERIN, ACUTE

Indications and Dose: On initial presentation to control ongoing ischemic pain: Sublingual nitroglycerin tablets (0.4 mg) or aerosol spray every 5 minutes × 3. Aerosol spray should not be shaken (affects metered dose). IV nitroglycerin acutely for persistent ischemic pain despite sublingual nitroglycerin and IV beta-blockers: Initial IV bolus of 10–20 mcg if systolic BP >100 mmHg, then infusion of 10–20 mcg/min. The infusion can be increased by 5–10 mcg/min every 5–10 minutes until ischemia is relieved, mean arterial pressure falls by 10% (or 30% if hypertensive), heart rate increases by 10 bpm, or pulmonary artery end-diastolic pressure decreases by 10% to 30%. Do not allow systolic BP to fall below 90 mmHg or heart rate to exceed 110 bpm. Doses in excess of 200 mcg/min are generally not recommended. IV nitroglycerin × 24–48 hours for acute MI or high-risk unstable angina with hypertension, recurrent ischemia, or heart failure: see dose given earlier.

Contraindications: Systolic BP <90 mmHg; severe bradycardia (<50 bpm) or tachycardia;

RV infarction; severe hypovolemia. Avoid if sildenafil (Viagra) or vardenafil (Levitra) is used within 24 hours, or if tadalafil (Cialis) is used within 48 hours (may cause severe hypotension or MI).

Clinical Trials: IV nitroglycerin reduced infarct size and death in patients treated within 4 hours of anterior MI in a meta-analysis of 10 small trials, but ISIS-4 and GISSI-3 failed to show a mortality benefit. There are no large randomized trials of IV nitroglycerin for unstable angina.

Comments: Nitroglycerin yields nitric oxide, a smooth-muscle relaxant that increases myocardial blood flow and decreases myocardial oxygen consumption. IV administration is preferred over nonparenteral (oral, dermal) routes acutely, due to the ease of titration and predictable bioavailability; long-acting oral nitrate preparations should be avoided early. Nitrates should be decreased or discontinued if blood pressure-lowering effects preclude use of beta-blockers/ACE inhibitors. Common side effects include hypotension and headaches. Nitroglycerin can worsen V/Q mismatch and cause hypoxemia in COPD patients who rely on hypoxic pulmonary vasoconstriction to maintain oxygenation. Tolerance (lack of response) to anti-ischemic effects can occur after 1 day of continuous therapy, requiring an increase in dose or a nitrate-free interval (~12 hours). Supplemental antioxidants (e.g., vitamin C) may also prevent nitrate tolerance. Nitrates can reduce the sensitivity to heparin: Higher heparin doses may be needed during nitrate administration and lower heparin doses may be needed once nitrates are stopped (follow ACT/aPTT).

NITROGLYCERIN, CHRONIC

Indications and Dose: To prevent recurrent angina: Isosorbide dinitrate sustained-release: start at 40 mg PO qd; may increase to 160 mg qd (18-hour nitrate-free interval is recommended). Isosorbide mononitrate immediate-release (Ismo): 20 mg PO bid (doses given 7 hours apart). Isosorbide mononitrate extended-release (Imdur): 30–60 mg PO q24h titrated to ~120 mg q24h.

Clinical Trials: Oral nitrates starting on day 1 following acute MI had no impact on mortality at 1 month in ISIS-4 or GISSI-3.

Comments: Not routinely recommended after successful reperfusion or revascularization. Patients receiving IV nitroglycerin should not be switched to oral/transdermal therapy until they have been free from ischemia for 12–24 hours. A nitrate-free interval of at least 10–12 hours is required with oral/transdermal therapy to maintain anti-ischemic effects. All ACS patients should receive sublingual nitroglycerin prior to discharge and instructions for use, including avoidance within at least 24 hours of sildenafil (Viagra) or vardenafil (Levitra) and within 48 hours of tadalafil (Cialis).

NITROPRUSSIDE

Indications and Dose: Hypertensive emergencies; acute heart failure; afterload reduction for acute mitral or aortic regurgitation: IV infusion of 0.3–0.5 mcg/kg/min, titrated every 3–5 minutes to desired effect (usual dose 0.5–8.0 mcg/kg/min). Use lowest effective dose. Maximum dose of 10 mcg/kg/min IV should not be used for longer than 10 minutes. Taper gradually upon discontinuation.

Comments: Nitroprusside improves cardiac output in heart failure primarily through vasodilation (afterload reduction), but it can also decrease ischemia by reducing myocardial work and improving diastolic relaxation. Adverse effects include headache, nausea, vomiting, and abdominal discomfort. Nitroprusside can worsen V/Q mismatch and cause hypoxemia in COPD patients who rely on hypoxic pulmonary vasoconstriction to maintain oxygenation. Excessive administration can cause hypotension, tachycardia, and myocardial ischemia. Thiocyanate toxicity (tinnitus, blurred vision, mental status changes, abdominal pain, and seizures) is uncommon, but is more likely to occur with higher (>2 mcg/kg/min) doses, prolonged (>2 day) infusions, or renal failure. Thiocyanate levels should be monitored; levels <l0 mg/l00 mL are usually considered safe. Cyanide toxicity is treated with 3% sodium nitrite followed immediately by sodium thiosulfate. Protect drug reservoir and tubing from light with aluminum foil to avoid deterioration. Hemodynamic monitoring is required to avoid excessive hypotension.

OXYGEN

Indications: Oxygen is often given by convention for ACS, but there are no clear data to support its routine use. Supplemental oxygen is best reserved for patients with respiratory distress or hypoxemia to maintain SaO_2 >90%.

Comments: Its use can increase vascular resistance as well as induce hypoventilation and respiratory acidosis in patients with COPD who rely on hypoxic drive for ventilation.

PRASUGREL

Indications and Dose: Acute coronary syndrome patients that are managed with PCI: Patients presenting with unstable angina, NSTE-ACS, or STEMI who undergo planned PCI may be treated with the oral thienopyridine prasugrel. The loading dose of prasugrel is 60mg, followed by a daily maintenance dose of 10mg daily. However, vulnerability to bleeding with the current dosing recommendations among specific patient populations, including patients ≥75 years of age or patients those weighing less than 60 kg, may result in excess harm, thus patient selection may be critical when considering the use of prasugrel. Since the evidence and experience with lower doses and broader patient populations are not available, prasugrel may not be appropriate for these patients until further studies are performed. Based on the available evidence, the duration of dual antiplatelet therapy with prasugrel may be extended to a minimum of 15 months.

Precautions: The concomitant use of prasugrel and aspirin with NSAIDs or anticoagulants is not advised, given the increasing risk for hemorrhage. Patients with a prior history of cerebrovascular disease (e.g., stroke or transient ischemic attack) have demonstrated higher risks of intracranial hemorrhage and should not be treated with prasugrel. Patients scheduled for cardiac surgery should have prasugrel discontinued for 7–10 days prior to their scheduled procedure to reduce the risk of perioperative bleeding. This longer duration of thienopyridine cessation prior to cardiac surgery is based on higher perioperative bleeding rates among prasugrel treated patients as compared with clopidogrel treated patients.

Clinical Trials: The FDA approval of prasugrel was based on the findings from the TRITON-TIMI 38 study, a randomized controlled trial comparing prasugrel to clopidogrel among moderate to high-risk ACS patients undergoing planned PCI. The primary composite endpoint of cardiovascular death, non-fatal MI, or non-fatal stroke was significantly lower among prasugrel treated patients when compared with clopidogrel (9.9% versus 12.1%). In addition, prasugrel treated patients were observed to have a marked reduction in the incidence of probable stent thrombosis (1.1%) compared with clopidogrel treated patients (2.4%). The incidence on non-CABG related major bleeding, including life-threatening and fatal bleeding, was higher in the prasugrel group. These serious bleeding complications were greatest among subgroups of patients previously demonstrated to be at higher hemorrhagic risk: patients ≥75 years of age, patients weighing <60kg, and those with prior cerebrovascular disease.

Comments: Similar to clopidogrel, prasugrel inhibits platelet activation and aggregation by irreversibly binding to the platelet $P2Y_{12}$ receptor and impairing ADP-mediated activation of the platelet GP IIb/IIIa receptor complex. However, the greater potency and less response variability of prasugrel compared with that of clopidogrel has been attributed to its greater efficiency during drug metabolism in generating the active compound. The rates of serious adverse events not related to bleeding were shown to be similar between prasugrel and clopidogrel from TRITON-TIMI 38; there were significantly higher rates of colonic cancers detected in the prasugrel treated patients but more patients in the prasugrel group had gastrointestinal bleeding preceeding the diagnosis of neoplasia. Diabetic patients treated with prasugrel compared with clopidogrel from TRITON-TIMI 38 had greater reductions in cardiovascular events, suggesting patients at higher atherothrombotic risk and lower bleeding risk may have the most to gain from more intensive platelet inhibition mediated by the $P2Y_{12}$ receptor. There are ongoing studies evaluating the safety and efficacy of dual antiplatelet therapy with prasugrel on the clinical outcomes of patients who are not acutely revascularized after an ACS event (i.e., the medically managed).

PROCAINAMIDE

Indications and Dose: For refractory VF or VT, 100-mg IV bolus doses repeated every 5 minutes can be used. For other indications (stable wide QRS complex tachycardia, SVT resistant to adenosine and vagal maneuvers, rate control of atrial fibrillation in WPW syndrome): 20 mg/min IV infusion until the arrhythmia is suppressed, hypotension develops, QRS widens by 50%, or a total dose of 17 mg/kg is given, followed by an IV maintenance infusion of 1–4 mg/min.

Contraindications: Avoid in patients with a prolonged QT interval or torsade de pointes. Use with caution in conjunction with other drugs that prolong the QT interval. Do not use in patients with CrCl <20 mL/min.

Comments: Its use can induce torsade de pointes, especially in patients with renal insufficiency, hypokalemia, or hypomagnesemia. For patients with heart failure or renal insufficiency, the loading dose should be reduced to 12 mg/kg and the maintenance dose reduced to 1–2 mg/min. Blood pressure and ECG should be monitored continuously during IV administration, because sharp drops in blood pressure can occur with rapid infusion, especially in patients with LV dysfunction. Follow blood levels (procainamide & NAPA) in renal failure and during prolonged use (>3 mg/min × 24 hours).

STATINS (HMG COA REDUCTASE INHIBITORS)

Indications: All ACS patients (see the discussion on pp. 104–106).

Clinical Trials: Statins reduced early recurrent ischemia when initiated during hospitalization for NSTE-ACS in MIRACL. In PROVE IT, in-hospital initiation of atorvastatin 80 mg/d (intensive LDL-lowering therapy; mean LDL 62 mg/dL) improved early (30-day) and late (2-year) cardiovascular outcomes compared to pravastatin 40 mg (standard LDL-lowering therapy; mean LDL 95 mg/dL) (see Table 9.8, p. 105). High-dose statin therapy was well-tolerated. Statins improve long-term event-free survival in patients with coronary artery disease, even if cholesterol levels are within "normal" range. Trials are underway to evaluate the use of statins immediately on presentation versus after 6 weeks.

Comments: Clinical benefits occur long before changes in plaque morphology, suggesting salutary effects beyond cholesterol lowering and plaque regression. Intensive LDL lowering is recommended for all ACS patients. See the discussion on pp. 104–106.

WARFARIN

Indications and Dose: LV thrombus or chronic risk of thromboembolic complications (e.g., atrial fibrillation, prolonged immobilization, low cardiac output): Initial dose of 2.5–10 mg PO daily × 2–4 days, then titrated to maintain an INR of 2.0–3.0. Dosage should be individualized.

Contraindications: Active bleeding; when risk of bleeding exceeds the benefit of anticoagulation; pregnancy; surgery of CNS or eye; malignant hypertension; lack of patient cooperation. Use with caution in renal or hepatic dysfunction.

Clinical Trials: Long-term anticoagulation with warfarin reduced the risk of recurrent MI or death in ACS patients not receiving aspirin. However, in trials of warfarin versus aspirin, warfarin resulted in more bleeding without reducing reocclusion after successful or death. Recent ACS trials (OASIS-2, CARS, CHAMP) failed to show benefit for the combination of low-intensity warfarin plus aspirin versus aspirin alone. In contrast, studies utilizing higher intensity anticoagulation (INR 2.0–2.5) have demonstrated benefit for aspirin plus warfarin compared to aspirin alone, including 25% to 50% reductions in death, MI, or stroke in ASPECT-2 and WARIS-2, and less reocclusion after fibrinolysis in APRICOT-2.

Comments: Warfarin inhibits synthesis of vitamin K–dependent clotting factors (II, VII, IX, X) and proteins C and S. Warfarin has no direct effect on existing thrombus but can prevent propagation and embolism of clot. Numerous factors including travel, environment, physical state, and medications can influence the response to therapy. Warfarin interacts with many drugs; check tertiary source for listing. Warfarin's anticoagulant effects can be reversed by vitamin K, fresh whole blood, or fresh frozen plasma (200–500 mL). Studies have shown that systematic follow-up of patients through anticoagulation clinics results in better compliance and control. Recent trials have suggested that pharmacogenomics may play a role in dose prediction and adjustment.

Footnote:
Dosages assume normal renal and hepatic function, unless otherwise specified. Check other drug references for complete prescribing information, including dosage adjustments, drug interactions, adverse effects, and safety in pregnancy.

REFERENCES

Chapter 1

Brouwer MA, Martin JS, Maynard C, et al., for the MITI Project Investigators. Influence of early prehospital thrombolysis on mortality and event-free survival: the Myocardial Infarction Triage and Intervention Randomized Trial. *Am J Cardiol* 1996;78:497–502.

Fath-Ordoubadi F, Al-Mohammad A, Huehns TY, et al. Meta-analysis of randomised trials of prehospital versus hospital thrombolysis. *Circulation* 1994;90:325.

Kastrati A, Dibra A, Spaulding C, et al. Meta-analysis of randomized trials on drug-eluting stents versus bare-metal stents in patients with acute myocardial infarction. *Eur Heart J* 2007;28(22):2706–2713.

Lamfers EJ, Hooghoudt TE, Uppelschoten A, et al. Effect of prehospital thrombolysis on aborting acute myocardial infarction. *Am J Cardiol* 1999;84:928–930.

Rioufol G, Finet G, Ginon I, et al. Multiple atherosclerotic plaque rupture in acute coronary syndrome. A three-vessel intravascular ultrasound study. *Circulation* 2002. http://circ.ahajournals.org/.

Chapter 2

Alpert JS, Thygesen K, Antman E, et al. Myocardial infarction redefined—a consensus document of The Joint European Society of Cardiology/American College of Cardiology Committee for the redefinition of myocardial infarction. *J Am Coll Cardiol* 2000;36:959–969.

Antman EM, Tanasijevic MJ, Thompson B, et al. Cardiac-specific troponin I levels to predict the risk of mortality in patients with acute coronary syndromes. *N Engl J Med* 1996;335:1342–1347.

Barron HV, Bowlby LJ, Breen T, et al. Use of reperfusion therapy for acute myocardial infarction in the United States: data from the National Registry of Myocardial Infarction 2. *Circulation* 1998;97:1150–1156.

The ECG Criteria Book. Eds: O'Keefe J, Hammill S, Freed M, Pogwizd S. Physicians' Press, Royal Oak, MI, 2002.

Fibrinolytic Therapy Trialists' (FTT) Collaborative Group. Indications for fibrinolytic therapy in suspected acute myocardial infarction: collaborative overview of early mortality and major morbidity results from all randomized trials of more than 1000 patients. *Lancet* 1994;343:311–322.

Galvani M, Ottani F, Ferrini D, et al. Prognostic influence of elevated values of cardiac troponin I in patients with unstable angina. *Circulation* 1997;95: 2053–2059.

Hamm CW, Goldmann BU, Heeschen C, et al. Emergency room triage of patients with acute chest pain by means of rapid testing for cardiac troponin T or troponin I. *N Engl J Med* 1997;337:1648–1653.

Hamm CW, Heeschen C, Goldmann B, et al. Benefit of abciximab in patients with refractory unstable angina in relation to serum troponin levels. *N Engl J Med* 1999;340:1623–1629.

Heeschen C, Hamm CW, Goldmann B. Troponin concentrations for stratification of patients with acute coronary syndromes in relation to therapeutic efficacy of tirofiban. *Lancet* 1999;354:1757–1762.

Heidenreich PA, Alloggiamento T, Melsop K, et al. The prognostic value of troponin in patients with non-ST-elevation acute coronary syndromes: a meta-analysis. *J Am Coll Cardiol* 2001;38:478–485.

Kannel WB, Abbott RD. Incidence and prognosis of unrecognized myocardial infarction: an update on the Framingham Study. *N Engl J Med* 1984;311: 1444–1447.

Kontos MC, Anderson FP, Schmidt KA, et al. Early diagnosis of acute myocardial infarction in patients without ST-segment elevation. *Am J Cardiol* 1999;83:155–158.

Lee TH, Cook EF, Weisberg MC, et al. Impact of the availability of a prior electrocardiogram on the triage of the patient with acute chest pain. *J Gen Intern Med* 1990;5:381–388.

Mair J, Morandell D, Genser N, et al. Equivalent early sensitivities of myoglobin, creatine kinase MB mass, creatine kinase isoform ratios, and cardiac troponins I and T for acute myocardial infarction. *Clin Chem* 1995;41:1266–1272.

Margolis JR, Kannel WS, Feinleib M, et al. Clinical features of unrecognized myocardial infarction—silent and symptomatic. Eighteen year follow-up: the Framingham study. *Am J Cardiol* 1973;32:I–7.

Matetzky S, Freimark D, Feinberg MS, et al. Acute myocardial infarction with isolated ST-segment elevations revealing acute posterior infarction. *J Am Coll Cardiol* 1999;34:748–753.

McElroy JB. Angina pectoris with coexisting skeletal chest pain. *Am Heart J* 1963;66:96–99.

Morrow DA, Cannon CP, Nader R, et al., for the TACTICS-T1MI 18 Investigators. Ability of minor elevations of troponins I and T to predict benefit from an early invasive strategy in patients with unstable angina and non-ST-elevation myocardial infarction. *JAMA* 2001;286:2405–2412.

Ohman EM, Armstrong PW, Christenson RH, for the GUSTO IIA Investigators. Cardiac troponin T levels for risk stratification in acute myocardial ischemia. *N Engl J Med* 1996;335:1333–1341.

Pettijohn TL, Doyle T, Spiekerman AM, et al. Usefulness of positive troponin-T and negative creatine kinase levels in identifying high-risk patients with unstable angina pectoris. *Am J Cardiol* 1997;80:510–511.

Puleo PR, Meyer D, Wathen C, et al. Use of a rapid assay for subforms of creatine kinase-MB to diagnose or rule out acute myocardial infarction. *N Engl J Med* 1994;331:561–566.

Tierney WM, Fitzgerald J, McHenry R. Physician estimates of the probability of myocardial infarction in emergency room patients with chest pain. *Med Decision Making* 1986;6:12–17.

Tsung SH. Several conditions causing elevation of serum CK-MB and CK-BB. *Am J Clin Pathol* 1981;75:711–715.

Zaninotto M, Altinier S, Lachin M, et al. Strategies for the early diagnosis of acute myocardial infarction using biochemical markers. *Am J Clin Pathol* 1999; 111:399–405.

Chapter 3

Amadeo B, Masotti M. Optimal reperfusion in evolving myocardial infarction. Does abciximab improve outcomes in stent treated patients? 2002;39(Supp B):7B.

American Diabetes Association. Standards of medical care for patients with diabetes mellitus. *Diabetes Care* 2000;23(Suppl 1):S32–S42.

Antiplatelet Trialists' Collaboration. Collaborative overview of randomized trials of antiplatelet therapy, I: prevention of death, myocardial infarction, and stroke by prolonged antiplatelet therapy in various categories of patients. *BMJ* 1994;308:81–106.

Antiplatelet Trialists' Collaboration. Secondary prevention of vascular disease by prolonged antiplatelet treatment. *BMJ* (Clin Res Ed) 1988;296:320–331.

Antman EA, Anbe TD, Armstrong PW, et al. ACC/AHA Guidelines for the Management of Patients with ST-Elevation Myocardial Infarction—executive summary. *J Am Coll Cardiol* 2004;44:671–719. Full-text guidelines available at www.acc.org/clinical/guidelines/stemi/index.pdf.

Boersma E. The primary coronary angioplasty versus thrombolysis—2 trialists' collaborative G. Does time matter? A pooled analysis of randomized clinical trials comparing primary percutaneous coronary intervention and in-hospital fibrinolysis in acute myocardial infarction patients. *Eur Heart J* 2006;27(7):779–788.

Brouwer MA, Martin JS, Maynard C, et al., for the MITI Project Investigators. Influence of early prehospital thrombolysis on mortality and event-free survival: the Myocardial Infarction Triage and Intervention Randomized Trial. *Am J Cardiol* 1996;78:497–502.

Cannon CP, Braunwald E, McCabe CH, et al. Comparison of intensive and moderate lipid lowering with statins after acute coronary syndromes. *N Engl J Med* 2004;350.

Cox DA, Stone GW, Grines CL, et al. Outcomes of optimal or "stent-like" balloon angioplasty in acute myocardial infarction: the CADILLAC Trial. *J Am Coll Cardiol* 2003;42:971–977.

Davies MJ, Thomas AC. Plaque fissuring: the cause of acute myocardial infarction, sudden ischaemic death, and crescendo angina. *Br Heart J* 1985;53:363–373.

DeWood MA, Fisher MJ, for the Spokane Heart Research Group. Direct PTCA versus intravenous rtPA in acute myocardial infarction: preliminary results from a prospective randomized trial. *Circulation* 1989;80: II-418.

DeWood MA, Spores J, Notske R, et al. Prevalence of total coronary occlusion during the early hours of transmural myocardial infarction. *N Engl J Med* 1980; 303:897–902.

Eagle KA, Nallamothu BK, Mehta RH, et al., for the Global Registry of Acute Coronary Events I. Trends in acute reperfusion therapy for ST-segment elevation myocardial infarction from 1999 to 2006: we are getting better but we have got a long way to go. *Eur Heart J* 2008;29(5):609–617.

Elizaga J, Garcia EJ, Delcan JL, et al. Primary coronary angioplasty versus systemic thrombolysis in acute anterior myocardial infarction: in-hospital results from a prospective randomized trial. Circulation 1993;88:I-411.

Falk E. Plaque rupture with severe preexisting stenosis precipitating coronary thrombosis: characteristics of coronary atherosclerotic plaques underlying fatal occlusive thrombi. Br Heart J 1983;50:127–134.

Fath-Ordoubadi F, Al-Mohammad A, Huehns TY, et al. Meta-analysis of randomised trials of prehospital versus hospital thrombolysis. Circulation 1994;90:325.

Fox K. Efficacy of perindopril in reduction of cardiovascular events among patients with stable coronary artery disease (the EUROPA study). Lancet 2003;362:782–788.

Franzosi MG, Santoro E, De Vita C, et al. Ten-year follow-up of the first megatrial testing thrombolytic therapy in patients with acute myocardial infarction: results of the Gruppo Italiano per lo Studio della Sopravvivenza nell' Infarto-1 study. The GISSI Investigators. Circulation 1998;98:2659–2965.

Gibbons RJ, Holmes DR, Reeder GS, et al. Immediate angioplasty compared with the administration of a thrombolytic agent followed by conservative treatment for myocardial infarction. N Engl J Med 1993;328:685–691.

Gibson CM, Pride YB, Frederick PD, et al. Trends in reperfusion strategies, door-to needle and door-to-balloon times, and in-hospital mortality among patients with ST-segment elevation myocardial infarction enrolled in the National Registry of Myocardial Infarction from 1990 to 2006. American Heart Journal 2008;156(6):1035–1044.

Grines CL, Browne KF, Marco J, et al. A comparison of immediate angioplasty with thrombolytic therapy for acute myocardial infarction. N Engl J Med 1993;328:673–679.

Hambrecht R, Neibauer J, Marburger C, et al. Various intensities of leisure time physical activity in patients with coronary artery disease: effects on cardiorespiratory fitness and progression of coronary atherosclerotic lesions. J Am Coll Cardiol 1993;22:468–477.

Kastrati A, Dibra A, Spaulding C, et al. Meta-analysis of randomized trials on drug-eluting stents versus bare-metal stents in patients with acute myocardial infarction. Eur Heart J 2007;28(22):2706–2713.

Keeley EC, Boura JA, Grines CL. Primary angioplasty versus intravenous thrombolytic therapy for acute myocardial infarction: a quantitative review of 23 randomised trials. Lancet 2003;361(9351):13–20.

Kris-Etherton P, Eckel RH, Howard BV, et al. Lyon diet heart study. Benefits of a Mediterranean-style, National Cholesterol Education Program/American Heart Association Step I dietary pattern on cardiovascular disease. Circulation 2001;103:1823–1825.

Krumholtz HM, Cohen BJ, Tsevat J, et al. Cost-effectiveness of a smoking cessation program after myocardial infarction. J Am Coll Cardiol 1993;22:1697–1702.

Lamfers EJ, Hooghoudt TE, Uppelschoten A, et al. Effect of prehospital thrombolysis on aborting acute myocardial infarction. Am J Cardiol 1999;84:928–930.

Magid DJ, Calonge BN, Rumsfeld JS, et al. Relation between hospital primary angioplasty volume and mortality for patients with acute MI treated with primary angioplasty vs. thrombolytic therapy. JAMA 2000;284:3131–3138.

Michels KB, Yusuf S. Does PTCA in acute myocardial infarction affect mortality and reinfarction rates? A quantitative overview (meta-analysis) of the randomized clinical trials. Circulation 1995;91:476–485.

Mori TA, Beilin LJ, Burke V, et al. Interactions between dietary fat, fish, and fish oils and their effects on platelet function in men at risk of cardiovascular disease. Arterioscler Thromb Vasc Biol 1997;17:279–286.

NCEP Report. Implications of recent clinical trials for the National Cholesterol Education Program Adult Treatment Panel III Guidelines. Circulation 2004;110:227–239.

Nieuwlaat R, Lenzen M, Crijns HJGM, et al. Which factors are associated with the application of reperfusion therapy in ST-elevation acute coronary syndromes? Cardiology 2006;106(3):137–146.

O'Connor GT, Burning JE, Yusuf S, et al. An overview of randomized trials of rehabilitation with exercise after myocardial infarction. Circulation 1989;80:234–244.

O'Neill WW, Timmis GC, Bourdillon PD, et al. A prospective randomized clinical trial of intracoronary streptokinase versus coronary angioplasty for acute myocardial infarction. N Engl J Med 1986;341:812–818.

Oldridge NB, Guyatt GH, Fischer ME, et al. Cardiac rehabilitation after myocardial infarction: combined experience of randomized clinical trials. JAMA 1988;260:945–950.

Randomised trial of cholesterol lowering in 4444 patients with coronary heart disease: the Scandinavian Simvastatin Survival Study (4S). Lancet 1994; 344:1383–1389.

Rentrop KP, Blanke H, Karsch KR, et al. Acute myocardial infarction: intracoronary application of nitroglycerin and streptokinase. Clin Cardiol 1979;2:354–363.

Rentrop P, Blanke H, Karsch KR, et al. Selective intracoronary thrombolysis in acute myocardial infarction and unstable angina pectoris. *Circulation* 1981;63:307–317.

Ribeiro EE, Silva LA, Carneiro R, et al. Randomized trial of direct coronary angioplasty versus intravenous streptokinase in acute myocardial infarction. *J Am Coll Cardiol* 1993;22:376–380.

Rosengren A, Hawken S, Ounpuu S, et al. Association of psychosocial risk factors with risk of acute myocardial infarction in 11119 cases and 13648 controls from 52 countries (the INTERHEART study): case-control study. *Lancet* 2004;364:953–962.

Smith SC, Blair SN, Bonow RO, et al. AHA/ACC guidelines for preventing heart attack and death in patients with atherosclerotic cardiovascular disease: 2001 update; a statement for health care professionals from the American Heart Association and the American College of Cardiology. *J Am Coll Cardiol* 2001;38:1581–1583.

Stone GW, Grines CL, Cox DA, et al. Comparison of angioplasty with stenting, with or without abciximab, in acute myocardial infarction. *N Engl J Med* 2002;346:957–966.

Stone GW, Lansky AJ, Pocock SJ, Gersh BJ, Dangas G, Wong SC, Witzenbichler B, Guagliumi G, Peruga JZ, Brodie BR, Dudek D, Möckel M, Ochala A, Kellock A, Parise H, Mehran R; HORIZONS-AMI Trial Investigators. Paclitaxel-eluting stents versus bare-metal stents in acute myocardial infarction. *N Engl J Med*. 2009 May 7;360(19):1946–1959.

The Heart Outcomes Prevention Evaluation Study Investigators. Effects of an angiotensin-coverting-enzyme inhibitor, ramipril, on cardiovascular events in high-risk patients. *N Engl J Med* 2000;342:145–153.

The Sixth Report of the Joint National Committee on Detection, Evaluation, and Treatment of High Blood Pressure (JNC VI). *Arch Intern Med* 1997;157:2413–2446.

Timolol-induced reduction in mortality and reinfarction in patients surviving acute myocardial infarction. *N Engl J Med* 1981;304:801–807.

Valgimigli M, Campo G, Percoco G, et al., for the Multicentre Evaluation of Single High-Dose Bolus Tirofiban Versus Abciximab with Sirolimus-Eluting Stent or Bare Metal Stent in Acute Myocardial Infarction Study I. Comparison of angioplasty with infusion of tirofiban or abciximab and with implantation of sirolimus-eluting or uncoated stents for acute myocardial infarction: the MULTISTRATEGY Randomized Trial. *JAMA* 2008;299(15):1788–1799.

van't Hof AWJ, ten Berg J, Heestermans T, et al. Prehospital initiation of tirofiban in patients with ST-elevation myocardial infarction undergoing primary angioplasty (On-TIME 2): a multicentre, double-blind, randomized controlled trial. *Lancet* 2008;372(9638):537–546.

Weaver WD, Simes RJ, Ellis SG, et al. Comparison of primary coronary angioplasty and intravenous thrombolytic therapy for acute myocardial infarction. A quantitative review. *JAMA* 1997;278:2093–2098.

Zijlstra F, Jan de Boaer M, Hoorntje JCA, et al. A comparison of immediate coronary angioplasty with intravenous streptokinase in acute myocardial infarction. *N Engl J Med* 1993;328:680–684.

Chapter 4

Amadeo B, Masotti M. Optimal reperfusion in evolving myocardial infarction. Does abciximab improve outcomes in stent treated patients? 2002;39(Supp B):7B.

Antoniucci D, Rodriguez A, Hempel A, et al. A randomized trial comparing primary infarct artery stenting with or without abciximab in acute myocardial infarction. *J Am Coll Cardiol* 2003;42:1879–1885.

Antoniucci D, Santoro GM, Bolognese L, et al. A clinical trial comparing primary stenting of the infarct-related artery with optimal primary angioplasty of acute myocardial infarction. Results from the Florence Randomized Elective Stenting in Acute Coronary Occlusions (FRESCO) trial. *J Am Coll Cardiol* 1998;3:1234–1239.

Assessment of the Safety and Efficacy of a New Treatment Strategy with Percutaneous Couronary Intervention (ASSENT-4 PCI) Investigators. Primary versus tenecteplase-facilitated percutaneous coronary intervention in patients with ST- segment elevation acute myocardial infarction (ASSENT-4 PCI): randomised trial. *Lancet* 2006;367(9510):569–578.

Bakhai A, Stone GW, Grines CL, et al. Cost-effectiveness of coronary stenting and abciximab for patients wi th acute myocardial infarction: Results from the CADILLAC *Circulation* 2003;108:2857–2863.

Berkowitz SD, Sane DC, Sigmon KN, et al. Occurrence and clinical significance of thrombocytopenia in a population undergoing high-risk percutaneous coronary revascularization. *J Am Coll Cardiol* 1998;32:311–319.

Direct Inhibition of delta-Protein Kinase C Enzyme to Limit Total Infarct Size in Acute Myocardial Infraction (DELTA MI) Investigators: Bates E, Bode C, Costa M, Gibson CM, Granger C, et al. Direct inhibition of protein kinase CEtLTISiAMII. Intracoronary KAI-9803 as an adjunct to primary percutaneous coronary intervention for acute STsegment elevation myocardial infarction. *Circulation* 2008;117(7):886–896.

Disler L, Haitas B, Benjamin J, et al. Cardiogenic shock in evolving myocardial infarction: treatment by angioplasty and streptokinase. *Heart Lung* 1987;16:649.

Ellis SG, Tendera M, de Belder MA, et al., the FI. Facilitated PCI in patients with ST-elevation myocardial infarction. *N Engl J Med* 2008;358(21):2205–2217.

Grines CL, Cox DA, Stone GW, et al. Coronary angioplasty with or without stent implantation for acute myocardial infarction. *N Engl J Med* 1999;341:1949–1956.

Hochman JS, Boland J, Sleeper LA, et al., and the SHOCK Registry Investigators. Current spectrum of cardiogenic shock and effect of early revascularization on mortality. *Circulation* 1995;91:372–388.

Hochman JS, Sleeper LA, White HW, et al. One-year survival following early revascularization for cardiogenic shock. *JAMA* 2001;285:190–192.

Holmes DR, Bates EF, Kleiman NS, et al. Contemporary reperfusion therapy for cardiogenic shock: the GUSTO-I trial experience. *J Am Coll Cardiol* 1995;26:668–674.

Kandzari DE, Hasselblad V, Tcheng JE, et al. *Improved clinical outcomes with abciximab therapy in acute myocardial infarction: A systematic overview of randomized clinical trials.* Accepted for presentation at ACC 2003.

Kastrati A, Mehilli J, Dirschinger J, et al. Myocardial salvage after coronary stenting plus abciximab versus fibrinolysis plus abciximab in patients with acute myocardial infarction: a randomized trial. *Lancet* 2002;359:920–925.

Keeley EC, Boura JA, Grines CL. Comparison of primary and facilitated percutaneous coronary interventions for ST-elevation myocardial infarction: quantitative review of randomised trials. *Lancet* 367(9510):579–588.

Laarman GJ, Suttorp MJ, Dirksen MT, et al. Paclitaxeleluting versus uncoated stents in primary percutaneous coronary intervention. *N Engl J Med* 2006;355(11):1105–1113.

Lansky AJ, Stone GW. Percutaneous intervention for acute coronary syndromes. Eds: Safian, RD, Freed, MS. In: *The Manual of Interventional Cardiology*, 3rd Edition. Physicians' Press, Royal Oak, MI, 2001.

Lee L, Erbel R, Brown TM, et al. Multicenter registry of angioplasty therapy of cardiogenic shock: initial and long-term survival. *J Am Coll Cardiol* 1991;17:599–603.

Lemos PA, Lee CH, Degertekin M, et al. Early outcome after sirolimus-eluting stent implantation in patients with acute coronary syndromes: insights from the Rapamycin-Eluting Stent Evaluation at Rotterdam Cardiology Hospital (RESEARCH) registry. *J Am Coll Cardiol* 2003;41:2093–2099.

Maillard L, Hamon M, Khalife K, et al. A comparison of systematic stenting and conventional balloon angioplasty during primary percutaneous transluminal coronary angioplasty for acute myocardial infarction. *J Am Coll Cardiol* 2000;35:1729–1736.

Menichelli M, Parma A, Pucci E, et al. Randomized Trial of Sirolimus-Eluting Stent Versus Bare-Metal Stent in Acute Myocardial Infarction (SESAMI). *Journal of the American College of Cardiology* 2007;49(19):1924–1930.

Montalescot G, Barragan P, Wittenberg O, et al. Platelet glycoprotein IIb/IIIa inhibition with coronary stenting for acute myocardial infarction. *N Engl J Med* 2001;344:1895–1903.

Montalescot G, Wiviott SD, Braunwald E, et al. Prasugrel compared with clopidogrel in patients undergoing percutaneous coronary intervention for ST-elevation myocardial infarction (TRITON-TIMI 38): double-blind, randomised controlled trial. *Lancet* 2009;373(9665):723–731.

O'Neill WW, Erbel R, Laufer N, et al. Coronary angioplasty therapy of cardiogenic shock complicating acute myocardial infarction. *Circulation* 1995;72:III-309.

O'Neill WW, Martin JL, Dixon SR, et al. Acute Myocardial Infarction with Hyperoxemic Therapy (AMIHOT): A prospective, randomized trial of intracoronary hyperoxemic reperfusion after percutaneous coronary intervention. *Journal of the American College of Cardiology* 2007;50(5):397–405.

Piot C, Croisille P, Staat P, et al. Effect of cyclosporine on reperfusion injury in acute myocardial infarction. *N Engl J Med* 2008;359(5):473–481.

Saia F, Lemos PA, Lee CH, et al. Sirolimus-eluting stent implantation in ST-elevation acute myocardial infarction. *Circulation* 2003;108:1927–1929.

Saito S, Hosokawa G, Tanaka S, Nakamura S. Primary stem implantation is superior to balloon angioplasty in acute myocardial infarction: final results the primary angioplasty versus stent implantation in acute myocardial infarction (PASTA) trial. *Cathet Cardiovasc Intervent* 1999;48:262–268.

Spaulding C, Henry P, Teiger E, et al., the TI. Sirolimuseluting versus uncoated stents in acute myocardial infarction. *N Engl J Med* 2006;355(11):1093–1104.

Steinhubl SR, Berger PB, Mann JT III, et al. Early and sustained dual oral antiplatelet therapy following percutaneous coronary intervention. The CREDO trial. *JAMA* 2002;288:2411–2420.

Stone GW, Grines CL, Cox DA, et al. Comparison of angioplasty with stenting, with or without abciximab, in acute myocardial infarction. *N Engl J Med* 2002;346:957–966.

Stone GW, Lansky AJ, Pocock SJ, Gersh BJ, Dangas G, Wong SC, Witzenbichler B, Guagliumi G, Peruga JZ, Brodie BR, Dudek D, Möckel M, Ochala A, Kellock A, Parise H, Mehran R; HORIZONS-AMI Trial Investigators. Paclitaxel-eluting stents versus bare-metal stents in acute myocardial infarction. *N Engl J Med* 2009 May 7;360(19):1946–1959.

Stone GW, Witzenbichler B, Guagliumi G, et al., the H-AMITI. Bivalirudin during primary PCI in acute myocardial infarction. *N Engl J Med* 2008;358(21):2218–2230.

Svilaas T, Vlaar PJ, van der Horst IC, et al. Thrombus aspiration during primary percutaneous coronary intervention. *N Engl J Med* 2008;358(6):557–567.

Timmers L, Henriques JPS, de Kleijn DPV, et al. Exenatide reduces infarct size and improves cardiac function in a porcine model of ischemia and reperfusion injury. *Journal of the American College of Cardiology* 2009;53(6):501–510.

Valgimigli M, Campo G, Percoco G, et al., for the Multicentre Evaluation of Single High-Dose Bolus Tirofiban Versus Abciximab with Sirolimus-Eluting Stent or Bare Metal Stent in Acute Myocardial Infarction Study I. Comparison of angioplasty with infusion of tirofiban or abciximab with implantation of sirolimus-eluting or uncoated stents for acute myocardial infarction: MULTISTRATEGY Randomized Trial. *JAMA* 2008;299(15):1788–1799.

Vlaar PJ, Svilaas T, van der Horst IC, et al. Cardiac death and reinfarction after 1 year in the Thrombus Aspiration During Percutaneous Coronary Intervention in Acute Myocardial Infarction Study (TAPAS). A 1-year follow-up study. *Lancet* 2008;371(9628):1915–1920.

Zhu MM, Feit A, Chadow H, et al. Primary stent implantation compared with primary balloon angioplasty for acute myocardial infarction: a meta-analysis of randomized clinical trials. *American Journal of Cardiology* 2001;88(3):297–301.

Chapter 5

1SIS-3 (Third International Study of Infarct Survival) Collaborative Group. A randomized comparison of streptokinase vs. tissue plasminogen activator vs. anistreplase and of aspirin plus heparin vs. aspirin alone among 41,299 cases of suspected acute myocardial infarction: ISIS-3. *Lancet* 1992;339:753–770.

Adamian MG, Stone GW, Mehran R, et al. Have the outcomes of rescue angioplasty after failed thrombolytic therapy in acute myocardial infarction improved in the stent era? *J Am Coll Cardiol* 2002;39(Suppl A):309A.

Andersen HR. *Danish trial in acute myocardial infarction (DANAMI) 2*. Presented at American College of Cardiology Scientific Sessions, Atlanta, GA, March, 2002.

Anderson JL. Overview of patency as an endpoint of thrombolytic therapy. *Am J Cardiol* 1991;67:11–16E.

Antman EA, Anbe TD, Armstrong PW, et al. ACC/AHA Guidelines for the Management of Patients with ST-Elevation Myocardial Infarction—executive summary. *J Am Coll Cardiol* 2004;44:671–719. Full-text guidelines available at www.acc.org/clinical/guidelines/stemi/index.pdf.

Antman EM, Gibson CM, de Lemos JA, et al. Combination reperfusion therapy with abciximab and reduced dose reteplase: results from TIMI 14. The Thrombolysis in Myocardial Infarction (TIMI) 14 Investigators. *Eur Heart J* 2000;21:1944–1953.

Armstrong PW, Collen D. Fibrinolysis for acute myocardial infarction. *Circulation* 2001;103:2862–2866.

Antman EM, Louwerenburg HW, Baars HF, et al., for the E-TI. Enoxaparin as adjunctive antithrombin therapy for ST-elevation myocardial infarction: results of the ENTIRE Thrombolysis in Myocardial Infarction (TIMI) 23 Trial. *Circulation* 2002;105(14):1642–1649.

Antman EM, Morrow DA, McCabe CH, et al., for the ExTRACT-TIMI 25 investigators. Enoxaparin versus unfractionated heparin with fibrinolysis for ST-elevation myocardial infarction. *N Engl J Med* 2006;354:1477–1488.

ASSENT-2 Investigators. Single-bolus tenecteplase compared with front-loaded alteplase in acute myocardial infarction: the ASSENT-2 double blind randomized trial. *Lancet* 1999;354:716–722.

The Assessment of the Safety and Efficacy of a New Thrombolytic Regimen (ASSENT)-3 Investigators. Efficacy and safety of tenecteplase in combination with enoxaparin, abciximab, or unfractionated heparin: the ASSENT-3 randomized trial in acute myocardial infarction. *Lancet* 2001;358:605–613.

The Assessment of the Safety and Efficacy of a New Treatment Strategy with Percutaneous Couronary Intervention (ASSENT-4 PCI) Investigators. Primary versus tenecteplase-facilitated percutaneous coronary intervention in patients with ST-segment elevation acute myocardial infarction (ASSENT-4 PCI): randomised trial. *Lancet* 2006;367(9510):569–578.

Bonnefoy E, Lapostolle F, Leizorovicz A, et al. Primary angioplasty versus prehospital fibrinolysis in acute myocardial infarction: a randomised study. *Lancet* 2002;360(9336):825–829.

Chen ZM, Jiang LX, Chen YP, et al. Addition of clopidogrel to aspirin in 45,852 patients with acute myocardial infarction: randomised placebo-controlled trial. *Lancet* 2005;366(9497):1607–1621.

The CORAMI Study Group. Outcome of attempted rescue coronary angioplasty after failed thrombolysis for acute myocardial infarction. *Am J Cardiol* 1994;74:172–174.

Dalby M, Bouzamondo A, Lechat P, et al. Transfer for primary angioplasty versus immediate thrombolysis in acute myocardial infarction: a meta-analysis. *Circulation* 2003;108:1809–1814.

Davies MJ, Thomas AC. Plaque fissuring: the cause of acute myocardial infarction, sudden ischaemic death, and crescendo angina. *Br Heart J* 1985;53:363–373.

Di Mario C, Dudek D, Piscione F, et al. Immediate angioplasty versus standard therapy with rescue angioplasty after thrombolysis in the Combined Abciximab REteplase Stent Study in Acute Myocardial Infarction (CARESS-in-AMI): an open, prospective, randomised, multicentre trial. *Lancet* 2008;371(9612):559–568.

Dubois CL, Belmans A, Granger CB, et al. Outcome of urgent and elective percutaneous coronary interventions after pharmacologic reperfusion with tenecteplase combined with unfractionated heparin, enoxaparin, or abciximab. *J Am Coll Cardiol* 2003;42:1178–1185.

Ellis SG, Ribeiro da Silva E, Heyndrickx G, et al. Randomized comparison of rescue angioplasty with conservative management of patients with early failure of thrombolysis for acute anterior myocardial infarction. *Circulation* 1994;90:2280–2284.

Ellis SG, Tendera M, de Belder MA, et al., the FI. Facilitated PCI in patients with ST-elevation myocardial infarction. *N Engl J Med* 2008;358(21):2205–2217.

Fernandcz-Aviles F, Alonso JJ, Castro-Beiras AC, et al. Routine invasive strategy within 24 hours of thrombolysis versus ischaemia-guided conservative approach for acute myocardial infarction with ST-segment elevation (GRACIA-1): a randomised controlled trial. *Lancet* 2004;364:1045–1053.

Galvani M, Ottani F, Ferrini D, et al. Patency of the infarct-related artery and left ventricular function as the major determinants of survival after Q-wave acute myocardial infarction. *Am J Cardiol* 1993;71:1–7.

Gershlick A. Presented at the American Heart Association Meeting, November, 2004, New Orleans, LA.

Gibson CM, Cannon CP, Piana RN, et al. Rescue PTCA in the TIMI 4 trial. *J Am Coll Cardiol* 1994;1A–48A:225A.

Giugliano RP, Roe MT, Harrington RA, et al. Combination reperfusion therapy with eptifibatide and reduced-dose tenecteplase for ST-elevation myocardial infarction. *J Am Coll Cardiol* 2003;41:1251–1260.

The GUSTO investigators. An international randomized trial comparing four thrombolytic strategies for acute myocardial infarction. *N Engl J Med* 1993;329:673–682.

The GUSTO V Investigators. Reperfusion therapy for acute myocardial infarction with fibrinolytic therapy or combination reduced fibrinolytic therapy and platelet glycoprotein IIb/IIIa inhibition: the GUSTO V randomized trial. *Lancet* 2001;357:1905–1914.

The GUSTO III Investigators. A comparison of reteplase with alteplase for acute myocardial infarction. *N Engl J Med* 1997;337:1124–1130.

Herrmann HC, Moliterno DJ, Ohman EM, et al. Facilitation of early percutaneous coronary intervention after reteplase with or without abciximab in acute myocardial infarction: results from the SPEED (GUSTO-4 Pilot) trial. *J Am Coll Cardiol* 2000;36:1489–1496.

The Hirulog and Early Reperfusion or Occlusion (HERO)-2 Trial Investigators. Thrombin-specific anticoagulation with bivalirudin versus heparin in patients receiving fibrinolytic therapy for acute myocardial infarction: the HERO-2 randomized trial. *Lancet* 2001; 358:1855–1863.

Hochman JS, Lamas GA, Buller CE, et al., for the Occluded Artery Trial I. Coronary intervention for persistent occlusion after myocardial infarction. *N Engl J Med* 2006;355(23):2395–2407.

Ito H, Okamura A, Iwakura K, et al. Myocardial perfusion patterns related to thrombolysis in myocardial infarction perfusion grades after coronary angioplasty in patients with acute anterior wall myocardial infarction. *Circulation* 1996;93:1993–1999.

Kleiman N, Ohman E, et al. Profound inhibition of platelet aggregation with monoclonal antibody 7E3Fab after thrombolytic therapy: results from the Thrombolysis and Angioplasty in myocardial infarction (TAMI) 8 pilot study. *J Am Coll Cardiol* 1993;22:381–389.

Madsen J, Grande P, et al. Danish multi-center randomized study of invasive versus conservative treatment in patients with inducible ischemia after thrombolysis in acute myocardial infarction (DANAM1). *Circulation* 1997;96:748–755.

Maggioni AP, Franzosi MG, Santoro E, et al. The risk of stroke in patients with acute myocardial infarction after thrombolytic and antithrombotic treatment. Gruppo italiano per lo Studio della Sopravvivenza nell'Infarto Miocardico II (GISSI-2), and The International Study Group. *N Engl J Med* 1992;327:1–6.

McKendall GR, Antman EM, Braunwald E, et al. What is the clinical outcome and impact of revascularization of TIMI 2 flow following acute myocardial infarction? *J Am Coll Cardiol* 1997;29:389A.

Miller JM, Smalling R, Ohman EM, Bode C, Betriu A, Kleiman NS, Schildcrout JS, Bastos E, Topol EJ, Califf RM. Effectiveness of early coronary angioplasty and abciximab for failed thrombolysis (reteplase or alteplase) during acute myocardial infarction (results from the GUSTO-III trial). Global Use of Strategies To Open occluded coronary arteries. *Am J Cardiol* 1999;84:779–784.

Ohman E, Kleiman N, et al. Combined accelerated tissue plasminogen activator and platelet glycoprotein IIb/IIIa integrin receptor blockade in acute myocardial infarction: results of a randomized placebo controlled dose ranging trial. *Circulation* 1997;95:846–854.

The PARADIGM Investigators. Combined thrombolysis with the platelet glycoprotein IIb/IIIa inhibitor lamifiban: results of the platelet aggregation receptor antagonist dose investigation and reperfusion gain in myocardial infarction (PARADIGM) trial. *J Am Coll Cardiol* 1998;32:2003–2010.

Rogers WJ, Baim DS, Fore JM, et al., for the TIMI-IIA investigators. Comparison of immediate invasive, delayed invasive, and conservative strategies after tissue-type plasminogen activator. *Circulation* 1990;81: 1457–1476.

Ross AM, Coyne KS, Reiner JS, et al. A randomized trial comparing primary angioplasty with a strategy of short acting thrombolysis and immediate planned rescue angioplasty in acute myocardial infarction: the PACT trial. *J Am Coll Cardiol* 1999;34:1954–1962.

Ross AM, Reiner JS, Thompson MA, et al. Immediate and follow-up procedural outcome of 214 patients undergoing rescue PTCA in the GUSTO trial: no effect of the lytic agent. *Circulation* 1993;88(Suppl I):I-410(abstr.).

Sabatine MS, Cannon CP, Gibson CM, et al., the C-TI. Addition of clopidogrel to aspirin and fibrinolytic therapy for myocardial infarction with ST-segment elevation. *N Engl J Med* 2005;352(12):1179–1189.

Simoons ML, Arnold AET, Bertriu A, et al. Thrombolysis with tissue plasminogen activator in acute myocardial infarction: no additional benefit from immediate percutaneous coronary angioplasty. *Lancet* 1988;1:197–202.

Stone GW, Lansky AJ, Pocock SJ, Gersh BJ, et al. Paclitaxel-eluting stents versus bare-metal stents in acute myocardial infarction. HORIZONS-AMI Trial Investigators. *N Engl J Med* 2009 May 7;360(19):1946–1959.

Suttan AG, Campbell PG, Graham R, et al. A randomized trial of rescue angioplasty versus a conservative appeal for failed fibrinolysis in ST-segment elevation myocardial infarction: the Middlesbrough Early Revascularization to Limit Infarction (MERLIN) trial.

Topol E, Ohman EM, Armstrong PW, et al., for the GUSTO III Investigators. Survival outcomes one year after reperfusion therapy with either alteplase or reteplase for AMI: results from GUSTO III trial. *Circulation* 2000;102:1761–1765.

Topol EJ, Califf RM, George BS, et al., and the Thrombolysis and Angioplasty in Myocardial Infarction Study Group. A randomized trial of immediate versus delayed elective angioplasty after intravenous tissue plasminogen activator in acute myocardial infarction. *N Engl J Med* 1987;317:581–588.

Topol EJ, Califf RM, Vandormael M, et al., and the Thrombolysis and Angioplasty in Myocardial Infarction-6 Study Group. A randomized trial of late reperfusion therapy for acute myocardial infarction. *Circulation* 1992;85:2090–2099.

Topol EJ, Ohman EM, Armstrong PW, et al. Survival outcomes 1 year after reperfusion therapy with either alteplase or reteplase for acute myocardial infarction: results from the Global Utilization of Streptokinase and t-PA for Occluded Coronary Arteries (GUSTO) III Trial. *Circulation* 2000;102:1761–1765.

Van de Werf F. Discrepancies between the effects of coronary reperfusion on survival and left ventricular function. *Lancet* 1989;I:1367–1369.

Widimsky P, Groch L, Zelizko M, et al. Multicentre randomized trial comparing transport to primary angioplasty vs. immediate thrombolysis vs. combined strategy for patients with acute myocardial infarction presenting to a community hospital without a catheterization laboratory: the PRAGUE study. *Eur Heart J* 2000;21:823–831.

Widminsky P. *PRAGUE-2 study.* Presented at the European Society of Cardiology meeting, Berlin, Germany, Sept. 2002.

Wnqk A, Krupa H, Gasior M, et al. *Results of rescue-angioplasty after unsuccessful intracoronary streptokinase therapy in patients with acute myocardial infarction.* European Congress of Cardiology, abstract, 1995.

Yusuf, S. Presented at the American Heart Association Meeting, November, 2004, New Orleans, LA.

Zeymer U, Ubis R, Vogt A, et al. Randomized comparison of percutaneous transluminal angioplasty and medical therapy in stable survivors of acute myocardial infarction with single vessel disease: a study of ALKK. *Circulation* 2003;108:1324–1328.

Zijlstra F, Patel A, Jones M, et al. Clinical characteristics and outcome of patients with early (<2 h), intermediate (2–4 h) and late (>4 h) presentation treated by primary coronary angioplasty or thrombolytic therapy for acute myocardial infarction. *Eur Heart J* 2002;23:550–557.

Chapter 6

Antman EM, Cohen M, Bernink PJ , et al. The TIMI risk score for unstable angina/non-ST-elevation MI: a method for prognostication and therapeutic decision making. *JAMA* 2000;284:835–842.

Antman EM, Tanasijevic MJ, Thompson B, et al. Cardiac-specific troponin I levels to predict the risk of mortality in patients with acute coronary syndromes. *N Engl J Med* 1996;335:1342–1349.

Anderson JL, Adams CD, Antman EM , et al. ACC/AHA 2007 guidelines for the management of patients with unstable angina/non-ST-elevation myocardial infarction: a report of the American College of Cardiology/American Heart Association Task Force on Practice Guidelines (Writing Committee to Revise the 2002 Guidelines for the Management of Patients with Unstable Angina/Non-ST-Elevation Myocardial Infarction) developed in collaboration with the American College of Emergency Physicians, the Society for Cardiovascular Angiography and Interventions, and the Society of Thoracic Surgeons endorsed by the American Association of Cardiovascular and Pulmonary Rehabilitation and the Society for Academic Emergency Medicine. *J Am Coll Cardiol* 2007;50:e1–e157.

Braunwald E. Unstable angina classification. *Circulation* 1989;80:410–414.

Cannon CP, McCabe CH, Stone PH, et al. The electrocardiogram predicts one-year outcome of patients with unstable angina and non-Q wave myocardial infarction: results of the TIMI III registry ECG ancillary study. *J Am Coll Cardiol* 1997;30:133–140.

de Zwaan C, Bar FW, Janssen JH, et al. Angiographic and clinical characteristics of patients with unstable angina showing an ECG pattern indicating critical narrowing of the proximal LAD coronary artery. *Am Heart J* 1989;117:657–665.

Eagle KA, Lim MJ, Dabbous OH , et al. A validated prediction model for all forms of acute coronary syndrome: estimating the risk of 6-month postdischarge death in an international registry. *JAMA* 2004;291:2727–2733.

The ECG Criteria Book. Eds: O'Keefe J, Hammill S, Freed M, Pogwizd S. Physicians' Press, Royal Oak, MI, 2002.

Galvani M, Ottani F, Ferrini D, et al. Prognostic influence of elevated values of cardiac troponin I in patients with unstable angina. *Circulation* 1997;95:2053–2059.

Hamm CW, Heeschen C, Goldmann B, et al. Benefit of abciximab in patients with refractory unstable angina in relation to serum troponin levels. *N Engl J Med* 1999;340:1623–1629.

Heeschen C, Hamm CW, Goldmann B. Troponin concentrations for stratification of patients with acute coronary syndromes in relation to therapeutic efficacy of tirofiban. *Lancet* 1999;354:1757–1762.

Heidenreich PA, Alloggiamento T, Melsop K, et al. The prognostic value of troponin in patients with non-ST-elevation acute coronary syndromes: a meta-analysis. *J Am Coll Cardiol* 2001;38:478–485.

Morrow DA, Cannon CP, Nader R, et al., for the TACTICS-TIMI 18 Investigators. Ability of minor elevations of troponins I and T to predict benefit from an early invasive strategy in patients with unstable angina and non-ST-elevation myocardial infarction. *JAMA* 2001;286:2405–2412.

Ohman EM, Armstrong PW, Christenson RH, for the GUSTO IIA Investigators. Cardiac troponin T levels for risk stratification in acute myocardial ischemia. *N Engl J Med* 1996;335:1333–1341.

Pettijohn TL, Doyle T, Spiekerman AM, et al. Usefulness of positive troponin-T and negative creatine kinase levels in identifying high-risk patients with unstable angina pectoris. *Am J Cardiol* 1997;80:510–511.

Roberts R, Fromm RE. Management of acute coronary syndromes based on risk stratification by biochemical markers: an idea whose time has come. *Circulation* 1998;98:1831–1833.

Ryan TJ, Anderson JL, Antman EM, Braniff BA, et al. ACC/AHA guidelines for the management of patients with acute myocardial infarction: a report of the American College of Cardiology/American Heart Association Task Force on Practice Guidelines (Committee on Management of Acute Myocardial Infarction). *J Am Coll Cardiol* 1996;28:1328–1428.

Slater DK, Hlatky MA, Mark DB, et al. Outcome in suspected acute myocardial infarction with normal or minimally abnormal admission electrocardiographic findings. *Am J Cardiol* 1987;60:766–770.

Chapter 7

American Diabetes Association. Standards of medical care for patients with diabetes mellitus. *Diabetes Care* 2000;23(Suppl 1):S32–S42.

Anderson JL, Adams CD, Antman EM , et al. ACC/AHA 2007 guidelines for the management of patients with unstable angina/non-ST-elevation myocardial infarction: a report of the American College of Cardiology/American Heart Association Task Force on Practice Guidelines (Writing Committee to Revise the 2002 Guidelines for the Management of Patients with Unstable Angina/Non-ST-Elevation Myocardial Infarction) developed in collaboration with the American College of Emergency Physicians, the Society for Cardiovascular Angiography and Interventions, and the Society of Thoracic Surgeons endorsed by the American Association of Cardiovascular and Pulmonary Rehabilitation and the Society for Academic Emergency Medicine. *J Am Coll Cardiol* 2007;50:e1–e157.

Antiplatelet Trialists' Collaboration. Collaborative overview of randomized trials of antiplatelet therapy, I: prevention of death, myocardial infarction, and stroke by prolonged antiplatelet therapy in various categories of patients. *BMJ* 1994;308:81–106.

Antiplatelet Trialists' Collaboration. Secondary prevention of vascular disease by prolonged antiplatelet treatment. *BMJ* (Clin Res Ed) 1988;296:320–331.

Berger PB, Steinhubl S. Clinical implications of percutaneous coronary intervention-clopidogrel in unstable angina to prevent recurrent events (PCICURE) study: A US perspective. *Circulation* 2002;106:2284–2287.

Cannon CP, Braunwald E, McCabe CH, et al. Comparison of intensive and moderate lipid lowering with statins after acute coronary syndromes. *N Engl J Med* 2004;350.

Cannon CP, Weintraub WS, Demopoulos LA, et al. Comparison of early invasive and conservative strategies in patients with unstable coronary syndromes treated with the glycoprotein IIb/IIIa inhibitor tirofiban. *N Engl J Med* 2001;344:1879–1887.

The CAPTURE Investigators. Randomized placebo-controlled trial of abciximab before and during coronary intervention in refractory unstable angina: the CAPTURE study. *Lancet* 1997;349:2429–2435.

Cheithn ME, Hutter AM, Brindis RG, et al. Use of sildenafil (Viagra) in patients with cardiovascular disease. AHA/ACC expert consensus document. *J Am Coll Cardiol* 1999;33:273–482.

The EPISTENT Investigators. Randomized placebo-controlled and balloon-angioplasty-controlled trial to assess safety of coronary stenting with use of platelet glycoprotein IIb/IIIa blockade. *Lancet* 1998;352: 87–92.

Fox et al. Efficacy of perindopril in reduction of cardiovascular events among patients with stable coronary artery disease (the EUROPA study). *Lancet* 2003;362:782–788.

Fox KA. Mehta SA, Peters R, et al. Benefits and risks of the combination of clopidogrel and aspirin in patients undergoing surgical revascularization for non-ST-elevation acute coronary syndrome. *Circulation* 2004;110:1202–1208.

Gibbons RJ, Chatterjee K, Daley J, et al. ACC/AHA/ACP-ASIM guidelines for the management of patients with chronic stable angina. *J Am Coll Cardiol* 1999;33:2092–2197.

Gibson CM, Goel M, Cohen DJ, et al. Six-month angiographic and clinical follow-up of patients prospectively randomized to receive either tirofiban or placebo during angioplasty in the RESTORE trial. *J Am Coll Cardiol* 1998;32:28–34.

Hambrecht R, Neibauer J, Marburger C, et al. Various intensities of leisure time physical activity in patients with coronary artery disease: effects on cardiorespiratory fitness and progression of coronary atherosclerotic lesions. *J Am Coll Cardiol* 1993;22:468–477.

The Heart Outcomes Prevention Evaluation Study Investigators. Effects of an angiotensin-coverting-enzyme inhibitor, ramipril, on cardiovascular events in high-risk patients. *N Engl J Med* 2000;342:145–153.

The IMPACT-II Investigators. Randomized placebo-controlled trial of effect of eptifibatide on complications of percutaneous coronary intervention: IMPACT-II. *Lancet* 1997;349:1422–1428.

Kris-Etherton P, Eckel RH, Howard BV, et al. Lyon diet heart study. Benefits of a Mediterranean-style, National Cholesterol Education Program/American Heart Association Step I dietary pattern on cardiovascular disease. *Circulation* 2001;103:1823–1825.

Krumholtz HM, Cohen BJ, Tsevat J, et al. Cost-effectiveness of a smoking cessation program after myocardial infarction. *J Am Coll Cardiol* 1993;22:1697–1702.

Mori TA, Beilin LJ, Burke V, et al. Interactions between dietary fat, fish, and fish oils and their effects on platelet function in men at risk of cardiovascular disease. *Arterioscler Thromb Vasc Biol* 1997;17:279–286.

NCEP Report. Implications of recent clinical trials for the National Cholesterol Education Program Adult Treatment Panel III Guidelines. *Circulation* 2004;110:227–239.

O'Connor GT, Burning JE, Yusuf S, et al. An overview of randomized trials of rehabilitation with exercise after myocardial infarction. *Circulation* 1989;80: 234–244.

O'Shea JC, Buller CE, Cantor WJ, et al. Long-term efficacy of platelet glycoprotein IIb/IIIa integrin blockade with eptifibatide in coronary stent intervention. *JAMA* 2002;287:618–621.

Oldridge NB, Guyatt GH, Fischer ME, et al. Cardiac rehabilitation after myocardial infarction: combined experience of randomized clinical trials. *JAMA* 1988;260:945–950.

The PURSUIT Trial Investigators. Inhibition of platelet glycoprotein IIb/IIIa with eptifibatide in patients with acute coronary syndromes. *N Eng J Med* 1998;339:436–443.

Randomised trial of cholesterol lowering in 4444 patients with coronary heart disease: the Scandinavian Simvastatin Survival Study (4S). *Lancet* 1994; 344:1383–1389.

Report of The Holland Interuniversity Nifedipine/Metoprolol Trial (HINT) Research Group. Early treatment of unstable angina in the coronary care unit: a randomized, double blind, placebo controlled comparison of recurrent ischemia in patients treated with nifedipine or metoprolol or both. *Br Heart J* 1986;56:400–413.

The RESTORE Investigators. Effects of platelet glycoprotein IIb/IIIa blockade with tirofiban on adverse cardiac event in patients with unstable angina or acute myocardial infarction undergoing coronary angioplasty. *Circulation* 1997;96:1445–1453.

Rosengren A, Hawken S, Ounpuu S, et al. Association of psychosocial risk factors with risk of acute myocardial infarction in 11,119 cases and 13,648 controls from 52 countries (the INTERHEART) study: case-controlled study. *Lancet* 2004.

Sixth Report of the Joint National Committee on Detection, Evaluation, and Treatment of High Blood Pressure (JNC VI). *Arch Intern Med* 1997;157:2413–446.

Smith SC, Blair SN, Bonow RO, et al. AHA/ACC guidelines for preventing heart attack and death in patients with atherosclerotic cardiovascular disease: 2001 update; a statement for health care professionals from the American Heart Association and the American College of Cardiology. *J Am Coll Cardiol* 2001;38:1581–1583.

Stone GW, Moliterno DJ, Bertrand M, et al. Impact of clinical syndrome acuity on the differential response to 2 glycoprotein IIb/IIIa inhibitors in patients undergoing coronary stenting: the TARGET Trial. *Circulation* 2002;105:2347–2354.

TIMI IIIB Trial Investigators. Effects of tissue plasminogen activator and a comparison of early invasive and conservative strategies in unstable angina and non-Q-wave myocardial infarction. Results of the TIMI IIIB trial. *Circulation* 1994;89:1545–1556.

Timolol-induced reduction in mortality and reinfarction in patients surviving acute myocardial infarction. *N Engl J Med* 1981;304:801–807.

Yusuf S, Mehta SR, Chrolavicius S, et al. Comparison of fondaparinux and enoxaparin in acute coronary syndromes. *N Engl J Med* 2006;354(14):1464–1476.

Chapter 8

Anstrom KJ, Kong DF, Shaw LK , et al. Long-term clinical outcomes following coronary stenting. *Arch Intern Med* 2008;168:1647–1655.

Blazing MA, de Lemos JA, White HD, et al. Safety and efficacy of enoxaparin vs. unfractionated heparin in patients with non-ST-segment elevation acute coronary syndromes who receive tirofiban and aspirin: a randomized controlled trial. *JAMA* 2004;292:55–64.

Boden W. O'Rourke R, et al. Outcomes in patients with acute non-Q-wave myocardial infarction randomly assigned to an invasive as compared with a conservative management strategy. *N Engl J Med* 1998;338:1785–1792.

Cannon CP, Weintraub WS, Demopoulos LA, et al. Comparison of early invasive and conservative strategies in patients with unstable coronary syndromes treated with the glycoprotein IIb/IIIA inhibitor tirofiban. *N Engl J Med* 2001;344:1879–1887.

The CAPTURE Investigators. Randomized placebo-controlled trial of abciximab before and during coronary intervention in refractory unstable angina: the CAPTURE study. *Lancet* 1997;349:2429–2435.

Eisenstein EL, Anstrom KJ, Kong DF , et al. Clopidogrel use and long-term clinical outcomes after drug-eluting stent implantation. *JAMA* 2007;297:159–168.

The EPISTENT Investigators. Randomized placebo-controlled and balloon-angioplasty-controlled trial to assess safety of coronary stenting with use of platelet glycoprotein IIb/IIIa blockade. *Lancet* 1998;352:87–92.

Fox KA, Poole-Wilson PA, Henderson RA, et al. Interventional versus conservative treatment for patients with unstable angina or non-ST-elevation myocardial infarction: the British Heart Foundation RITA 3 randomized trial. *Lancet* 2002;360:743–751.

Fragmin and Fast Revascularization during Instability in Coronary artery disease (FRISC II) Investigators. Long-term low-molecular-mass heparin in unstable coronary-artery disease: FRISC II prospective randomized multicenter study. *Lancet* 1999;354:701–707.

Gibbons RJ, Chatterjee K, Daley J, et al. ACC/AHA/ACP-ASIM guidelines for the management of patients with chronic stable angina. *J Am Coll Cardiol* 1999;33:2092–2197.

Gibson CM, Goel M, Cohen DJ, et al. Six-month angiographic and clinical follow-up of patients prospectively randomized to receive either tirofiban or placebo during angioplasty in the RESTORE trial. *J Am Coll Cardiol* 1998;32:28–34.

Giugliano RP, White JA, Bode C , et al. Early versus delayed, provisional eptifi batide in acute coronary syndromes. *N Engl J Med* 2009;360(21):2237–2240.

Glaser R, Herrmann HC, Murphy SA, et al. Benefit of an early invasive management strategy in women with acute coronary syndromes. *JAMA* 2002;288: 3124–3129.

The IMPACT-II Investigators. Randomized placebo-controlled trial of effect of eptifibatide on complications of percutaneous coronary intervention: IMPACT-II. *Lancet* 1997;349:1422–1428.

Lagerqvist B, Husted S, Kontny F, et al. Long-term perspective on the protective effects of an early invasive strategy in unstable coronary disease. Two-year follow-up of the FRISC-II invasive study. *J Am Coll Cardiol* 2002;40:1902–1914.

Neumann FJ, Kastrati A, Pogatsa-Murray G, et al. Evaluation of prolonged antithrombotic pretreatment ('cooling-off' strategy) before intervention in patients with unstable coronary syndromes: a randomized controlled trial. *JAMA* 2003;290;1593–1599.

O'Shea JC, Buller CE, Cantor WJ, et al. Long-term efficacy of platelet glycoprotein IIb/IIIa integrin blockade with eptifibatide in coronary stent intervention. *JAMA* 2002;287:618–621.

Pfisterer M, Brunner-La Rocca HP, Buser PT , et al. Late clinical events after clopidogrel discontinuation may limit the benefit of drug-eluting stents: an observational study of drug-eluting versus bare-metal stents. *J Am Coll Cardiol* 2006;48:2584–2591.

PRISM-PLUS Study Investigators. Inhibition of the platelet glycoprotein IIb/IIIa receptor with tirofiban in unstable angina and non-Q-wave myocardial infarction. *N Engl J Med* 1998;338:1488–1497.

The PURSUIT Trial Investigators. Inhibition of platelet glycoprotein IIb/IIIa with eptifibatide in patients with acute coronary syndromes. *N Eng J Med* 1998; 339:436–443.

The RESTORE Investigators. Effects of platelet glycoprotein IIb/IIIa blockade with tirofiban on adverse cardiac event in patients with unstable angina or acute myocardial infarction undergoing coronary angioplasty. *Circulation* 1997;96:1445–1453.

Singh M, Holmes DR, Garratt KN, et al. Stents versus conventional PTCA in unstable angina. *J Am Coll Cardiol* 1999;33–29A.

Stone GW, Moliterno DJ, Bertrand M, et al. Impact of clinical syndrome acuity on the differential response to 2 glycoprotein IIb/IIIa inhibitors in patients undergoing coronary stenting: the TARGET Trial. *Circulation* 2002;105:2347–2354.

TIMI-3B Investigators. Effects of tissue plasminogen activator and a comparison of early invasive and conservative strategies in unstable angina and non-Q-wave myocardial infarction. *Circulation* 1994;89:1545–1556.

Topol EJ, Mark DB, Lincoff AM, et al. Outcomes at 1 year and economic implications of platelet glycoprotein IIb/IIIa blockade in patients undergoing coronary stenting: results from a multicenter randomized trial. EPISTENT Investigators. Evaluation of platelet IIb/IIIa inhibitor for stenting. *Lancet* 1999;354:2019–2024.

Chapter 9

Alexander JH, Ohman EM, Harrington RA. Platelet GP IIb/IIIa inhibitors in acute MI: pathophysiology and clinical effects. *Acute Coronary Syndromes* 1998;1:46–51.

Alvarez JM. Emergency coronary bypass grafting for failed percutaneous coronary artery stenting: increased costs and platelet transfusion requirements after the use of abciximab. *J Thorac Cardiovasc Surg* 1998;115:472–473.

Antman EM, Cohen M, McCabe C, et al., for the TIMI 11B and ESSENCE Investigators. Enoxaparin is superior to unfractionated heparin for preventing clinical events at 1-year follow-up of TIMI 11B and ESSENCE. *Eur Heart J* 2002;23:308–314.

Antman EM, Cohen M, Radley D, et al. Assessment of the treatment effect of enoxaparin for unstable angina/non-Q-wave myocardial infarction. TIMI 11B-ESSENCE meta-analysis. *Circulation* 1999;100:1602–1608.

Antman EM, McCabe CH, Gurfinkel EP, et al. Enoxaparin prevents death and cardiac ischemic events in unstable angina/non-Q-wave myocardial infarction: results of the Thrombolysis In Myocardial Infarction (TIMI) 11B trial. *Circulation* 1999;100:1593–1601.

Antman EM. The search for replacements for unfractionated heparin. *Circulation* 2001;103:2310–2314.

Ballantyne CM, Blasing MA, King TR, et al. Efficacy and safety of ezetimibe co-administered with simvastatin compared with atorvastatin in adults with hypercholesterolemia. *Am J Cardiol* 2004;93:1487–1494.

Beinart S, Kolm P, Veledar E, et al. *Short and long-term cost effectiveness of early and sustained dual oral antiplatelet therapy with clopidogrel following percutaneous coronary intervention: Results from CREDO.* American Heart Association Scientific Sessions 203. Abstract 3495.

Bennett CL, Connors JM, Carwile JM, et al. Thrombotic thrombocytopenia purpura associated with clopidogrel. *N Engl J Med* 2000;342(24):1773–1777.

Bennett CL, Weinberg PD, Rozenberg-Ben-Dror K, et al. Thrombotic thrombocytopenia purpura associated with ticlopidine: a review of 60 cases. *Ann Intern Med* 1998;128:541–544.

Bertrand ME, Rupprecht H-J, Urban P, et al., for the CLASSICS Investigators. Double-blind study of the safety of clopidogrel with and without a loading dose in combination with aspirin compared with ticlopidine in combination with aspirin after coronary stenting. The Clopidogrel Aspirin Stent International Cooperative Study (CLASSICS). *Circulation* 2000;102:642–629.

Bhatt DL. Presented at the American Heart Association meeting, Anaheim, CA, November, 2001.

Bhatt DL, Fox KA, Hacke W, et al. Clopidogrel and aspirin versus aspirin alone for the prevention of atherothrombotic events. *N Engl J Med* 2006;354(16):1706–1717.

Bijsterveld NR, Peters RJ, Murphy SA, et al. Recurrent cardiac ischemic events early after discontinuation of short-term heparin treatment in acute coronary syndromes. *J Am Coll Cardiol* 2003;42:2083–2089.

Blazing MA, de Lemos JA, White HD, et al. Safety and efficacy of enoxaparin vs. unfractionated heparin in patients with non-ST-segment elevation acute coronary syndromes who receive tirofiban and aspirin: a randomized controlled trial. *JAMA* 2004;292:55–64.

Boersma E, Harrington RA, Moliterno DJ, et al. Platelet glycoprotein IIb/IIIa inhibitors in acute coronary syndromes: a meta-analysis of all major randomised clinical trials. *Lancet* 2002;359:189–198.

Boneu B, Destelle G. Platelet anti-aggregating activity and tolerance of clopidogrel in atherosclerotic patients. *Thromb Haemost* 1996;76:939–943.

Cannon CP, Antman EM, Crawford MH. Heparin and low-molecular-weight heparin in acute coronary syndromes and angioplasty. In: Crawford MH, editor. *Cardiology Clinics: Annual of Drug Therapy.* Philadelphia: WB Saunders;1997;105–119.

Cannon CP, Braunwald E, McCabe CH, et al. Comparison of intensive and moderate lipid lowering with statins after acute coronary syndromes. *N Engl J Med* 2004;350.

The CAPRIE steering committee. A randomized blinded trial of clopidogrel versus aspirin in patients at risk of ischemic events. (CAPRIE) *Lancet* 1996;348:1329–1339.

The CAPTURE Investigators. Randomized placebo-controlled trial of abciximab before and during coronary intervention in refractory unstable angina: the CAPTURE study. *Lancet* 1997;349:2429–2435.

Cohen M, Demers C, Gurfinkel EP, et al., for the Efficacy and Safety of Subcutaneous Enoxaparin in Non-Q-Wave Coronary Events Study Group. A comparison of low-molecular-weight heparin with unfractionated heparin for unstable coronary artery disease. *N Engl J Med* 1997;337:447–452.

Cohen M. Initial experience with the low-molecular-weight heparin, enoxaparin, in combination with the platelet glycoprotein IIb/IIIa blocker, tirofiban, in patients with non-ST segment elevation acute coronary syndromes. *J Invasive Cardiol* 2000;12 (Suppl E):E5–E9; discussion E25–E28.

Coller BS. Potential non-glycoprotein IIb/IIIa effects of abciximab. *Am Heart J* 1999;138:S1–S5.

Dalli E, Martinez A, Herrera G, et al. *Platelet P-selectin expression after clopidogrel discontinuation in stenting patients.* Presented at American Heart Association Scientific Session, abstract 2603, November 2003, Orlando, FL.

Direct Thrombin Inhibitor Trialists' Collaborative Group. Direct thrombin inhibitors in acute coronary syndromes: principal results of a meta-analysis based on individual patients' data. *Lancet* 2002;359:294–302.

The EPIC Investigators. Use of a monoclonal antibody directed against the platelet glycoprotein IIb/IIIa receptor in high-risk coronary angioplasty. *N Engl J Med* 1994;330:956–961.

The EPILOG Investigators. Platelet glycoprotein IIb/IIIa receptor blockade and low-dose heparin during percutaneous coronary revascularization. *N Engl J Med* 1997;336:1689–1696.

The EPISTENT Investigators. Randomized placebo-controlled and balloon-angioplasty-controlled trial to assess safety of coronary stenting with use of platelet glycoprotein IIb/IIIa blockade. *Lancet* 1998;352:87–92.

Fareed J, Hoppensteadt DA, Bick RL. An update on heparins at the beginning of the new millenium. *Semin Thromb Hemost* 2000;26:5–21.

Ferguson JJ, Califf RM, Antman EM, et al. Enoxaparin vs. unfractionated heparin in high-risk patients with non-ST segment elevation acute coronary syndromes managed with an intended early invasive strategy: primary results of the SYNERGY randomized trial. *JAMA* 2004;292:45–54.

Ferguson JJ. Combining low-molecular-weight heparin and glycoprotein IIb/IIIa antagonists for the treatment of acute coronary syndromes: the NICE 3 story. National Investigators Collaborating on Enoxaparin. *J Invasive Cardiol* 2000;12(Suppl E):E10–E13; discussion E25–E28.

Fourth American College of Chest Physicians Consensus Conference on Antithrombotic Therapy. *Chest* 1995; 108(suppl):225S–522S.

Fox KA, Mehta SA, Peters R, et al. Benefits and risks of the combination of clopidogrel and aspirin in patients undergoing surgical revascularization for non-ST-elevation acute coronary syndrome. *Circulation* 2004;110:1202–1208.

FRAXIS Study Group. Comparison of two treatment durations (6 days and 14 days) of a low molecular weight heparin with a 6-day treatment of unfractionated heparin in the initial management of unstable angina or non-Q-wave myocardial infarction: FRAXIS (Fraxiparine in Ischaemic Syndrome). *Eur Heart J* 1999;20:1553–1562.

Gammie JS, Zenati M, Kormos RL, et al. Abciximab and excessive bleeding in patients undergoing emergency cardiac operations. *Ann Thorac Surg* 1998;65:465–469.

Greinacher A, Lubenow N. Recombinant hirudin in clinical practice: focus on lepirudin. *Circulation* 2001;103:1479–1484.

Gum PA, Kottke-Marchant K, Poggio ED, et al. Profile and prevalence of aspirin resistance among patients with heart disease: a prospective, comprehensive assessment. *Circulation* 2000;18:II-418.

Harrington RA, Kleiman NS, Kottke-Marchant K, et al. Immediate and reversible platelet inhibition after intravenous administration of a peptide glycoprotein IIb/IIIa inhibitor during percutaneous coronary intervention. *Am J Cardiol* 1995;76:1222–1227.

Heeschen C, Hamm CW, Laufs U, et al., for the Platelet Receptor Inhibition in Ischemic Syndrome Management (PRISM) Investigators. Withdrawal of statins increases event rates in patients with acute coronary syndromes. *Circulation* 2002;105:1446–1452.

Heidenreich PA, Alloggiamento T, Melsop K, et al. The prognostic value of troponin in patients with non-ST-elevation acute coronary syndromes: a meta-analysis. *J Am Coll Cardiol* 2001;38:478–485.

Henderson W, Goldman S, Copeland J, et al. Antiplatelet or anticoagulant therapy after coronary artery bypass surgery: a meta-analysis of clinical trials. *Ann Intern Med* 1989;111:743–750.

Hirsh J, Anand SS, Halperin JL, et al. Guide to anticoagulant therapy: heparin. A statement for healthcare professionals from the American Heart Association. *Circulation* 2001;103:2994–3018.

Jones P, Kafonek S, Lauoroa I, et al. Comparative dose efficacy study of atorvastatin vs. simvastatin, pravastatin, lovastatin, and fluvastatin in patients with hypercholesterolemia (the CURVES study). *Am J Cardiol* 1998;81:582–587.

Jones PH, Davidson MA, Stein EA, et al. Comparison of the efficacy and safety of rosuvastatin compared versus atorvastatin, simvastatin and pravastatin across doses (STELLAR trial). *Am J Cardiol* 2003;92:152–160.

Karvouni E, Katritsis DG, Ioannidis JPA. Intravenous glycoprotein IIb/IIIa receptor antagonists reduce mortality after percutaneous coronary interventions. *J Am Coll Cardiol* 2003;41:26–32.

Kastrati A, Mehilli J, Schuhlen H, et al. A clinical trial of abciximab in elective percutaneous coronary intervention after pretreatment with clopidogrel. *N Engl J Med* 2004;350:232–238.

Kereiakes DJ, Grines C, Fry E, et al. Enoxaparin and abciximab adjunctive pharmacotherapy during percutaneous coronary intervention. *J Invasive Cardiol* 2001;13:272–278.

Klein W, Buchwald A, Hillis SE, et al. Comparison of low-molecular-weight heparin with unfractionated heparin acutely and with placebo for 6 weeks in the management of unstable coronary artery disease: Fragmin in coronary artery disease study (FRIC). *Circulation* 1997;96:61–68.

Lefkovits J, Plow EF, Topol EJ. Platelet glycoprotein IIb/IIIa receptors in cardiovascular medicine. *N Engl J Med* 1995;332:1553–1559.

Lefkovits J, Topol E. Direct thrombin inhibitors in cardiovascular medicine. *Circulation* 1994;90:1522–1536.

Lincoff AM, Bittl JA, Harrington RA, et al. Bivalirudin and provisional glycoprotein IIb/IIIa blockade compared with heparin and planned glycoprotein IIb/IIIa blockade during percutaneous coronary intervention. *JAMA* 2003;289:853–863.

Mahoney EM, Mehta S, Lamy A, et al. *Long-term cost effectiveness of platelet inhibition with clopidogrel in patients undergoing PCI after presenting with an acute coronary syndrome: Results from PCI-CURE.* American Heart Association Scientific Sessions 203. Abstract 2625.

Medical Economics. Lovenox. In: *Physicians' Desk Reference*, 56th edition. 2002, p. 750.

Mehta SR, Yusuf S, Peters RJ, et al. Effects of pretreatment with clopidogrel and aspirin followed by long-term therapy in patients undergoing percutaneous coronary intervention: the PCI-CURE study. *Lancet* 2001;358:527–533.

Mitsios, JV Papathanasiou AI. Rodis F, et al. Atorvastatin does not affect the antiplatelet potency of clopidogrel when it is administered concomitantly for 5 weeks in patients with acute coronary syndromes. *Circulation* 2004;109:1335–1338.

Mufson L, Black A, Roubin G, et al. A randomized trial of aspirin in PTCA: effect of high vs. low dose aspirin on major complications and restenosis. *J Am Coll Cardiol* 1988;11:236A.

NCEP Report. Implications of recent clinical trials for the National Cholesterol Education Program Adult Treatment Panel III Guidelines. *Circulation* 2004;110: 227–239.

Newby LK, Ohman EM, Christenson RH, et al. Benefit of glycoprotein IIb/IIIa inhibition in patients with acute coronary syndromes and troponin T-positive status: the Paragon-B troponin T substudy. *Circulation* 2001;103:2891–2896.

Peters RJ, Mehta SR, Fox KA, et al. Effects of aspirin dose when used alone or in combination with clopidogrel in patients with acute coronary syndromes. *Circulation* 2003;108:1682–1687.

Phillips DR., Scarborough RM. Clinical pharmacology of eptifibatide. *Am J Cardiol* 1997;80:11B–20B.

Presented at the American College of Cardiology meeting, Atlanta, GA, March, 2002.

Pulcinelli FM, Pignatelli P, Celestini A, et al. Inhibition of platelet aggregation by aspirin progressively decreases in long-term treated patients. *J Am Coll Cardiol* 2004;43:979–984.

Quinn MJ, Aronow HD, Califf RM, et al. Aspirin dose and six-month outcome after an acute coronary syndrome. *J Am Coll Cardiol* 2004;43:972–978.

Ryan TJ, Anderson JL, Antman EM, et al. ACC/AHA guidelines for the management of patients with acute myocardial infarction: a report of the American College of Cardiology/American Heart Association Task Force on Practice Guidelines (Committee on Management of Acute Myocardial Infarction). *J Am Coll Cardiol* 1996;28:1328–1428.

Savi P. Heilmann E, Nurden P, et al. Clopidogrel: an antithrombic drug acting on the ADP-dependant activation pathway of human platelets. *Clin Appl Thromb/Hemost* 1996;2:35–42.

Schrör K. The basic pharmacology of ticlopidine and clopidogrel. *Platelets* 1993;4:252–261.

Schwartz GG, Olsson AG, Ezekowitz MD, et al. Effects of atorvastatin on early recurrent ischemic events in acute coronary syndromes. *JAMA* 2001;285:1711–1718.

Schwartz L, Bourassa MG, Lesperance J, et al. Aspirin and dipyridamole in the prevention of restenosis after percutaneous transluminal coronary angioplasty. *N Engl J Med* 1988;318:1714–1719.

Serbruany V, Midei M, Malinin A, et al. *Atorvastatin does not inhibit clopidogrel in patients undergoing coronary stenting in prospective data from the INTERACTION Study.* Presented at American Heart Association Scientific Sessions, Abstract 3065, November 2003, Orlando, FL.

Slater DK, Hlatky MA, Mark DB, et al. Outcome in suspected acute myocardial infarction with normal or minimally abnormal admission electrocardiographic findings. *Am J Cardiol* 1987;60:766–770.

Steinhubl SR, Berger PB, Mam JT, et al. Early and sustained oral antiplatelet therapy following percutaneous coronary intervention: a randomized control trial. *JAMA* 2002;288:2411–2420.

Stone GW, McLaurin BT, Cox DA, et al. Bivalirudin for patients with acute coronary syndromes. *N Engl J Med* 2006;355(21):2203–2216.

Stone GW, Ware JH, Bertrand ME, et al., Antithrombotic strategies in patients with acute coronary syndromes undergoing early invasive management: one-year results from the ACUITY trial. *JAMA* 2007;298(21):2497–2506.

Tam SH, Sassoli PM, Jordan RE, Nakada MT. Abciximab (ReoPro, chimeric 7E3 Fab) demonstrates equivalent affinity and functional blockade of glycoprotein IIb/IIIa and $a_v\beta_3$, integrins. *Circulation* 1998;98:1085–1091.

Theroux P. Tirofiban. *Drugs of Today* 1999;35:59–73.

Topol EJ, Byzova TV, Plow EF. Platelet GPIIb-IIIa blockers. *Lancet* 1999;353:227–231.

Weintraub WS, Mahoney EM, Lamy A, et al. *Long-term cost effectiveness of platelet inhibition with clopidogrel in patients presenting with acute coronary syndromes: Results from the CURE trial.* Presented at American Heart Association Scientific Sessions, abstract 1925, November 2003, Orlando, FL.

Weitz JI. Low-molecular-weight heparins [published erratum appears in *N Engl J Med* 1997;337:1567]. *N Engl J Med* 1997;337:688–698.

White CW, Chaitman B, Knudtson ML, et al. Antiplatelet agents are effective in reducing the acute ischemic complications of angioplasty but do not prevent restenosis: results from the ticlopidine trial. *Coronary Artery Dis* 1991;2:757.

Wiviott SD, Braunwald E, McCabe CH, et al. Prasugrel versus clopidogrel in patients with acute coronary syndromes. *N Engl J Med* 2007;357(20):2001–2015.

Young JJ, Kereiakes DJ, Grines CL. Low-molecular-weight heparin therapy in percutaneous coronary intervention: the NICE 1 and NICE 4 trials. National Investigators Collaborating on Enoxaparin Investigators. *J Invasive Cardiol* 2000;12(Suppl E):E14–E18; discussion E25–E28.

Yusuf S, Mehta SR, Chrolavicius S, et al. Comparison of fondaparinux and enoxaparin in acute coronary syndromes. *N Engl J Med* 2006;354(14):1464–1476.

Yusuf S, Zhao F, Mehta SR, et al. Effects of clopidogrel in addition to aspirin in patients with acute coronary syndromes without ST-segment elevation. *N Engl J Med* 2001;345:494–502.

Chapter 10

Alexander KP, Chen AY, Roe MT, et al. Excess dosing of antiplatelet and antithrombin agents in the treatment of non-ST-segment elevation acute coronary syndromes. *JAMA* 2005;294:3108–3116.

Alexander KP, Newby LK, Cannon CP, et al. Acute coronary care in the elderly, part I: Non-ST-segment elevation acute coronary syndromes: a scientific statement for healthcare professionals from the American Heart Association Council on Clinical Cardiology: in collaboration with the Society of Geriatric Cardiology. *Circulation* 2007;115:2549–2569.

The BARI Investigators. Seven-year outcome in the Bypass Angioplasty Revascularization Investigation (BARI) by treatment and diabetic status. *J Am Coll Cardiol* 2000;35:1122–1129.

Boersma E, Harrington RA, Moliterno DJ, et al. Platelet glycoprotein IIb/IIIa inhibitors in acute coronary syndromes: a meta-analysis of all major randomized clinical trials. *Lancet* 2002;359:189–98.

Brogan WC, Lange RA, Kim AS, et al. Alleviation of cocaine-induced coronary vasoconstriction by nitroglycerin. *J Am Coll Cardiol* 1991;18:581–586.

Chahine RA, Feldman RL, Giles TD, et al. Randomized placebo controlled trial of amlodipine in vasospastic angina. *J Am Coll Cardiol* 1993;21:1365–1370.

Chen L, Theroux P, Lesperance J, et al. Angiographic features of vein grafts versus ungrafted coronary arteries in patients with unstable angina and previous bypass surgery. *J Am Coll Cardiol* 1996;28:1493–1499.

Fava S, Azzopardi J, Agium-Muscat H. Outcome of unstable angina in patients with diabetes mellitus. *Diabet Med* 1997;14:209–213.

Hollander JE. The management of cocaine-associated myocardial ischemia. *N Engl J Med* 1995;33:1267–1272.

Hulley S, Grady D, Bush T, et al. Randomized trial of estrogen plus progestin for secondary prevention of coronary heart disease in postmenopausal women. Heart and estrogen/progestin replacement study (HERS) research group. *JAMA* 1998;280:605–613.

Isner JM, Chokshi SK. Cardiovascular complications of cocaine. *Curr Probl Cardiol* 1991;16:89–123.

Isner JM, Chokshi SK. Cocaine and vasospasm. *N Engl J Med* 1989;321:1604–1606.

Kip KE, Faxon DP, Detre KM, et al. Coronary angioplasty in diabetic patients: the National Heart, Lung, and Blood Institute percutaneous transluminal coronary angioplasty registry. *Circulation* 1996;94:1818–1825.

Kleiman NS, Anderson HV, Rogers WJ, et al. Comparison of outcome of patients with unstable angina and non-Q-wave acute myocardial infarction with and without prior coronary artery bypass grafting (Thrombolysis in Myocardial Ischemia III Registry). *Am J Cardiol* 1996;77:227–231.

Opie LH. Calcium channel antagonists in the management of anginal syndromes: changing concepts in relation to the role of coronary vasospasm. *Prog Cardiovasc Dis* 1996;38:291–314.

Robertson RM. Women and cardiovascular disease: the misconception and the need for action. *Circulation* 2001;103:2318–2320.

Silva JA, White CJ, Collins TJ, Ramee SR. Morphologic comparison of atherosclerotic lesions in native coronary arteries and saphenous vein grafts with intracoronary angioscopy in patients with unstable angina. *Am Heart J* 1998;136:156–163.

Ryan TJ, Anderson JL, Antman EM, et al. ACC/AHA guidelines for the management of patients with acute myocardial infarction: a report of the American College of Cardiology/American Heart Association Task Force on Practice Guidelines (Committee on Management of Acute Myocardial Infarction). *J Am Coll Cardiol* 1996;28:1328–1428.

Waters DD, Walling A, Roy D, Theroux P. Previous coronary artery bypass grafting as an adverse prognostic factor in unstable angina pectoris. *Am J Cardiol* 1986;58:465–469.

Yao SS, Spindola-Franco H, Menegus M, et al. Successful intracoronary thrombolysis in cocaine-induced acute myocardial infarction. *Cathet Cardiovasc Diagn* 1997;42:294–297.

Chapter 11

Andersen HR. *Danish trial in acute myocardial infarction (DANAMI) 2*. Presented at: American College of Cardiology Scientific Sessions, Atlanta, GA, March, 2002.

Antman EA, Anbe TD, Armstrong PW, et al. ACC/AHA Guidelines for the Management of Patients with ST-Elevation Myocardial Infarction—executive summary. *J Am Coll Cardiol* 2004;44:671–719. Full-text guidelines available at www.acc.org/clinical/guidelines/stemi/index.pdf.

The BARI Investigators. Seven-year outcome in the Bypass Angioplasty Revascularization Investigation (BARI) by treatment and diabetic status. *J Am Coll Cardiol* 2000;35:1122–1129.

Buxton AE, Lee KL, Fisher JD, et al., for the Multicenter Unsustained Tachycardia Trial Investigators. A randomized study of the prevention of sudden death in patients with coronary artery disease. *N Engl J Med* 1999;341:1882–1890.

Califf RM, Topol EJ, Stack RS, et al. Evaluation of combination thrombolytictherapy and timing of cardiac catheterization in acute myocardial infarction. Results of Thrombolysis and Angioplasty in Myocardial Infarction–phase 5 randomized trial. TAMI Study Group. *Circulation* 1991;83:1543–1556.

Detre KM, Lombardero MS, Brooks MM, et al. The effect of previous coronary artery bypass surgery on the prognosis of patients with diabetes who have acute myocardial infarction. *N Engl J Med* 2000;342:989–997.

Dreifus LS, Fisch C, Griffin JC, et al. Guidelines for implantation of cardiac pacemakers and antiarrhythmia devices: a report of the American College of Cardiology/American Heart Association task force on assessment of diagnostic and therapeutic cardiovascular procedures (committee on pacemaker implantation). *J Am Coll Cardiol* 1991;18:1–13.

Freed M, Grines C. In: *Essentials of Cardiovascular Medicine*, Physicians' Press, Royal Oak, MI, 1994.

Hochman JS, Lamas GA, Buller CE, et al. Coronary intervention for persistent occlusion after myocardial infarction. *N Engl J Med* 2006;355:2395–2407.

Moss AJ, Hall WJ, Cannom DS, et al., for the Multicenter Automatic Defibrillator Implantation Trial Investigators. Improved survival with an implanted defibrillator in patients with coronary disease at high risk for ventricular arrhythmia. *N Engl J Med* 1996;335:1933–1940.

Moss AJ, Zareba W, Hall WJ, et al. Prophylactic implantation of a defibrillator in patients with myocardial infarction and reduced ejection fraction. *N Engl J Med* 2002;346:877–883.

Ohman EM, George BS, White CJ, et al., for the Randomized IABP Study Group. Use of aortic counterpulsation to improve sustained coronary artery patency during acute myocardial infarction: results of a randomized trial. *Circulation* 1994;90:792–799.

Presented at the American College of Cardiology Meeting, March, 2004, New Orleans, LA.

Stone GW, Marsalese D, Brodie BR, et al. A prospective, randomized evaluation of prophylactic intraaortic balloon counterpulsation in high risk patients with acute myocardial infarction treated with primary angioplasty. Second Primary Angioplasty in Myocardial Infarction (PAMI-II) Trial Investigators. *J Am Coll Cardiol* 1997;29:1459–1467.

Stone GW, Ohman EM, Miller MF, et al. Contemporary utilization and outcomes of intra-aortic balloon counterpulsation in acute myocardial infarction. *J Am Coll Cardiol* 2003;41:1940–1945.

Widimsky P, Groch L, Zelizko M, et al. Multicentre randomized trial comparing transport to primary angioplasty vs. immediate thrombolysis vs. combined strategy for patients with acute myocardial infarction presenting to a community hospital without a catheterization laboratory: the PRAGUE study. *Eur Heart J* 2000;21:823–831.

Chapter 12

Buxton AE, Lee KL, Fisher JD, et al., for the Multicenter Unsustained Tachycardia Trial Investigators. A randomized study of the prevention of sudden death in patients with coronary artery disease. *N Engl J Med* 1999;341:1882–1890.

Jain A, Myers GH, Sapin PM, O'Rourke RA. Comparison of symptom-limited and low level exercise tolerance tests early after myocardial infarction. *J Am Coll Cardiol* 1993;22:1816–1820.

Chapter 13

Antman EA, Anbe TD, Armstrong PW, et al. ACC/AHA Guidelines for the Management of Patients with ST-Elevation Myocardial Infarction—executive summary. *J Am Coll Cardiol* 2004;44:671–719. Full-text guidelines available at www.acc.org/clinical/guidelines/stemi/index.pdf.

Antman EM, Berlin JA. Declining incidence of ventricular fibrillation in myocardial infarction: implications for the prophylactic use of lidocaine. *Circulation* 1992;86:764–773.

Behar S, Goldbourt U, Reicher-Reiss H, Kaplinsky E. Prognosis of acute myocardial infarction complicated by primary ventricular fibrillation: principal investigators of the SPRINT study. *Am J Cardiol* 1990;66:1208–1211.

Behar S, Zahavi Z, Goldbourt U, Reicher-Reiss H. Long-term prognosis of patients with paroxysmal atrial fibrillation complicating acute myocardial infarction: SPRINT study group. *Eur Heart J* 1992;13:45–50.

Berger PB, Rucco NA Jr, Ryan TJ, et al. Incidence and prognostic implications of heart block complicating inferior myocardial infarction treated with thrombolytic therapy: Results from TIMI II. *J Am Coll Cardiol* 1992;20:533.

Berisso MZ, Carratino L, Ferroni A, et al. Frequency, characteristics and significance of supraventricular tachyarrhythmias detected by 24-hour electrocardiographic recording in the late hospital phase of acute myocardial infarction. Am J Cardiol 1990;65:1064.

Bernard SA, Gray TW, Buist MD, et al. Treatment of comatose survivors of out-of-hospital cardiac arrest with induced hypothermia. N Engl J Med 2002;346(8):557–563, 2002;346:549–556.

Brilakis ES, Wright RS, Kobecky SL, et al. Bundle branch block as a predictor of long-term survival after acute myocardial infarction. Am J Cardiol 2001;88:205–9.

Campbell RW, Murray A, Julian DG. Ventricular arrhythmias in trials of thrombolytic therapy for acute myocardial infarction: natural history study. Br Heart J 1981;46:351–357.

Campbell RWF. Arrhythmias. In: Julian DG, Braunwald E, eds. Management of Acute Myocardial Infarction. London, England: WB Saunders Co Ltd; 1994;223–240.

Clemmensen P, Bates ER, Califf RM, et al. Complete atrioventricular block complicating inferior wall acute myocardial infarction treated with reperfusion therapy: TAMI study group. Am J Cardiol 1991;67:225.

Crenshaw BS, Ward SR, Granger CB, et al. Atrial fibrillation in the setting of acute myocardial infarction: the GUSTO-I experience. Global Utilization of Streptokinase and TPA for Occluded Coronary Arteries. J Am Coll Cardiol 1997;30:406–13.

Crenshaw BS, Ward SR, Stebbins AL, et al. Risk factors and outcomes in patients with atrial fibrillation following acute myocardial infarction. Circulation 1995;92(suppl):I-777.

Crimm A, Severance HW, Coffey K, et al. Prognostic significance of isolated sinus tachycardia during the first three days of acute myocardial infarction. Am J Med 1984;976:983.

Denes P. Am J Cardiol 1991;68(9):887–896. PMID: 1718158.

DeSanctis RW, Block P, Hutter AM. Tachyarrhythmias in myocardial infarction. Circulation 1972;45:681.

Dhurandhar RW. MacMillan RL, Brown KW. Primary ventricular fibrillation complicating acute myocardial infarction. Am J Cardiol 1971;27:347–351.

DOI: 10.1161/CIRCULATIONAHA.105.166557 2005;112; IV-58IV-66; originally published online Nov 28, 2005; Circulation Part 7.2: Management of Cardiac Arrest.

The ECG Criteria Book. Eds: O'Keefe J, Hammill S, Freed M, Pogwiz S. Physicians' Press, Royal Oak, MI, 2002.

Eldar M, Sievner Z, Goldbourt U, et al. Primary ventricular tachycardia in acute myocardial infarction: clinical characteristics and mortality. The SPRINT study group. Ann Intern Med 1992;117:31.

Fibrinolytic Therapy Trialists' (FTT) Collaborative Group. Indications for fibrinolytic therapy in suspected acute myocardial infarction: collaborative overview of early mortality and major morbidity results from all randomized trials of more than 1000 patients. Lancet 1994;343:311–322.

Goldberg RJ, Seeley D, Becker RC, et al. Impact of atrial fibrillation on the in-hospital and long-term survival of patients with acute myocardial infarction: a community-wide perspective. Am Heart J 1990;119:996–1001.

Graner LE, Gershen BJ, Orlando MM, et al. Bradycardia and its complications in the pre-hospital phase of acute myocardial infarction. Am J Cardiol 1973;32:607–611.

Guidelines 2000 for Cardiopulmonary Resuscitation and Emergency Cardiovascular Care. Circulation 2000;102: I86–I203.

Higham PD, Adams PC, Murray A, Campbell RW. Plasma potassium, serum magnesium and ventricular fibrillation: a prospective study. Q J Med 1993;86:609–617.

Hindman MC, Wagner GS, Jaro M, et al. The clinical significance of bundle branch block complicating acute myocardial infarction. 1. Clinical characteristics, hospital mortality, and one-year follow-up. Circulation 1978;58:679.

Hindman MC, Wagner GS, Jaro M, et al. The clinical significance of bundle branch block complicating acute myocardial infarction. 2. Indications for temporary and permanent pacemaker insertion. Circulation 1978;58:689.

Hypothermia After Cardiac Arrest Study Group. Mild therapeutic hypothermia to improve the neurologic outcome after cardiac arrest. N Engl J Med 2002; 346: 612–613

Klein RC, Vera Z, Mason DT. Intraventricular conduction defects in acute myocardial infarction: incidence, prognosis and therapy. Am Heart J 1984;108:1007.

Koren G, Weiss AT, Ben-David J, et al. Bradycardia and hypotension following reperfusion with streptokinase (Bezold-Jarish reflex): a sign of coronary thrombolysis and myocardial salvage. Am Heart J 1986;112:468.

Kostuk WJ, Beanlands DS. Complete heart block associated with acute myocardial infarction. Am J Cardiol 1970;26:380.

Kyriakidis M, Barbetseas J, Antonopoulos A, et al. Early atrial arrhythmias in acute myocardial infarction: role of the sinus node artery. Chest 1992;101:944–947.

Lie KI, Wellens HJ, Durrer D. Characteristics and predictability of primary ventricular fibrillation. Eur J Cardiol 1974;1:379–384.

Lopes RD. *Heart* 2008;94:873–876. PMID: 18332062.

Mark AL. The Bezold-Jarisch reflex revisted: clinical implications of inhibitory reflexes originating in the heart. *J Am Coll Cardiol* 1983;1:90.

McDonald K, O'Sullivan JJ, Conroy RM, et al. Heart block as a predictor of in-hospital death in both acute inferior and acute anterior myocardial infarction. *Q J Med* 1990;74:277.

McMachon S, Collins R, Koster RW, Yusuf S. Effects of prophylactic lidocaine in suspected acute myocardial infarction: an overview of results from the randomized, controlled trials. *JAMA* 1988;260:1910–1916.

Mullins CB, Atkins JM. Prognoses and management of ventricular conduction blocks in acute myocardial infarction. *Mod Concepts Cardiovasc Dis* 1976;45:129.

Nordehaug JE, von der Lippe G. Hypokalaemia and ventricular fibrillation in acute myocardial infarction. *Br Heart J* 1983;50:525–529.

Pantridge JF, Adgey AAJ. Pre-hospital coronary care: the mobile coronary care unit. *Am J Cardiol* 1969; 624:666.

Part 7.5: Postresuscitation Support 2005 American Heart Association Guidelines for Cardiopulmonary Resuscitation and Emergency Cardiovascular Care. *Circulation* 2005;112:IV-84–IV-88. Published online before print November 28, 2005, doi:10.1161/CIRCULATIONAHA.105.166560.

Ricou F, Nicod P, Gilpin E, et al. Influence of a right bundle branch block on short-and long-term survival after acute anterior myocardial infarction. *J Am Coll Cardiol* 1991;17:858.

Ricou F, Nicod P, Gilpin E, et al. Influence of a right bundle branch block on short-and long-term survival after inferior Q-wave myocardial infarction. *Am J Cardiol* 1991;67:1143.

Scheinman MM, Gonzalez RP. Fascicular block and acute myocardial infarction. *JAMA* 1980;224:2646.

Serrano CV, Ramires JAF, Mansur AP, et al. Importance of the time of onset of supraventricular tachyarrhythmias on prognosis of patients with acute myocardial infarction. *Clin Cardiol* 1995;18:84.

Soloman SD, Ridker PM, Amman EM. Ventricular arrhythmias in trials of thrombolytic therapy for acute myocardial infarction: a meta-analysis. *Circulation* 1993;88:2575–2581.

Volpi A, Cavalli A, Santoro E, Tognoni G. Incidence and prognosis of secondary ventricular fibrillation in acute myocardial infarction: evidence for a protective effect of thrombolytic therapy. GISSI Investigators. *Circulation* 1990;82:1279–1288.

Weisfeldt ML, Becker LB. Resuscitation after cardiac arrest: a 3-phase time-sensitive model. *JAMA* 2002;288(23):3035–3038. PMID: 12479769.

Wenzel V, Krismer AC, Arntz HR, et al. A comparison of vasopressin and epinephrine for out-of-hospital cardiopulmonary resuscitation. *N Engl J Med* 2004;350:105–113.

Chapter 14

Abrams DL, Edelist A, Lruia MH, et al. Ventricular aneurysm: a reappraisal based on a study of 65 consecutive autopsied cases. *Circulation* 1963;27:164.

Anderson HR, Falk E, Nielsen D. Right ventricular infarction: frequency, size and topography in coronary heart disease: a prospective study comprising 107 consecutive autopsies from a coronary care unit. *J Am Coll Cardiol* 1987;10:1223–1232.

Antman EA, Anbe TD, Armstrong PW, et al. ACC/AHA Guidelines for the Management of Patients with ST-Elevation Myocardial Infarction—executive summary. *J Am Coll Cardiol* 2004;44:671–719.

Balakumaran K, Verbaan CJ, Essed CE, et al. Ventricular free wall rupture: sudden, subacute, slow, sealed and stabilized varieties. *Eur Heart J* 1984;5:282–288.

Berger PB, Ruocco NA Jr, Ryan TJ, et al. Frequency and significance of right ventricular dysfunction during inferior wall left ventricular myocardial infarction treated with thrombolytic therapy (results from the Thrombolysis in Myocardial Infarction [TIMI] II trial): the TIMI research group. *Am J Cardiol* 1993;71:1148–1152.

Berman J, Haffajee CI, Alpert JS. Therapy of symptomatic pericarditis after myocardial infarction: retrospective and prospective studies of aspirin, indomethacin, prednisone, and spontaneous resolution. *Am Heart J* 1981;101:750–753.

Blanche C, Khan SS, Chaux A, Matloff JM. Postinfarction ventricular septal defect in the elderly: analysis and results. *Ann Thorac Surg* 1994;57:91–98.

Blanche C, Khan SS, Matloff JM, et al. Results of early repair of ventricular septal defect after an acute myocardial infarction. *J Thorac Cardiovasc Surg* 1992;104:961–965.

Brown EJ Jr, Kloner RA, Schoen FJ, et al. Scar thinning due to ibuprofen administration after experimental myocardial infarction. *Am J Cardiol* 1983;51:877.

Brown SL, Gropler RJ, Harris KM. Distinguishing left ventricular aneurysm from pseudoaneurysm. A review of the literature. *Chest* 1997;111:1403–1409.

Bulkey BH, Roberts WC. Steroid therapy during acute myocardial infarction: a cause of delayed healing and of ventricular aneurysm. *Am J Med* 1974;56:244–250.

Califf RM, Bengtson JR. Cardiogenic shock. *N Engl J Med* 1994;330:1724–1730.

Carney RM, Freedland KE, Sheline YI, et al. Depression and coronary heart disease: a review for cardiologists. *Clin Cardiol* 1997;20:196–200.

Clements SD Jr, Story WE, Hurst JW, et al. Ruptured papillary muscle, a complication of myocardial infarction: clinical presentation, diagnosis and treatment. *Clin Cardiol* 1985;8:93–103.

Cohn JN. Hormones, drugs, remodeling and outcome in heart failure and after myocardial infarction. *Cardiovasc Drugs Ther* 2001;15:9–10.

Crenshaw BS, Granger CB, Bir Baum Y, et al. Risk factors, angiographic patterns, and outcomes in patients with ventricular septal defect complicating acute myocardial infarction. *Circulation* 2000;101:27–32.

Dargie HJ. Effect of carvedilol on outcome after myocardial infarction in patients with left-ventricular dysfunction: the CAPRICORN randomised trial. *Lancet* 2001;357:1385–1390.

Dell'Italia LJ, Starling MR, Blumhardt R, et al. Comparative effects of volume loading, dobutamine, and nitroprusside in patients with predominant right ventricular infarction. *Circulation* 1985;72:1327–1335.

Di Donato M, Sabatier M, Montiglio F, et al. Outcome of left ventricular aneurysmectomy with patch repair in patients with severely depressed pump function. *Am J Cardiol* 1995;76:557–561.

Disler L, Haitas B, Benjamin J, et al. Cardiogenic shock in evolving myocardial infarction: treatment by angioplasty and streptokinase. *Heart Lung* 1987;16:649.

Dressler W. The post-myocardial infarction syndrome: a report of forty-four cases. *Arch Intern Med* 1959;103:28.

Fijewski TR, Pollack ML, Chan TC, Brady WJ. Electrocardiographic manifestations: right ventricular infarction. *J Emerg Med* 2002;22:189–194.

Frances C, Romero A, Grady D. Left ventricular pseudoaneurysm. *J Am Coll Cardiol* 1998;32:557–561.

Friedman PL, Brown EJ Jr, Gunther S, et al. Coronary vasoconstrictor effect of indomethacin in patients with coronary-artery disease. *N Engl J Med* 1981; 305:1171–1175. Full-text guidelines available at www.acc.org/clinical/guidelines/stemi/index.pdf.

Gattis WA, O'Conner CM, Gallup DS, et al. Predischarge initiation of carvedilol in patients hospitalized for decompensated heart failure: results of the Initiation Management Predischarge: Process for Assessment of Carvedilol Therapy in Heart Failure (IMPACT-HF) trial. *J Am Coll Cardiol* 2004;43: 1534–1541.

Gershlick A, Stephens-Lloyd A, Hughes S, et al. Rescue angioplasty after failed thrombolytic therapy for acute myocardial infarction. *N Engl J Med* 2005; 353:2758–2768.

Glassman AH, O'Connor CM, Califf RM, et al., for the Sertraline Antidepressant Heart Attack Randomized Trial (SADHART) Group. Sertraline treatment of major depression in patients with acute MI or unstable angina. *JAMA* 2002;288:701–709.

The GUSTO investigators. An international randomized trial comparing four thrombolytic strategies for acute myocardial infarction. *N Engl J Med* 1993;329:673–682.

Haji SA, Movahed A. Right ventricular infarction—diagnosis and treatment. *Clin Cardiol* 2000;23:473–482.

Halperin JL, Fuster V. Left ventricular thrombi and cerebral embolism. *N Engl J Med* 1989;320:392.

Halperin JL, Peterson P. Thrombosis in the cardiac chambers: ventricular dysfunction and atrial fibrillation. In: Fuster V, and Verstraete M (eds). *Thrombosis in Cardiovascular Disorders*. Philadelphia, WB Saunders Company, 1992, p. 215.

Hammerman H, Schoen FJ, Braunwald E, Kloner RA. Drug-induced expansion of infarct: morphologic and functional correlations. *Circulation* 1984;69:611–617.

Hochman JS, Sleeper LA, White HW, et al. One-year survival following early revascularization for cardiogenic shock. *JAMA* 2001;285:190–192.

Hollenberg SM, Kavinsky CJ, Parrillo JE. Cardiogenic shock. *Ann Intern Med* 1999;131:47–59.

Hutchins GM, Bulkley BH. Infarct expansion versus extension: two different complications of acute myocardial infarction. *Am J Cardiol* 1978;41:1127–1132.

Jacobs AK, Leopold JA, Bates E, et al. Cardiogenic shock caused by right ventricular infarction. *J Am Coll Cardiol* 2003;41:1273–1279.

Jones RH, Velazquez EJ, Michler RE, et al., the STICH Hypothesis 2 Investigators. Coronary bypass surgery with or without surgical ventricular reconstruction. *N Engl J Med* 2009; PMID: 19329820.

Keeley EC, Hillis LD. Left ventricular mural thrombus after acute myocardial infarction. *Clin Cardiol* 1996;19:83.

Khan AH. The postcardiac injury syndromes. *Clin Cardiol* 1992;15:67.

Kishon Y, Oh JK, Schaff HV, et al. Mitral valve operation in post-infarction rupture of a papillary muscle: immediate results and long-term follow-up of 22 patients. *Mayo Clin Proc* 1992;67:1023–1030.

Kloner RA, Fishbein MC, Lew H, Maroko PR, Braunwald E. Mummification of the infarcted myocardium by high dose of corticosteroids. *Circulation* 1978;57:56–73.

Komeda M, David TE, Malik A, et al. Operative risks and long-term results of operation for left ventricular aneurysm. *Ann Thorac Surg* 1992;53:22–58.

Lemery R, Smith HC, Guiliani ER, Gersh BJ. Prognosis in rupture of the ventricular septum after acute myocardial infarction and the role of early surgical intervention. *Am J Cardiol* 1992;70:147–151.

Lichstein E, Arsura E, Hollander G, et al. Current incidence of postmyocardial infarction (Dressler's) syndrome. *Am J Cardiol* 1982;50:1269.

Lilavie CJ, Gersh PJ. Mechanical and electrical complications of acute myocardial infarction. *Mayo Clin Proc* 1990;65:709–730.

Lim ST, Goldstein JA. Right Ventricular Infarction. Current treatment options in cardiovascular medicine. 2001;3:95–101.

Lupi-Herrera E, Lasses LA, Cosio-Aranda J, et al. Acute right ventricular infarction: clinical spectrum, results of reperfusion therapy and short-term prognosis. *Coron Artery Dis* 2002;13:57–64.

Madsen J, Grande P, et al. Danish multi-center randomized study of invasive versus conservative treatment in patients with inducible ischemia after thrombolysis in acute myocardial infarction (DANAM1). *Circulation* 1997;96:748–755.

Mehta SR, Eikelboom JW, Natarajan MK, et al. Impact of right ventricular involvement on mortality and morbidity in patients with inferior myocardial infarction. *J Am Coll Cardiol* 2001;37:37–43.

Meizlish JL, Berger HJ, Plankey M, et al. Functional left ventricular aneurysm formation after acute anterior transmural myocardial infarction: incidence, natural history, and prognostic implications. *N Engl J Med* 1984;311:1001.

Packer M. Heart failure. In: Goldman L, and Bennett JC (eds) *Cecil Textbook of Medicine.* WB Saunders Co, Philadelphia, 2000, pp. 215–225.

Pfeffer MA, McMurray JJ, Velazquez EJ, et al. Valsartan, captopril, or both in myocardial infarction complicated by heart failure, left ventricular dysfunction, or both. *N Engl J Med* 2003;349:1893–1906.

Pitt B, Remme W, Zannad F, et al. Eplerenone, a selective aldosterone blocker, in patients with left ventricular dysfunction after myocardial infarction. *N Engl J Med* 2003;348:1309–1321.

Pollak H, Nobis H, Mlczoch J. Frequency of left ventricular free wall rupture complicating acute myocardial infarction since the advent of thrombolysis. *Am J Cardiol* 1994;74:184–186.

Prieto A, Eisenberg J, Thakur RK. Nonarrhythmic complications of acute myocardial infarction. *Emerg Med Clin North Am* 2001;19:397–415, xii–xiii.

Rankin JS, Livesey SA, Smith LR, et al. Trends in the surgical treatment of ischemic mitral regurgitation: effects of mitral valve repair on hospital mortality. *Semin Thorac & Cardiovasc Surg* 1989;1:149–163.

Reardon MJ, Carr CL, Diamond A, et al. Ischemic left ventricular free wall rupture: prediction, diagnosis and treatment. *Ann Thoracic Surg* 1997;64:1509–1513.

Robalino BD, Whitlow PL, Underwood DA, Salcedo EE. Electrocardiographic manifestations of right ventricular infarction. *Am Heart J* 1989;118:138–144.

Sanborn TA, Sleeper LA, Webb JG, et al. Correlates of one-year survival in patients with cardiogenic shock complicating acute myocardial infarction. *J Am Coll Cardiol* 2003;42:1373–1379.

Silverman HW, and Pfeifer ME. Relation between use of anti-inflammatory agents and left ventricular free wall rupture during acute myocardial infarction. *Am J Cardiol* 1987;59:363.

Skillington PD, Davies RH, Luff AJ, et al. Surgical treatment for infarct-related ventricular septal defects: improved early results combined with analysis of late functional status. *J Thorac Cardiovasc Surg* 1990;99:798–808.

Steg PG, Dabbous OH, Feldman LJ, et al. Determinants and prognostic impact of heart failure complicating acute coronary syndromes. *Circulation* 2004;109:494–499.

STEMI guidelines Antman JACC 2004 PMID: 15358047.

Tcheng JE, Jackman JD Jr, Nelson CL, et al. Outcome of patients sustaining acute ischemic mitral regurgitation during myocardial infarction. *Ann Intern Med* 1992;117:18–24.

Tepe NA, Edmunds LH Jr. Operation for acute postinfarction mitral insufficiency and cardiogenic shock. *J Thorac Cardiovasc Surg* 1985;89:525–530.

Tikiz H. *Int J Cardiol* 2002; PMID: 11786151.

Topaz O, Taylor AL. Interventricular septal rupture complicating acute myocardial infarction: from pathophysiologic features to the role of invasive and noninvasive diagnostic modalities in current management. *Am J Med* 1992;93:683–688.

Visser CA, Kan G, Meltzer RS, et al. Incidence, timing and prognostic value of left ventricular aneurysm formation after myocardial infarction; a prospective, serial echocardiographic study of 158 patients. *Am J Cardiol* 1985;57:729–732.

Weisman HF, Healy B. Myocardial infarct expansion, infarct extension, and reinfarction: pathophysiologic concepts. *Prog Cardiovasc Dis* 1987;30:73–110.

Writing Committee for the ENRICHD Investigators. Effects of treating depression and low perceived social support on clinical events after myocardial infarction: The enhancing recovery in coronary heart disease patients (ENRICHD) randomized trial. *JAMA* 2003;289:3106–3116.

Yusuf S, Wittes J, Friedman L. Overview of results of randomized clinical trials in heart disease: I. Treatments following myocardial infarction. *JAMA* 1988;260:2088–2093.

Zehender M, Kasper W, Kauder E, et al. Right ventricular infarction as an independent predictor of prognosis after acute inferior myocardial infarction. *N Engl J Med* 1993;328:981–988.

Chapter 15

2007 Focused Update of the ACC/AHA 2004 Guidelines for the Management of Patients with ST-Elevation Myocardial Infarction. *J Am Coll Cardiol* 2008;51(2):210–247.

Alexander KP, Chen AY, Roe MT, et al., CRUSADE investigators. Excess dosing of antiplatelet and antithrombin agents in the treatment of non-ST segment elevation acute coronary syndromes. *JAMA* 2005;294(24):3108–3116.

Anderson JL, et al. 2007 ACC/AHA Guidelines for the Management of Patients with Unstable Angina/Non-ST-Elevation Myocardial Infarction. *J Am Coll Cardiol* 2007;50:652–726.

Antman EM, Tanasijevic MJ, Thompson B, et al. Cardiac-specific troponin I levels to predict the risk of mortality in patients with acute coronary syndromes. *N Engl J Med* 1996;335:1342–7.9.

Armstrong PW, Fu Y, Chang WC, et al. Acute coronary syndromes in the GUSTO-IIb trial: prognostic insights and impact of recurrent ischemia. The GUSTO-IIb Investigators. *Circulation* 1998;98:1860–1868.

Barron HV, Bowlby LJ, Breen T, et al. Use of reperfusion therapy for acute myocardial infarction in the United States: data from the National Registry of Myocardial Infarction 2. *Circulation* 1998;97:1150–1156.

Beinart S, Kolm P, Veledar E, et al. *Short and long-term cost effectiveness of early and sustained dual oral antiplatelet therapy with clopidogrel following percutaneous coronary intervention: Results from CREDO.* American Heart Association Scientific Sessions 203. Abstract 3495.

Beta Blocker Heart Attack Study Group. The beta-blocker heart attack trial. *JAMA* 1981;246:2073–2074.

Breaking Clinical Trial IV: Arrhythmias/CHF. American College of Cardiology 2009 Scientific Sessions, Orlando, FL, March 31, 2009.

Cannon CP, Braunwald E, McCabe CH, et al. Comparison of intensive and moderate lipid lowering with statins after acute coronary syndromes. *N Engl J Med* 2004;350.

Canto JG, Shlipak MG, Rogers WJ, et al. Prevalence, clinical characteristics, and mortality among patients with myocardial infarction presenting without chest pain. *JAMA* 2000;283:3223–3229.

Carney RM, Freedland KE, Sheline YI, et al. Depression and coronary heart disease: a review for cardiologists. *Clin Cardiol* 1997;20:196–200.

Centers for Disease Control and Prevention. Receipt of outpatient cardiac rehabilitation among heart attack survivors—United States, 2005. *MMWR* 2008;57(4):89–94. PMID: 18235423.

Chen ZM, Pan HC, Chen YP, et al., for the COMMIT (ClOpidogrel and Metoprolol in Myocardial Infarction Trial) collaborative group. Early intravenous then oral metoprolol in 45,852 patients with acute myocardial infarction: randomised placebo-controlled trial. *Lancet* 2005;366(9497):1622–1632.

Cockcroft DW, Gault MH. Prediction of creatinine clearance from serum creatinine. *Nephron* 1976; 16:31–41.

Coronary Artery Bypass Graft (CABG) Patch Trial Investigators. Prophylactic use of implanted cardiac defibrillators in patients at high risk for ventricular arrhythmias after coronary-artery bypass graft surgery. *N Engl J Med* 1997;337(22):1569–1575. PMID: 9371853.

Eagle KA, Goodman SG, Avezum A. Practice variation and missed opportunities for reperfusion in ST-segment-elevation myocardial infarction: findings from the Global Registry of Acute Coronary Events (GRACE). *Lancet* 2002;359:373–377.

Eisenstein EL, Anstrom KJ, Kong DF, et al. Clopidogrel use and long-term clinical outcomes after drugeluting stent implantation. *JAMA* 2007;297(2):159–168. PMID: 17148711.

Fibrinolytic Therapy Trialists' (FTT) Collaborative Group. Indications for fibrinolytic therapy in suspected acute myocardial infarction: collaborative overview of early mortality and major morbidity results from all randomized trials of more than 1000 patients. *Lancet* 1994;343:311–322.

Franzosi MG, Santoro E, De Vita C, et al. Ten-year follow-up of the first megatrial testing thrombolytic therapy in patients with acute myocardial infarction: results of the Gruppo Italiano per lo Studio della Sopravvivenza nell' Infarto-1 study. The GISSI Investigators. *Circulation* 1998;98:2659–2665.

Galvani M, Ottani F, Ferrini D, et al. Prognostic influence of elevated values of cardiac troponin I in patients with unstable angina. *Circulation* 1997;95:2053–2059.

GISSI-3: Gruppo Italiano per lo Studio della Sopravvivenza nell'infarto Miocardico. Effects of lisinopril and transdermal glyceryl trinitrate singly and together on 6-week mortality and ventricular function after acute myocardial infarction. *Lancet* 1994;343:1115–1122.

Gottlieb SS, McCarter RJ, Vogel RA. Effect of beta-blockade on mortality among high-risk and low-risk patients after myocardial infarction. *N Engl J Med* 1998;339:489–497.

Granger CB, Hirsch J, Califf RM, et al. Activated partial thromboplastin time and outcome after thrombolytic therapy for acute myocardial infarction: results from the GUSTO-I trial. *Circulation* 1996;93:870–878.

Hamm CW, Heeschen C, Goldmann B, et al. Benefit of abciximab in patients with refractory unstable angina in relation to serum troponin levels. *N Engl J Med* 1999;340:1623–1629.

The Heart Outcomes Prevention Evaluation Study Investigators. Effects of an angiotensin-coverting-enzyme inhibitor, ramipril, on cardiovascular events in high-risk patients. *N Engl J Med* 2000;342:145–153.

Heeschen C, Hamm CW, Goldmann B. Troponin concentrations for stratification of patients with acute coronary syndromes in relation to therapeutic efficacy of tirofiban. *Lancet* 1999;354:1757–1762.

Heidenreich PA, Alloggiamento T, Melsop K, et al. The prognostic value of troponin in patients with non-ST-elevation acute coronary syndromes: a meta-analysis. *J Am Coll Cardiol* 2001;38:478–485.

Hjalmarson A, Elmfeldt D, Herlitz J, et al. Effect on mortality of metoprolol in acute myocardial infarction: a double-blind randomized trial. *Lancet* 1981;2:823–827.

Ho PM, Peterson ED, Wang L, et al. Incidence of death and acute myocardial infarction associated with stopping clopidogrel after acute coronary syndrome. *JAMA* 2008;299(5):532–539.

Hohnloser SH, Kuck KH, Dorian P, et al. DINAMIT investigators. Prophylactic use of an implantable cardioverter-defibrillator after acute myocardial infarction. *N Engl J Med* 2004;351(24):2481–2488. PMID: 15590950.

ISIS-2 (Second International Study of Infarct Survival) Collaborative Group. Randomized trial of intravenous streptokinase, oral aspirin, both, or neither among 17,187 cases of suspected acute myocardial infarction: ISIS-2. *Lancet* 1988;2:349–360.

ISIS-4 (Fourth International Study of Infarct Survival) Collaborative Group. ISIS-4: a randomized factorial trial assessing early oral captopril, oral mononitrate, and intravenous magnesium sulphate in 58,050 patients with suspected acute myocardial infarction. *Lancet* 1995;345:669–685.

Jolliffe JA, Rees K, Taylor RS, et al. Exercise-based rehabilitation for coronary heart disease. Cochrane Database Syst Rev. 2000;(4):CD001800. PMID: 11034729.

Mahoney EM, Mehta S, Lamy A, et al. Long-term cost effectiveness of platelet inhibition with clopidogrel in patients undergoing PCI after presenting with an acute coronary syndrome: Results from PCI-CURE. American Heart Association Scientific Sessions 203. Abstract 2625.

Mehta SR, Yusuf S, Peters RJ, et al. Effects of pretreatment with clopidogrel and aspirin followed by long-term therapy in patients undergoing percutaneous coronary intervention: the PCI-CURE study. *Lancet* 2001;358:527–533.

Melloni C, Peterson ED, Chen AY, et al. Cockcroft-Gault versus modification of diet in renal disease: importance of glomerular filtration rate formula for classification of chronic kidney disease in patients with non-ST-segment elevation acute coronary syndromes. *J Am Coll Cardiol* 2008;51(10):991–996. PMID: 18325437.

Morrow DA, Cannon CP, Nader R, et al., for the TACTICS-TIMI 18 Investigators. Ability of minor elevations of troponins I and T to predict benefit from an early invasive strategy in patients with unstable angina and non-ST-elevation myocardial infarction. *JAMA* 2001;286:2405–2412.

Moss AJ, Zareba W, Hall WJ, et al. Prophylactic implantation of a defibrillator in patients with myocardial infarction and reduced ejection fraction. *N Engl J Med* 2002;346:877–883.

Ohman EM, Armstrong PW, Christenson RH, for the GUSTO IIA Investigators. Cardiac troponin T levels for risk stratification in acute myocardial ischemia. *N Engl J Med* 1996;335:1333–1341.

Pettijohn TL, Doyle T, Spiekerman AM, et al. Usefulness of positive troponin-T and negative creatine kinase levels in identifying high-risk patients with unstable angina pectoris. *Am J Cardiol* 1997;80:510–511.

Pfisterer M, Brunner-La Rocca HP, Buser PT, et al., BASKET-LATE Investigators. Late clinical events after clopidogrel discontinuation may limit the benefit of drug-eluting stents: an observational study of drug-eluting versus bare-metal stents. *J Am Coll Cardiol* 2006;48(12):2584–2591. PMID: 17174201.

PMID: 15358047 & PMID: 18191746.

Presented at the American College of Cardiology Meeting, March. 2004, New Orleans, LA.

Rogers JR, Canto JG, Lambrew CT, et al. Temporal trends in the treatment of over 1.5 million patients with myocardial infarction in the US from 1990 through 1999. *J Am Coll Cardio* 2000;36:2056–2063.

Ryan TJ, Anderson JL, Antman EM, Braniff BA, et al. ACC/AHA guidelines for the management of patients with acute myocardial infarction: a report of the American College of Cardiology/American Heart Association Task Force on Practice Guidelines (Committee on Management of Acute Myocardial Infarction). *J Am Coll Cardiol* 1996;28:1328–1428.

Ryan TJ, Antman EM, Brooks NH, Califf RM, et al. 1999 update: ACC/AHA guidelines for the management of patients with acute myocardial infarction: a report of the American College of Cardiology/American Heart Association Task Force on Practice Guidelines (Committee on Management of Acute Myocardial Infarction). *J Am Coll Cardiol* 1999;34:890–911.

Saito S, Hosokawa G, Tanaka S, Nakamura S. Primary stem implantation is superior to balloon angioplasty in acute myocardial infarction: final results the primary angioplasty versus stent implantation in acute myocardial infarction (PASTA) trial. *Cathet Cardiovasc Intervent* 1999;48:262–268.

Saketkhou BB, Conte FJ, Noris M, et al. Emergency department use of aspirin in patients with possible acute myocardial infarction. *Ann Intern Med* 1997;127:126–129.

Steinbeck G. A randomized study of the effects of defibrillator implantation early after myocardial infarction in high-risk patients on optimal medical therapy. American College of Cardiology 2009 Scientific Sessions; March 31, 2009; Orlando, FL. Late Breaking Clinical Trial IV: Arrhythmias/CHF.

Steinhubl SR, Berger PB, Mam JT, et al. Early and sustained oral antiplatelet therapy following percutaneous coronary intervention: a randomized control trial. *JAMA* 2002;288:2411–2420.

Timolol-induced reduction in mortality and reinfarction in patients surviving acute myocardial infarction. *N Engl J Med* 1981;304:801–807.

Weintraub WS, Mahoney EM, Lamy A, et al. *Long-term cost effectiveness of platelet inhibition with clopidogrel in patients presenting with acute coronary syndromes: Results from the CURE trial.* Presented at American Heart Association Scientific Sessions, abstract 1925, November 2003, Orlando, FL.

Yusuf S, Collins R, MacMahon S, Peto R. Effect of intravenous nitrates on mortality in acute myocardial infarction: an overview of the randomized trials. *Lancet* 1988;1:1088–1092.

Yusuf S, Zhao F, Mehta SR, et al. Effects of clopidogrel in addition to aspirin in patients with acute coronary syndromes without ST-segment elevation. *N Engl J Med* 2001;345:494–502.

Chapter 16

2007 STEMI Guideline Update & 2007 ACC NSTEMI guidelines. *J Am Coll Cardiol* 2007;50:652–726.

A controlled comparison of aspirin and oral anticoagulants in prevention of death after myocardial infarction. *N Engl J Med* 1982;307:701–708.

Anderson JL, et al. *Circulation* 2007;116:2563–2570.

Ansell JE. Anticoagulation management as a risk factor for adverse events: grounds for improvement. *J Thromb Thrombolys* 1998;5(suppl):S13–S18.

Antiplatelet Trialists' Collaboration. Collaborative overview of randomized trials of antiplatelet therapy, I: prevention of death, myocardial infarction, and stroke by prolonged antiplatelet therapy in various categories of patients. *BMJ* 1994;308:81–106.

Antman E. *Magnesium in coronaries (MAGIC) trial.* Presented at the European Society of Cardiology meeting, Berlin, Germany, Sept. 2002.

Antman EM, Cohen M, Radley D, et al. Assessment of the treatment effect of enoxaparin for unstable angina/non-Q-wave myocardial infarction. TIMI 11B-ESSENCE meta-analysis. *Circulation* 1999;100:1602–1608.

Antman EM, Lau J, Kupelnick B, et al. A comparison of results of meta-analysis of randomized control trials and recommendations of clinical experts: treatments for myocardial infarction. *JAMA* 1992;268:240–248.

Antman EM, McCabe CH, Gurfinkel EP, et al. Enoxaparin prevents death and cardiac ischemic events in unstable angina/non-Q-wave myocardial infarction: results of the Thrombolysis In Myocardial Infarction (TIMI) 11B trial. *Circulation* 1999;100:1593–1601.

Antman EM. Magnesium in acute MI: timing is critical. *Circulation* 1995;92:2367–2372.

Arsenian MA. Magnesium and cardiovascular disease. *Prog Cardiovasc Dis* 1993;35:271–310.

ASPECT Research Group. Effect of long-term oral anticoagulant treatment on mortality and cardiovascular morbidity after myocardial infarction: Anticoagulants in the Secondary Prevention of Events in Coronary Thrombosis (ASPECT) research group. *Lancet* 1994;343:499–503.

The Assessment of the Safety and Efficacy of a New Thrombolytic Regimen (ASSENT)-3 Investigators. Efficacy and safety of tenecteplase in combination with enoxaparin, abciximab, or unfractionated heparin:

the ASSENT-3 randomized trial in acute myocardial infarction. *Lancet* 2001;358:605–613.

Bennett CL, Connors JM, Carwile JM, et al. Thrombotic thrombocytopenia purpura associated with clopidogrel. *N Engl J Med* 2000;342(24): 1773–1777.

Berger JS. PMID: 18086929 & *Ann Intern Med* PMID: 19293072.

Beta Blocker Heart Attack Study Group. The beta-blocker heart attack trial. *JAMA* 1981;246:2073–2074.

Bhatt DL. Presented at the American Heart Association meeting, Anaheim, CA, November, 2001.

Blazing MA, de Lemos JA, White HD, et al. Safety and efficacy of enoxaparin vs. unfractionated heparin in patients with non-ST-segment elevation acute coronary syndromes who receive tirofiban and aspirin: a randomized controlled trial. *JAMA* 2004;292:55–64.

Boden WE, van Gilst WH, Scheldewaert RG, et al., for the Incomplete Infarction Trial of European Research Collaborators Evaluating Prognosis post-Thrombolysis (INTERCEPT) group. Diltiazem in acute myocardial infarction treated with thrombolytic agents: a randomized placebo-controlled trial. *Lancet* 2000;355:1751–1756.

Brieger DB, Mak KH, Kottke-Marchant K, Topol EJ. Heparin induced thrombocytopenia. *J Am Coll Cardiol* 1998;31:1449–1459.

Brouwer MA, van den Bergh PJPC, Aengevaeren WRM, et al. Aspirin plus coumarin versus aspirin alone in the prevention of reocclusion after fibrinolysis for acute myocardial infarction. Results of the antithrombotics in the prevention of reocclusion in coronary thrombolysis (APRICOT)-2 trial. *Circulation* [doi: 10.1161/01. CIR.0000024408.81821.32]. 2002. Available at: www.circulationaha.org.

Cairns JA, Connolly SJ, Roberts R, et al. Randomized trial of outcome after myocardial infarction in patients with frequent or repetitive ventricular premature depolarizations. *Lancet* 1997;349:675–682.

CAPRIE steering committee. A randomized blinded trial of clopidogrel versus aspirin in patients at risk of ischemic events. (CAPRIE) *Lancet* 1996;348:1329–1339.

Catella-Lawson F, Reilly MP, Kapoor SC, et al. Cyclooxygenase inhibitors and the antiplatelet effects of aspirin. *N Engl J Med* 2001;345:1809–1817.

Chen ZM. *Lancet* 2005. PMID: 16271643.

CIBIS-II *Lancet* 1999;353(9146):9–13.

Cohen M. Initial experience with the low-molecular-weight heparin, enoxaparin, in combination with the platelet glycoprotein IIb/IIIa blocker, tirofiban, in patients with non-ST segment elevation acute coronary syndromes. *J Invasive Cardiol* 2000;12 (Suppl E):E5–E9; discussion E25–E28.

Coumadin Aspirin Reinfarction Study (CARS) Investigators. Randomized double-blind trial of fixed low-dose warfarin with aspirin after myocardial infarction. *Lancet* 1997;350:389–96.

Dargie HJ. Effect of carvedilol on outcome after myocardial infarction in patients with left-ventricular dysfunction: the CAPRICORN randomised trial. *Lancet* 2001;357:1385–1390.

Eikelboom JW, Anand SS, Malmberg K, et al. Unfractionated heparin and low-molecular-weight heparin in acute coronary syndrome without ST elevation: a meta-analysis. *Lancet* 2000;355:1936–1942.

Eisenstein. *JAMA* 2007. PMID: 17148711.

Ferguson JJ, Califf RM, Antman EM, et al. Enoxaparin vs. unfractionated heparin in high-risk patients with non-ST segment elevation acute coronary syndromes managed with an intended early invasive strategy: primary results of the SYNERGY randomized trial. *JAMA* 2004;292:45–54.

Ferguson JJ. Combining low-molecular-weight heparin and glycoprotein IIb/IIIa antagonists for the treatment of acute coronary syndromes: the NICE 3 story. National Investigators Collaborating on Enoxaparin. *J Invasive Cardiol* 2000;12(Suppl E):E10–E13; discussion E25–E28.

Fiore LD, Ezekowitz MD, Brophy MT, et al. Department of Veterans Affairs Cooperative Studies Program Clinical Trial comparing combined warfarin and aspirin with aspirin alone in survivors of acute myocardial infarction. *Circulation* 2002;105:557–563.

First International Study of Infarct Survival Collaborative Group. Randomized trial of intravenous atenolol among 16,027 cases of suspected acute myocardial infarction. ISIS-1. *Lancet* 1986;2:57–66.

Flather MD, Yusuf S, Kober L, et al. Long-term ACE-inhibitor therapy in patients with heart failure or left-ventricular dysfunction: a systematic overview of data from individual patients. *Lancet* 2000;355: 1575–1581.

Fourth American College of Chest Physicians Consensus Conference on Antithrombotic Therapy. *Chest* 1995;108(suppl):225S-522S.

Fox et al. Efficacy of perindopril in reduction of cardiovascular events among patients with stable coronary artery disease (the EUROPA study). *Lancet* 2003;362:782–788.

The FRAXIS Study Group. Comparison of two treatment durations (6 days and 14 days) of a low molecular weight heparin with a 6-day treatment of unfractionated heparin in the initial management of unstable angina or non-Q-wave myocardial infarction: FRAXIS

(Fraxiparine in Ischaemic Syndrome). *Eur Heart J* 1999;20:1553–1562.

Gattis WA, O'Conner CM, Gallup DS, et al. Predischarge initiation of carvedilol in patients hospitalized for decompensated heart failure: results of the Initiation Management Predischarge: Process for Assessment of Carvedilol Therapy in Heart Failure (IMPACT-HF) trial. *J Am Coll Cardiol* 2004;43:1534–1541.

Gibson RS, Boden WE, Theroux P, et al. Diltiazem and reinfarction in patients with non-Q-wave myocardial infarction: results of a double-blind randomized, multicenter trial. *N Engl J Med* 1986;315:423–429.

GISSI-3: Gruppo Italiano per lo Studio della Sopravvivenza nell'infarto Miocardico. Effects of lisinopril and transdermal glyceryl trinitrate singly and together on 6-week mortality and ventricular function after acute myocardial infarction. *Lancet* 1994;343:1115–1122.

Giugliano RP. *N Engl J Med* 2009.

Goldbourt U, Behar S, Reicher-Reiss H, et al. Early administration of nifedipine in suspected acute myocardial infarction: the Secondary Prevention Reinfarction Israel Nifedipine Trial 2 Study. *Arch Intern Med* 1993;153:345–353.

Gottlieb SS, McCarter RJ, Vogel RA. Effect of beta-blockade on mortality among high-risk and low-risk patients after myocardial infarction. *N Engl J Med* 1998;339:489–497.

Granger CB, McMurray JJ, Yusuf S, et al. Effects of candesartan in patients with chronic heart failure and reduced left-ventricular systolic function intolerant to angiotensin-converting-enzyme inhibitors: the CHARM-Alternative trial. *Lancet* 2003;362:772–776.

Greinacher A, Lubenow N. Recombinant hirudin in clinical practice. *Circulation* 2001;103:1479–1484.

Guidelines 2000 for Cardiopulmonary Resuscitation and Emergency Cardiovascular Care. *Circulation* 2000;102:I86–I203.

Gum PA, Kottke-Marchant K, Poggio ED, et al. Profile and prevalence of aspirin resistance among patients with heart disease: a prospective, comprehensive assessment. *Circulation* 2000;18:II-418.

The GUSTO Angiographic Investigators. The effects of tissue plasminogen activator, streptokinase or both on coronary-artery patency, ventricular function, and survival after acute myocardial infarction. *N Engl J Med* 1993;329:1615–1622.

The Heart Outcomes Prevention Evaluation Study Investigators. Effects of an angiotensin-coverting-enzyme inhibitor, ramipril, on cardiovascular events in high-risk patients. *N Engl J Med* 2000;342:145–153.

Hirsh J, Anand SS, Halperin JL, et al. Guide to anticoagulant therapy: heparin. A statement for healthcare professionals from the American Heart Association. *Circulation* 2001;103:2994–3018.

Hjalmarson A, Elmfeldt D, Herlitz J, et al. Effect on mortality of metoprolol in acute myocardial infarction: a double-blind randomized trial. *Lancet* 1981;2:823–827.

Hjalmarson A, et al. *JAMA* 2000;283:1295–1302.

Ho PM. *JAMA* 2009;301(9):937–944. PMID: 19258584.

The International Study Group. In-hospital mortality and clinical course of 20,891 patients with suspected acute myocardial infarction randomized between alteplase and streptokinase with or without heparin. *Lancet* 1990;336:71–75.

ISIS-2 (Second International Study of Infarct Survival) Collaborative Group. Randomized trial of intravenous streptokinase, oral aspirin, both, or neither among 17,187 cases of suspected acute myocardial infarction. *Lancet* 1988;2:349–360.

ISIS-3 (Third International Study of Infarct Survival) Collaborative Group. A randomized comparison of streptokinase vs. tissue plasminogen activator vs. anistreplase and of aspirin plus heparin vs. aspirin alone among 41,299 cases of suspected acute myocardial infarction: ISIS-3. *Lancet* 1992;339:753–770.

ISIS-4 (Fourth International Study of Infarct Survival) Collaborative Group. ISIS-4: a randomized factorial trial assessing early oral captopril, oral mononitrate, and intravenous magnesium sulphate in 58,050 patients with suspected acute myocardial infarction. *Lancet* 1995;345:669–685.

Jessup M. PMID: 19324967.

Julian DG, Camm AJ, Frangin G, et al. Randomized trial of effect of amiodarone on mortality in patients with left ventricular dysfunction after recent myocardial infarction. *Lancet* 1997;349:667–674.

Kereiakes DJ, Grines C, Fry E, et al. Enoxaparin and abciximab adjunctive pharmacotherapy during percutaneous coronary intervention. *J Invasive Cardiol* 2001;13:272–278.

Klein W, Buchwald A, Hillis SE, et al. Comparison of low-molecular-weight heparin with unfractionated heparin acutely and with placebo for 6 weeks in the management of unstable coronary artery disease: Fragmin in coronary artery disease study (FRIC). *Circulation* 1997;96:61–68.

Latini R, Maggioni AP, Flather M, et al. ACE-inhibitor use in patients with myocardial infarction: summary of evidence from clinical trials. *Circulation* 1995;92:3123–3137.

Latini R, Tognoni G, Maggioni A, et al., for the Angiotensin-converting Enzyme Inhibitor Myocardial Infarction Collaborative Group. Clinical effects of early angiotensin-converting enzyme inhibitor treatment for acute myocardial infarction are similar in the presence and absence of aspirin. Systematic overview of individual data from 96,712 randomized patients. *J Am Coll Cardiol* 2000;35:1801–1807.

Lopes RD, et al. *JACC* 2009;53:1021–1030.

MacMahon S, Collins R, Knight C, et al. Reduction in major morbidity and mortality by heparin in acute myocardial infarction. *Circulation* 1988;78(suppl II):II-98.

McMahon S, Collins R, Koster RW, Yusuf S. Effects of prophylactic lidocaine in suspected acute myocardial infarction: an overview of results from the randomized, controlled trials. *JAMA* 1988;260:1910–1916.

McMurray JJ, Ostergren J, Swedberg K, et al. Effects of candesartan in patients with chronic heart failure and reduced left-ventricular systolic function taking angiotensin-converting-enzyme inhibitors: the CHARM-Added trial. *Lancet* 2003;362:767–771.

Medical Economics. Lovenox. In; *Physicians' Desk Reference*, 56th edition. 2002, p. 750.

Mehta SR, Yusuf S, Peters RJ, et al. Effects of pretreatment with clopidogrel and aspirin followed by long-term therapy in patients undergoing percutaneous coronary intervention: the PCI-CURE study. *Lancet* 2001;358:527–533.

Meijer A, Verheugt FW, Werter CJ, et al. Aspirin versus coumadin in the prevention of reocclusion and recurrent ischemia after successful thrombolysis: a prospective placebo-controlled angiographic study. Results of the APRICOT study. *Circulation* 1993;87:1524–1530.

Mitsios JV, Papathanasiou AI, Rodis F, et al. Atorvastatin does not affect the antiplatelet potency of clopidogrel when it is administered concomitantly for 5 weeks in patients with acute coronary syndromes. *Circulation* 2004;109:1335–1338.

Muller JE, Morrison J, Stone PH, et al. Nifedipine therapy for patients with threatened and acute myocardial infarction: a randomized, double-blind placebo-controlled comparison. *Circulation* 1984;69:740–747.

The Multicenter Diltiazem Postinfarction Trial Research Group. The effect of diltiazem on mortality and reinfarction after myocardial infarction. *N Engl J Med* 1988;319:385–392.

N Eng J Med 2006; PMID: 16537663.

NCEP Report. Implications of recent clinical trials for the National Cholesterol Education Program Adult Treatment Panel III Guidelines. *Circulation* 2004;110:227–239.

Neri Semen GG, Roveli F, Gensini GF, et al. Effectiveness of low-dose heparin in prevention of myocardial reinfarction. *Lancet* 1987;1:937–942.

Neri Serneri GG, Gensini GF, Poggesi L, et al. Effect of heparin, aspirin, or alteplase in reduction of myocardial ischemia in refractory unstable angina. *Lancet* 1990;335:615–618.

Norris RM, Barnaby PF, Brown MA, et al. Prevention of ventricular fibrillation during acute myocardial infarction by intravenous propranolol. *Lancet* 1984;2:883–886.

Oliveira GB, et al. *Arch Intern Med* 2008;168:94–102.

Opie LH, Messerli FH. Nifedipine and mortality: grave defects in the dossier. *Circulation* 1995;92:1068–1073.

Organization to Assess Strategies for Ischemic Syndromes (OASIS-2) Investigators. Effects of recombinant hirudin (lepirudin) compared with heparin on death, myocardial infarction, refractory angina, and revascularization procedures in patients with acute myocardial ischemia without ST elevation: a randomized trial. *Lancet* 1999;353:429–438.

P.H.B, Zannad F, Remme WJ. The effect of spironolactone on morbidity and mortality in patients with severe heart failure. *N Engl J Med* 1999;341:709–717.

Pfeffer MA, McMurray JJ, Velazquez EJ, et al. Valsartan, captopril, or both in myocardial infarction complicated by heart failure, left ventricular dysfunction, or both. *N Engl J Med* 2003;349:1893–1906.

Pitt B, Remme W, Zannad F, et al. Eplerenone, a selective aldosterone blocker, in patients with left ventricular dysfunction after myocardial infarction. *N Engl J Med* 2003;348:1309–1321.

Presented at the American College of Cardiology meeting, Atlanta, GA, March, 2002.

Presented at the American Heart Association Meeting, November, 2004, New Orleans, LA.

Pulcinelli FM, Pignatelli P, Celestini A, et al. Inhibition of platelet aggregation by aspirin progressively decreases in long-term treated patients. *J Am Coll Cardiol* 2004;43:979–984.

Results of the second Warfarin-Aspirin Re-Infarction Study (WARIS II). Presented at the XXIII Congress of the European Society of Cardiology, Stockholm, Sweden, September, 2001.

The RISC Group. Risk of myocardial infarction and death during treatment with low dose aspirin and intravenous heparin in men with unstable coronary artery disease. *Lancet* 1990;336:827–830.

Roberts R, Rogers WJ, Mueller HS, et al. Immediate versus deferred beta-blockade following thrombolytic therapy in patients with acute myocardial infarction.

Results of the Thrombolysis in Myocardial Infarction (TIMI) II-B study. *Circulation* 1991;83:422–437.

Roux S, Christeller S, Ludin E. Effects of aspirin on coronary reocclusion and recurrent ischemia after thrombolysis: a meta-analysis. *J Am Coll Cardiol* 1992;19:671–677.

Sabatine M. *N Engl J Med* 2005. PMID: 15758000.

The SCATI (Studio sulla Calciparina nell'Angina e nella Thrombosi Ventricolare nell'Infarto) Group. Randomized controlled trial of subcutaneous calciumheparin in acute myocardial infarction. *Lancet* 1989;2:182–186.

Schwartz GG, Olsson AG, Ezekowitz MD, et al. Effects of atorvastatin on early recurrent ischemic events in acute coronary syndromes. *JAMA* 2001;285:1711–1718.

Schwartz L, Bourassa MG, Lesperance J, et al. Aspirin and dipyridamole in the prevention of restenosis after percutaneous transluminal coronary angioplasty. *N Engl J Med* 1988;318:1714–1719.

Serbruany V, Midei M, Malinin A, et al. *Atorvastatin does not inhibit clopidogrel in patients undergoing coronary stenting in prospective data from the INTERACTION Study.* Presented at American Heart Association Scientific Sessions, abstract 3065, November 2003, Orlando, FL.

Shechter M, Hod H, Chouraqui P, et al. Magnesium therapy in acute myocardial infarction when patients are not candidates for thrombolytic therapy. *Am J Cardiol* 1995;75:321–323.

Sigurdsson A, Swedberg K. Left ventricular remodeling, neurohormonal activation and early treatment with enalapril (CONSENSUS II) following myocardial infarction. *Eur Heart J* 1994;15(suppl B):14–19.

Song KH, Fedyk R, Hoover R. Interaction of ACE inhibitors and aspirin in patients with congestive heart failure. *Arm Pharmacother* 1999;33:375–377.

Steinhubl SR, Berger PB, Mann JT III, et al. Early and sustained dual oral antiplatelet therapy following percutaneous coronary intervention. The CREDO trial. *JAMA* 2002;288:2411–2420.

STEMI guideline update JACC. PMID: 18191746.

Stone GW. *N Engl J Med* 2006;355:2203–2216.

Teo KK, Yusuf S, Collins R, et al. Effects of intravenous magnesium in suspected acute myocardial infarction: overview of randomized trials. *BMJ* 1991;303:1499–1503.

Teo KK, Yusuf S, Furberg CD. Effects of prophylactic antiarrhythmic drug therapy in acute myocardial infarction: an overview of results from randomized controlled trials. *JAMA* 1993;270:1589–1595.

Theroux P, Ouirnet H, McCans J, et al. Aspirin, heparin, or both to treat acute unstable angina. *N Engl J Med* 1988;319:1105–1111.

Theroux P, Waters D, Lam J, et al. Reactivation of unstable angina after the discontinuation of heparin. *N Engl J Med* 1992;327:141–145.

Timolol-induced reduction in mortality and reinfarction in patients surviving acute myocardial infarction. *N Engl J Med* 1981;304:801–807.

van Es RF, Jonker JC, Verheugt FWA, et al. Aspirin and coumadin after acute coronary syndromes (the ASPECT-2) a randomised controlled trial. *Lancet* 2002;360:109–113.

Woods KL, Fletcher S, Roffe C, Haider Y. Intravenous magnesium sulphate in suspected acute myocardial infarction: results of the second Leicester Intravenous Magnesium Intervention Trial (LIMIT-2). *Lancet* 1992;339:1553–1558.

Woods KL, Fletcher S. Long-term outcome after intravenous magnesium sulphate in suspected acute myocardial infarction: the second Leicester Intravenous Magnesium Intervention Trial (LIMIT-2). *Lancet* 1994;343:816–819.

Woods KL. Possible pharmacological actions of magnesium in acute myocardial infarction. *Br J Clin Pharmacol* 1991;32:3–10.

Young JJ, Kereiakes DJ, Grines CL. Low-molecular-weight heparin therapy in percutaneous coronary intervention: the NICE 1 and NICE 4 trials. National Investigators Collaborating on Enoxaparin Investigators. *J Invasive Cardiol* 2000;12(Suppl E):E14–E18; discussion E25–E28.

Yusuf S, Collins R, MacMahon S, Peto R. Effect of intravenous nitrates on mortality in acute myocardial infarction: an overview of the randomized trials. *Lancet* 1988;l:1088–1092.

Yusuf S, Peto R, Lewis J, et al. Beta blockade during and after myocardial infarction: an overview of the randomized trials. *Prog Cardiovasc Dis* 1985;27:335–371.

Yusuf S, Wittes J, Friedman L. Overview of results of randomized clinical trials in heart disease, II: unstable angina, heart failure, primary prevention with aspirin, and risk factor modification. *JAMA* 1988;260:2259–2263.

Yusuf S, Zhao F, Mehta SR, et al. Effects of clopidogrel in addition to aspirin in patients with acute coronary syndromes without ST-segment elevation. *N Engl J Med* 2001;345:494–502.

Yusuf S. *JAMA* 2006; PMID: 16537725.

INDEX

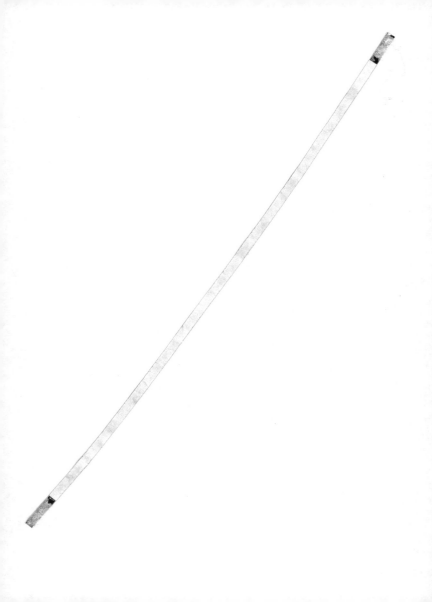